Group Theory/Process for Nursing Practice

Publishing Director: David Culverwell
Acquisitions Editor: Richard Weimer
Production Editor/Text Design: Eileen Baylus
Art Director/Cover Design: Don Sellers, AMI
Assistant Art Director: Bernard Vervin
Photographer: George Dodson

Indexer: William O. Lively
Typesetter: Graphic Visions Associates, Rockville, MD
Printer: Fairfield Graphics, Fairfield, PA
Typefaces: Souvenir demi-bold (display) and English Times (text)

Group Theory/Process for Nursing Practice

Margo Wilson RN, MS, CS

Brady Communications Company, Inc.
A Prentice-Hall Publishing Company
Bowie, MD 20715

Wilson, Margo, 1945-
  Group theory/process for nursing practice.
  Includes bibliographies and index.
  1. Nursing—Social aspects. 2. Small groups. 3. Interpersonal communication. 4. Social interaction. I. Title. [DNLM: 1. Group Processes—nurses' instruction. WY 87 W751g]
RT86.5.W54 1985   610.73   84-9213
ISBN 0-89303-500-9

Prentice-Hall International, Inc., *London*
Prentice-Hall Canada, Inc., Scarborough, *Ontario*
Prentice-Hall of Australia, Pty., Ltd., *Sydney*
Prentice-Hall India Private Limited, *New Delhi*
Prentice-Hall Japan, Inc., *Tokyo*
Prentice-Hall of Southeast Asia Pte. Ltd., *Singapore*
Whitehall Books, Limited, Petone, *New Zealand*
Editora Prentice-Hall Do Brasil LTDA., *Rio de Janeiro*
Prentice-Hall Hispanoamericana, S.A., *Mexico*

Printed in the United States of America

85 86 87 88 89 90 91 92 93 94 95 1 2 3 4 5 6 7 8 9 10

To my loving and patient family, my husband, Dave, and my children, Kimberly, Brett, and Colleen

Contents

Preface

I find leading or co-leading a group to be an exciting part of the practice of nursing. To be able to process the many elements of interaction occurring with any group of people at any one time is a skill that makes the nurse a more effective practitioner. The nurse with group skills may deal more effectively not only with groups of clients, but also with individual clients and with colleagues, especially when working in a multidisciplinary staff setting. This book was written to give nurses, working in a variety of roles and settings, a tool for communicating with groups of people and for facilitating their growth.

I do not expect everyone to share my enthusiasm about groups, but I do believe that all nurses must have a working knowledge of group dynamics and process, regardless of what professional role or area of expertise they choose to pursue. Not only is this knowledge helpful; it is essential to nursing practice. This book is a result of my experience in teaching nursing students group dynamics and process. I have drawn from a variety of sources to teach the theory and practice of group. I am an eclectic group leader, convinced that there is merit in using the ideas of a variety of theorists who have talked about human behavior. In this book, I present a number of theoretical approaches to group and attempt to illustrate their application in settings where nurses would most likely be working.

Although graduate preparation is essential for leading or co-leading an insight-oriented group and for using some of the therapeutic modalities discussed in the text, this book was also written for the nurse who does not have that preparation. As a participant in a variety of groups with both staff and clients, the nurse can use this text to become more knowledgeable and skilled in the role of member or leader. The nurse may function as a leader or co-leader of a supportive group for clients or as a member or leader of a staff task group.

To promote the transfer of learning from the book to actual nursing practice, I have developed a series of learning activities that attempt to apply most major concepts to clinical situations. The reader is asked to work on developing both a personal and a clinical acquaintance with the new concepts to make them part of his or her repertoire of skills.

The major thrust of my book is process. I spend many pages describing this elusive phenomenon and have included clinical examples to help the reader grasp this most important occurrence in groups. My swim instructor, who was trying to teach a group of us "nonswimmers" to tread water, said we would not "get it" on the first try. Learning to identify process is much like learning to tread water. It suddenly becomes apparent that there is a second, more sophisticated level of communication. The sudden awareness is often experienced as an "aha." I have experienced the "aha" of process, but I have yet to experience the "aha" of treading water. Several sections in the book have been included to promote process illumination for both the nurse group leader and the client.

In the book, I use the word "client" to describe a group member or individual who is seeking health care services and who is expected to take an active part in identifying needs and goals related to the consumption of care. Whether the individual actively works towards his own wellness will vary from person to person. However,

I believe strongly in giving the individual the message that this is the role I see that person taking. My orientation is one of partnership with the client in his response to illness.

The choices the nurse makes about how to structure a group will depend both on the skills mastered and on those interventions that the person finds most comfortable performing. Allowing oneself to be open means trying out a variety of different interventions and approaches to group. As the Gestalt therapist would say, "Will you give yourself permission to try on some new behaviors?" I invite nurses to approach this book in the same way, with some willingness to be open to a group approach to clients as an important part of nursing practice.

Acknowledgements

I would like to thank my undergraduate instructor in mental health nursing, Janet Rodgers, for pushing me to explore my own process as a necessary first step in working with clients. From my graduate work in group with Ellie White, I gained the knowledge and assurance that the nurse could be an effective group leader in professional practice. The many nursing students at Point Loma College to whom I taught group process responded with thoughtful feedback and enthusiasm in their newly-learned group skills. They allowed me to formulate and teach my perception of the nurse's role as a leader in group process. Finally, the many clients with whom I worked have furthered my understanding of interpersonal process and have convinced me that there is much merit in nurses structuring groups for clients.

As a novice writer, I appreciated the feedback and encouragement from Laura Mae Douglass, a widely-published author of several nursing texts. I would also like to thank Tracy Smith, a former regional editor at Brady, for her professional and personal support in the writing of this book.

Part One

Group Dynamics: The Basis for Understanding How a Group Functions

Section One
Theoretical Frameworks for Study Groups

The significance of groups in our culture cannot be overstated. Our identity as individuals meshes with our membership in a variety of groups. The family group is familiar to most of us as the primary source of our security, need fulfillment, social learning, and numerous other functions. It has particular properties that will be explored in more detail later. Even though some individuals cannot claim membership in a family, most people can identify a set of significant others who were influential in shaping their early development. Phipps (1982) discussed group membership in terms of primary, secondary, and reference groups. Appropriately, the family is labeled a primary group. The primary group is responsible for influencing the person's identity development, value structure, and way of interacting with the environment. Secondary groups tend to be less personal and more specialized in their purpose for being. A nurse may claim membership in such secondary groups as the set of peers or professional colleagues in the work setting, one or more social groups, various community organizations, and other formal and informal groups. Secondary groups form and are dissolved as their purpose for being no longer exists or their work is completed. A person also moves in and out of reference groups. Reference groups influence our attitudes and behaviors as well as our value system. However, their influence is less direct and obvious than that of the primary group. Reference groups become more influential during adolescence and through one's adult life. In fact, the adolescent's peer associations are a strong reference group. The women's movement has given birth to several reference groups who have fueled the controversy over a woman's right to decide what will happen to her body. This decade's struggle with the abortion issue is a prime example of how powerfully such groups can affect current mores and behaviors. Many women are not members of NOW or other similar organizations but identify strongly with these groups' beliefs, giving credence to the fact that formal membership is not a requisite for espousing the ideas of a reference group. The organized work force, religious groups, and various ethnic organizations may all be considered reference groups.

What do reference, secondary, and primary groups have to do with the theoretical frameworks presented in this first section of the book? It is helpful in interactions with clients, as individuals or in a group, to understand the context of the client's frame of reference. Probably one or more reference groups as well as the client's family have the most influence on how the client presents him or herself. There are many theories about how one develops the thoughts, feelings, and behaviors that

1

make up one's identity. Similarly, groups also have an identity. Chapter One describes the group's personality as a system interacting with and influenced by other systems in its environment. One such system is the individual member of the group. Further chapters will look more at the member's contribution to the group's identity. To summarize, primary, secondary, and reference groups may shape a person's identity, values, and behaviors, yet this same person, as a member of a group, influences the group's personality (*e.g.,* its leadership or executive structure, its values or normative structure, and its behaviors or process).

Some of the pioneers in the study of groups and group behavior suggested a close association between the individual member and the group itself. An individual's identity is shaped by groups which are the most significant to him (Cartwright and Zander, 1968). Wilfred Bion defined a group as an aggregate of individuals coming together to perform a certain function. He gave the example of a group of strangers on a beach who are nothing more than strangers until they respond to a swimmer in danger of drowning. At this point, they have a purpose or function for being together and are, therefore, a group (Bion, 1959; Rioch, 1972). Bion believed the individual cannot be understood apart from his affiliation with a group. Even when this person appears to be isolated from others, he should not be regarded as having no membership in a group (Bion, 1959; Kauff, 1979). In a similar idea, Kurt Lewin said that one needs to study a person's "life space"; *i.e.,* a person's perception of his internal and external world. The group(s) to which a person belongs is the source of his perceptions, feelings, and actions (Lewin, 1948, 1951; Sabin, 1981). Finally, Carl Rogers (1970) discussed the character of the group itself. "To me the group seems like an organism, having a sense of its own direction..." (p.44). Section One presents an overview of the contributors and concepts identified with each theoretical framework.

As nurses, we should be using a model for our group work with clients. Several nurses have described models for looking at a group and how it functions. The concepts presented through a model describe the structure of events or systems and specify relationships and processes (Lancaster and Lancaster, 1981). Janosik (1982) cited developmental theory as being the basis of the life cycle model for groups. Loomis (1979) developed a model for looking at group movement using objectives, structure, process, and outcome as criteria for assessment. As nurses work in the area of group practice, they are confronted with the influence of several theoretical frameworks for presenting the basis for the group's organization and leadership strategy (Janosik, 1982). Imogene King (1981) applied the framework of general systems theory to the nurse's interaction with both individuals and groups.

The major models used in nursing come from systems theory, developmental theory, and interactional theories (Bush, 1979). Rogers (1970) used a holistic approach in describing the way human beings function interactionally with their environment. Her ideas have a basis in general systems theory (Chance, 1982; Wilson and Kneisl, 1983). Orlando (1972) described the individual nurse as the basic unit of the nursing system. The nurse's interactions occur most often with three other systems: the client or clients, other nurses in staff or line positions, and professional and nonprofessional staff in other disciplines and facets of the health care system. Roy (1981) described the client as an adaptive system. She used concepts from role theory to discuss one's adaptation to illness.

It would seem that one cannot avoid the concept of the client and the nurse as interacting systems. The idea forms the basis for a look at the theoretical frameworks presented in Section One. A framework describes such elements in a group as the members' roles, the leadership of the group, and the boundaries of the group. Chapter One presents the group as a system. Since much of our discussion has focused on how several nursing models conceive the nurse and client as functioning in a systems framework, this seems an appropriate place to start. Chapter Two looks at the individual client, one part of the group's system, and considers the effect of one's experiences on interactions with others. "The study of the intrapsychic self, that is, of the human psyche in its totality, is essentially a systems approach." (von Bertalanffy, 1974). The group also has a collective internal process called the group psyche. Chapter Three continues the examination of the individual's internal process but emphasizes the person's freedom to resolve internal conflicts that affect present interactions with others. In Gestalt, one considers isolated behaviors as part of a whole. As the individual group member works on becoming more whole, the other group members participate in the emotional experience of this process. von Bertalanffy (1974) identified Gestalt theory as being conceptually related to systems theory. Chapter Four describes how one's environment, including other human systems, can influence one's actions. Many of the behaviors that occur in a group are the result of other actions by the group leader. Members learn how to behave in a group (group norms) partly because the leader reinforces these norms.

The structure and movement common to all groups and necessary for the group's task accomplishment is presented in Section Two of Part One. Part Two discusses the process of the group. Process is all those interactions that occur between the leader and its members and is an essential element for the nurse to understand. It is my bias that group texts for nurses have not adequately covered this area, and that process is at the "heart" of facilitating change for clients. The nurse as a group leader and the clients as group members take part in continuous interactions with one another. King (1981) described the practice of nursing as a series of interactions between interpersonal systems.

REFERENCES

Bion, W. *Experiences in Group.* New York: Basic Books, 1959.

Bush, H. "Models for Nursing," *Advances in Nursing Science,* 1, no. 2 (Jan., 1979), 13-21.

Cartwright, D. and A. Zander, eds. *Group Dynamics Research and Theory.* New York: Harper and Row, 1968.

Chance, K. "Nursing Models: A Requisite for Professional Accountability," *Advances in Nursing Science,* 4, no. 2 (Jan., 1982), 57-65.

Janosik, E. "Models of Group: Rationale and Typology," *Life Cycle Group Work in Nursing,* eds. E. Janosik and L. Phipps. Monterey, CA: Wadsworth Health Sciences Division, 1982.

Janosik, E. "Theoretical Frameworks: Intrapsychic Groups," *Life Cycle Group Work in Nursing,* eds. E. Janosik and L. Phipps. Monterey, CA: Wadsworth Health Sciences Division, 1982.

Kauff, P. "Diversity in Analytical Group Psychotherapy: The Relationship Between Theoretical Concepts and Technique," *International Journal of Group Psychotherapy,* 29, no. 1 (Jan., 1979), 51-65.

4

King, I. *A Theory for Nursing: Systems, Concepts, Process.* New York: John Wiley & Sons, Inc., 1981.

Lancaster, W. and J. Lancaster. "Models and Model Building in Nursing," *Advances in Nursing Science,* 3, no. 3 (April, 1981), 31-42.

Lewin, K. *Resolving Social Conflicts.* New York: Harper and Brothers, 1948.

Lewin, K. in *Field Theory in Social Science,* ed. D. Cartwright. New York: Harper and Brothers, 1951.

Loomis, M. *Group Process for Nurses.* St. Louis: C.V. Mosby Co., 1979.

Orlando, I. *The Discipline and Teaching of Nursing Process.* New York: G.P. Putnam's Sons, 1972.

Phipps, L. "Group Work: History and Overview," in *Life Cycle Group Work in Nursing,* eds. E. Janosik and L. Phipps. Monterey, CA: Wadsworth Health Sciences Division, 1982.

Rioch, M. "The Work of Wilfred Bion on Groups," in *Progress in Group and Family Therapy,* eds. G. Sager and H. Kaplan. New York: Brunner/Mazel, Inc., 1972.

Rogers, C. *Carl Rogers on Encounter Groups.* New York: Harper and Row, 1970.

Rogers, M. *An Introduction to the Theoretical Basis of Nursing.* Philadelphia: F.A. Davis Co., 1970.

Roy, Sr. C. and S. Roberts. *Theory Construction in Nursing: An Adaptation Model.* Englewood Cliffs, NY: Prentice-Hall, Inc., 1981.

Sabin, J. "Short-Term Group Psychotherapy: Historical Antecedents," in *Forms of Brief Therapy,* ed. S. Budman. New York: The Guilford Press, 1981.

von Bertalanffy, L. "General Systems Theory and Psychiatry," in *The American Handbook of Psychiatry Vol. I* (2nd ed.), ed. S. Arieti. New York: Basic Books, 1974.

Wilson, H. and C. Kneisl. *Psychiatric Nursing* (2nd ed.). Menlo Park, CA: Addison-Wesley Publishing Co., 1983.

The Group as an Interactional System

1

─────────────── Systems Theory ───────────────

The concept known as systems theory provides a framework for studying group phenomena. Systems theory describes the roles, behaviors, boundaries, and power of the communicants within the group. Systems theory has also become the basis for studying the primary group, the family. In Chapter One, general systems will be discussed with some specifics focused on how nurses work with systems in their interventions with groups of clients and with the primary group, the family. Identifying the client as a system provides options for this person's nursing care planning. A family assessment data sheet will be introduced later in the chapter to help the nurse view the client as the member of a family group. Learning activities at the end of Section One provide the reader with further opportunities to practice the application of systems theory to clinical nursing interventions.

The Properties of a System

A system is defined as a set of objects with attributes or properties whose inter-relationship ties the parts of the system together and to other systems (von Bertalanffy, 1972, 1974; Watzlawick, *et al.,* 1967). Most of us are familiar with mechanical systems such as the car engine and the chassis of a television set, and with living systems, such as the human body. Closed systems, such as the internal workings of a computer, would malfunction if any other matter permeated the "chips" or if they were removed. Closed systems, then, do not generally interact with other systems in their environment. This is true of most nonliving physical systems. Open systems or organic living things may interact with other systems within the environment (von Bertalanffy, 1972, 1974; Watzlawick, *et al.,* 1967). This occurs as a continuous, dynamic process (von Bertalanffy, 1974; King, 1981).

The principle of *equifinality* differentiates between a closed and an open system. In a closed system, such as an engine, operation is accomplished through a series of steps that must be the same each time the engine is started. With equifinality, the end result of a process may be reached independently of the conditions that initiated it (von Bertalanffy, 1974). Said simply, there is more than one way to reach a goal. The individual who is trying to lose weight has several options. This person might either reduce caloric intake or increase the amount of exercise each day. Some do both. Other options are to choose a quick weight loss diet, fast for one or more days, or enroll in a weight loss program. The final result will be some weight loss if the amount of calories expended is greater than that ingested. This process is an example of equifinality in an open system, the individual.

In King's (1981) theoretical model for nursing practice, she defined both the client and the nurse as *personal systems*. Each may act independently of the other as a total system. However, as the nurse and client interact, they become an *interpersonal system*. King identified the group as another interpersonal system with

5

characteristics that a group of two does not have. The nurse/client dyad may interact with a number of *social systems,* such as the family, the health care system, or a belief or religious system. The context of one's nursing practice, then, must include the awareness of both the self and the client as part of a multiple set of systems.

For purposes of studying groups, Watzlawick's (1967) definition of interactional systems will be used. He states that systems are "two or more communicants in the process of, or at the level of, defining the nature of their relationship." (p.121). Watzlawick (1967) identified certain attributes or properties which further define an interactional system.

1) A change in one part of a system will cause a change in all other parts and in the total system.

2) The whole is greater than the sum of its parts; *i.e.,* an interaction between any two or more parts in the system will yield another quality of the system entirely different than its interacting parts *(property of synergy).*

3) There is a circular quality to interactional systems which is called feedback *(property of circularity).* Bateson (1961; Jones, 1980) elaborated further on the feedback process. He saw the feedback loop as a way of maintaining stability in any biosocial system. The feedback loop allows informational exchanges to take place between systems, such as between the family and the social and economic environment surrounding it. The feedback model, therefore, facilitates interaction on interdisciplinary levels (von Bertalanffy, 1972). Wilson and Kneisl (1979) explained circularity as a process that occurs when each member in a system engages in behavior that influences the other members. This produces a cyclic phenomenon where such behavior becomes both the cause and the effect of the others' actions within the system.

Every system has boundaries which may be diffuse, clear, rigid, or conflicting. Boundaries identify the amount of differentiation permitted between members of a system and the amount of emotional investment present (Wilson and Kneisl, 1979). All systems' boundaries are "ultimately dynamic" or forever changing (von Bertalanffy, 1974). The boundaries of an open system must be permeable to allow for a continuous exchange of energy and information with other systems within the environment (King, 1981). The property of a system's boundaries is particularly meaningful in describing the family system.

Examining a Living System

The hospital is a complex interactional system and is part of a larger social system called the health care system. It is made up of smaller interactional units who maintain an interdependent relationship with other living systems. One of the most important systems that the hospital constantly interacts with is the client. Each is dependent on the other for actions that help maintain their systems. The client expects services that supply his basic needs of survival and security and that promote his health and well-being, such as the attention of knowledgeable, professional staff. In return, the hospital expects compliance with house rules, receipt of payment for services rendered, and behaviors that do not endanger the client or others.

The client in the hospital may experience a change in health status in a variety of ways. Equifinality allows for a condition of wellness to be reached with the help of many different hospital systems or very few. Recovery of a client's heart muscle after a myocardial infarction is due to many factors such as rest, decreased stress, increased ease of oxygenation, and a diet to promote tissue healing and new growth of collateral vessels feeding the heart muscle. The individual client may be visited by the dietitian, or the nurse may do diet teaching. As the client gains strength, he may attend a class, given by an exercise physiologist, on safe physical activity to increase the strength of the heart muscle. Someone from respiratory therapy may evaluate how the client's system is handling oxygenation. The client's degree of compliance with these health care measures also affects the end condition of wellness or illness. Such interactions between the client and hospital systems determine the outcome of his health status.

Departments operating within the hospital and those systems outside the hospital impacting on the institution's ability to deliver quality health care illustrate two properties of an interactional system. The effect of a change in the process of delivering nursing care alters the way other departments in the hospital operate. Consider the effects of a threatened or actual strike of registered nurses. The impetus for the job action is the values derived from the nurses' allegiance to one or more reference groups. A belief in primary nursing espoused by such reference groups as the set of undergraduate nursing faculties and the state nurse's association exert strong influence with the group of striking nurses. Hospital administrators cancel any elective admissions and make plans for transferring very acutely ill clients to other hospitals. A prolonged strike could lead to layoffs of other hospital personnel and affect local nursing programs which rely on the hospital for their clinical placements. Thus, a change in one part of the system (the nursing staff) has caused a change in other parts of the system (other hospital departments) and a change in the system as a whole (the delivery of health care). The feedback loops operating between the hospital, its departments, nurses, clients, and the educational institution are probably less functional.

To carry the example further, we can see the property of circularity in effect. If the nurses are striking over their belief in the need to give primary care, the hospital system must have, in some way, jeopardized their opportunity to do this. Perhaps the hospital administration put a freeze on hiring RNs or decided to replace vacant RN positions with auxiliary personnel. These behaviors caused the nurses' behavior, *i.e.,* the strike. The process of striking, in turn, led to new behaviors by the hospital administration, *i.e.,* canceling elective admissions, making arrangements for the transfer of acutely ill clients, and so forth. Such cause-and-effect interactions may proceed indefinitely in an interactional system.

The property of synergy is also illustrated by looking at the hospital system. A client who is given the wrong medication may or may not have untoward effects from this error. If she does, not only is an incident report made out, but the nurse's supervisor, the client's physician, hospital administration, and several other parts of the system must become involved. The relationship between the client and the nurse responsible for the error will change. It may be that the client will no longer trust the nurse nor accept medication from that person. The nurse may become more knowledgeable and careful about medication administration, or he may experience a loss of self-esteem and less status with his peers and supervisor. We could continue to speculate about changes in the character of the system as a result of this one interaction between the nurse and the client. If the client has no untoward effects from the error, quality assurance may still be questioned and suspect, especially if this is one of an excessive number of medication errors. An incident report may eventually lead to some studies on the occurrence of this type of error and a change in hospital policy or nursing procedures involving the administration of medications. The pharmacy might look at its procedures for labeling medications. Such quality assurance measures reflect a responsible hospital team and may change the character of the system or hospital as a whole.

Boundaries within the hospital system and between it and other systems are particularly fascinating. Traditionally, the relationship between the medical staff and the nursing staff may have been one of rigid boundaries. Roles and behaviors were well-defined between these two groups. With the many changes that have occurred primarily in nursing (*e.g.,* the advent of the nurse practitioner role, the expanded knowledge base and specialist preparation of nurses, and so forth), and as a result of other events (*e.g.,* the women's movement and the reduction in sexist views on occupational choices), the boundaries between medicine and nursing have become more diffuse. Within the nursing profession, the current controversy about the educational preparation for entry-level positions, *i.e.,* at the associate or baccalaureate level, creates boundary confusion among nurses. The American Nurses Association is one of the social systems wrestling with this issue. Some nurses would like boundaries between nurses of different educational preparation to be clear rather than diffuse. They see this as leading to more differentiation of their roles by other parts of the health care delivery system, such as physicians and hospital administrators, and by the client. We will explore the property of boundaries further when we talk about the family as a system.

─────── Communication: The Process That ─────── Connects Living Systems

The term "interaction" implies a reciprocal, mutual, dynamic process. Watzlawick (1967; Jones, 1980) offered several axioms about communications within a system.
1) All behavior is communication. One cannot not behave and one cannot not communicate. Even silence is a behavior.
2) Communication is the process that defines a relationship between persons and implies that a commitment between them exists.
3) One communicates verbally and nonverbally. Verbal communications deal with concepts but do not give as much information about the relationship of the communicants. A statement, "I'm sorry I hurt you," could mean the speaker is feeling guilty for causing pain to someone else or is apologizing because it is expedient to do so. Nonverbal communications present data about the relationship of the communicants but not the nature of their relationship. A smile toward someone may acknowledge that person's presence and invite interaction, or it may be a message of smugness or contempt. Thus, the verbal or nonverbal are generally incomplete used alone.
4) All communications are either symmetrical or complementary. In a symmetrical relationship, either party may take the lead. In a complementary relationship, one person exerts leadership over the other in the type of communications that exist.

Other systems theorists discuss communication with the same perspective as

Watzlawick. The process of communication between a dyad may be identified by observing the changing state of the two participants (King, 1981). Haley (1963; Jones, 1980) commented on how one's relationship with other individuals is influenced by the way one communicates. As two people interact, they begin to define the behaviors that will take place in their relationship. They also work on power or control issues; *i.e.,* who decides what behaviors will be allowed. This is similar to Watzlawick's idea of symmetrical and complementary relationships.

Levels of Communication

Haley (1963, 1980; Jones, 1980) also talked about communications as having a content level and a metacommunication level. The metacommunication level qualifies the content level. All nonverbal communications must be metacommunications, because all nonverbal (*e.g.,* a smile, a sigh, a handshake, a look away, and so forth) communications further define the meaning of a verbal message. A smile by a mother when she is rebuking her child is a very different communication than a frown with the same verbalization. We will discuss nonverbal communications in more depth in a later section of this chapter. Recall that Watzlawick defined the nonverbal communication as a comment on the relationship between the communicants. Satir (1967; Jones, 1980) also spoke of two levels of communications. Satir called them the literal, or denotative, level and the metacommunication level. Her definition of the metacommunication level expanded on what Haley and Watzlawick said by further explaining how a metacommunication affects the nature of the relationship between those communicating. Satir (1967) noted that there were both verbal and nonverbal metacommunications. Consider the following verbal metacommunications:

- "It was only a joke. I hope you aren't angry with me."
- "I just explained that to you. Didn't you understand?"
- "I really wasn't laughing at you. It's just such a ridiculous situation."

Verbal Channels

The connotative meaning of a word adds to our understanding of metacommunications. As differentiated from the denotative or literal meaning of a word, the connotative meaning refers to the feeling state or emotion surrounding a word. For example, "mother" may be defined denotatively as a female who has given birth to an offspring. Connotatively, "mother" elicits feelings of warmth, love, home, and even patriotism ("the Red-White-and-Blue, apple pie, and Mom"). "Mother-in-law," however, elicits some very negative responses. Yet, their denotative meanings are quite similar. Politicians frequently influence voters by choosing words with connotative meanings that will make their speeches more convincing and well-received. The politician, salesman, or other person who wants to define his or her relationship with us in a particular way is very conscious of the connotative meaning of words.

Related to our understanding of the meaning of words is what Sullivan (1953) called the three modes of experience. The prototaxic mode is the infant's first experience with life. At this point, the newborn cannot distinguish between itself and the rest of the world. The experience is tactile and would include the first encounters with the mothering person by way of the breast, nipple, and all tactile sensations of bonding. However, the infant feels these as sensations within its own body. The parataxic mode of experience is a sense of momentary encounters with one's environment but without any understanding of what this means for future encounters with the world outside oneself. There is no consensual validation of the real world. Such experience implies the existence of very personal meanings for one's way of looking at the world. A baby's utterances or "baby talk" would be a parataxic experience. It is rare that there is any relationship between a baby's talk and the denotative meanings of adult language (Sullivan, 1953). One must rely on the nonverbal level to understand communications in the parataxic mode. Finally, the syntaxic mode of experience is illustrated by words that can be consensually validated; that is, others should have the same denotative understanding of their use. If a connotative meaning is very personal, it may be in the parataxic mode. I have a lot of emotional attachment to the word "swimming." My inability to learn to swim, some negative experiences while trying, and my fear of the water all contribute to my feelings. Although another person may share some of my negative emotions around that word, they are probably not entirely the same. It is obvious that the meaning of a word has many ramifications for our communications with others. Nonverbal communications carry equal or greater importance.

Nonverbal Channels

Several theorists have highlighted the importance of the nonverbal channel in describing and defining the relationship of the communicants. Because nonverbal cues are linked to body physiology, they are considered to be less deceptive than verbalizations and are, therefore, given more validity (Kinseth, 1982). Less clearly defined, nonverbal cues require greater attentiveness (Satir, 1967). There are a variety of ways a person can express a message nonverbally. Wilson and Kneisl (1979) noted the following.

1) *Kinesics.* Kinesics deal with the body movements people put with most of their verbal communications. Facial expressions are the most important source of communicating nonverbally. This is evident when one watches another person's face for a clue as to how the communication is being received. Hand gestures, leg movements, and subtle movements such as tics are all part of kinesics.

2) *Paralanguage.* These are nonlanguage verbalizations such as sobbing, grunting, sighing, and so forth, as well as the voice quality of our speech.

3) *Proxemics.* Proxemics have to do with the space between ourselves and another person. Our potential space needs vary according to our current feeling state and to whom we are relating at the time. Generally, individuals demand less space from those with whom they are intimate. However, if one is angry at another person, there is a tendency to increase the space to a more impersonal distance.

4) *Touch.* This is an obvious nonverbal channel for relating. As with personal space, touch needs vary greatly with mood, the kind of message a person wants to express, the intimacy level between two people relating together, and so forth. Sexual and cultural taboos are also associated with the expression of touch.

5) *Cultural artifacts.* Nonverbal stimuli related to culture include the way of dressing, the style of grooming, the use of make-up and baubles, and other mannerisms culturally determined. Since nonverbal behaviors are the basis for defining

relationships with others, it is important to consider the many channels of communicating nonverbally.

The Message Unit

Reusch (1972) defined a message as a "series of statements which originate in one place and terminate in another" (p.173). The message unit illustrates the property of circularity and feedback loops within a living system in a more graphic way. Roy (1981) described a system as having input, internal and feedback processes, and output. Wilson and Kneisl (1979), in describing a communication model by J.E. Hulett, identified the phases of message sending and receiving. Several of these phases are not seen by the observer because they are internal processes. The sender is motivated to begin the process by a stimulus that requires the engagement of another person. During a period of what is called covert rehearsal, the sender is organizing the message by rehearsing what actions to take and considering possible reactions by the receiver. The sender processes information about himself, the receiver, and the social norms and structure, and weighs his self concept and role behaviors with those of the receiver. If he decides to send a message, this becomes the stimulus for the receiver. The receiver must then go through a phase of covert rehearsal before responding to the message from the sender. As each person responds by generating another message, a feedback loop is established. Ideally, both communicants should be correcting their own messages for further understanding while stimulating the other to do the same.

An individual's nonverbal behavior as he interacts with others gives cues to the covert rehearsal process preceding these behaviors. If I relate to others passively, allowing them to interrupt me, I have probably decided that I am not as worthy of being heard. A person's evaluation of his worth, his self-esteem, is directly tied to how he believes others perceive him; *i.e.,* the concept of public esteem (Yalom, 1975). His interactions with others, therefore, contribute to his worth as a person and to his self concept. As a group leader, I try to help clients look at the internal messages they are giving themselves. I use verbal as well as nonverbal cues that individuals allow to seep through during covert rehearsal. For example, I might point out a member's nonverbal behavior, such as a frown, and ask her how that "fit" with her perception of her relationship with others in the group. Even if the frown is a response to internal stimuli, such as a thought about an unpleasant incident that had occurred earlier in the day, the nonverbal also is a message to the group, *e.g.,* "What you are talking about is boring so I'm going to withdraw and think about me." The nonverbal may be directed to a particular member, *e.g.,* "When you said quiet people make you uncomfortable, I know you were talking about me." If I can get a client to make overt the covert rehearsal part of a message that might be incomplete, misinterpreted, too personalized, or meeting social norms rather than therapeutic norms, I can help this person become more adaptive in message generation.

The context in which a message is sent and received is important to its understanding. Satir (1967) defined the context of a communication as the circumstances, environment, setting, and past experiences which each communicant brings to the interaction. Any understood relationship between the communicants which occurred in the past is also part of the context. In looking at the covert phase of the message unit, the perceived roles of the sender and receiver as well as the social norms and structure may be considered context. Consider the context in the frequently repeated interaction that occurs when a nurse enters a client's hospital room.

1) *The Circumstances.* The client, Mrs. M., has been asking for more pain medication since her last injection three hours ago. This is the third time the nurse, Mr. B., has been in to make an assessment to determine the source of the pain and the presence of other stimuli contributing to the client's discomfort. Interventions up until now have been unsuccessful.

2) *The Environment.* The room is small and has four beds, all of them occupied with women experiencing various degrees of discomfort postsurgically. All of Mrs. M.'s roommates are asleep. The room is dimly lit, but light does creep in from the hallway.

3) *The Setting.* Mrs. M. is thrashing around in bed, hitting the siderails, and moaning. She pulls herself up slightly as the nurse walks in and over to her bedside. Mr. B. takes a chair next to the bed so that he is on a horizontal plane with her. He leans over and puts his hand on her arm.

4) *Past Experiences of Each Communicant.* Mrs. M. has had a long series of illnesses, all of which have caused her much pain. She is used to the medications not relieving her discomfort. Her doctor has told her she has a low tolerance for pain but has given in to her demands to try several different medications. Mrs. M. expects to always get her way. This is her first experience with a male nurse. Mr. B. has had similar responses from clients and has found that there can be a multitude of reasons for the medication's ineffectiveness. Since Mrs. M.'s doctor has tried several medications without success, Mr. B. feels that there may be some internal stimuli, such as concerns or fears related to other parts of her life, that are contributing to Mrs. M.'s response to pain.

5) *A Previous Understood Relationship Between the Communicants.* Mr. B. has cared one day for Mrs. M. He has felt frustrated interacting with her because he believes her requests for medication are masking other needs for attention, for control, and so forth. He communicated this by his clinical, impersonal attitude when describing to Mrs. M. the actions of the medication she is taking. Mrs. M. feels like a little child in Mr. B.'s presence. She has not perceived him as understanding her needs but as patronizing her.

The interactions that occur within the context of this scene are determined by the internal processing each communicant does prior to generating a message. If at least one of the communicants is able to assess the context of his message, there is a possibility this person can use that awareness to clarify his message to the other person. For example, Mr. B., the most likely person to assess the context in this situation, might share how frustrated he feels because he is not able to help Mrs. M. with her pain. He might talk to her about how powerless he would feel in the same situation and acknowledge the difficulty of coping with constant pain. These interactions change the context to one more conducive to self-disclosure by the client.

———— Dysfunctional Communications ————

Points of Breakdown in the Message Unit

Since the message unit is a circular process, any dysfunction along the feedback loop will affect all subsequent communications. Recall that the circularity property of living systems places each interactor as both the cause and effect of future processes that occur between them. It is important, therefore, to recognize dysfunctional parts of a message and to correct them as soon as possible. To consider dysfunction, we will examine the main parts of the message unit.

1) *Covert Rehearsal.* Since the context is part of the covert rehearsal process, misinterpreting the context will affect the individual's ability to generate a functional message. Preoccupation, fantasizing, strong negative or positive feelings, and physical discomfort are examples of intrapersonal stimuli shaping the context. Temperature, noise, and seating arrangements are environmental stimuli. Interpersonal stimuli include verbal and nonverbal cues from the other communicant that are part of the context. Any meaning an interactor chooses to give these stimuli may lead to a dysfunctional communication if it is not homologous with that of the other communicant. A possible dysfunction could occur if one communicant is using the parataxic mode of language. A private meaning for words will cause dysfunction if the uniqueness is not shared by others but is, instead, an autistic communication. In the process of covert rehearsal, a communicant may become dysfunctional using a language not understood by others.

2) *Message Generation.* A dysfunctional message may be generated on either the content level or the metacommunication level. The content sent may be incomplete. Satir (1967) identified several ways this could happen. A person may use vague pronouns such as "they, those, it, anyone..." "It really makes a difference when they tell us what to do," is not a clear message. What makes a difference? The communicant might be talking about her feelings being different, the outcome being different, or a combination of the two. She could be feeling badly about the situation or very positive. "They" would also cause confusion. Making incomplete sentences or leaving out a connecting sentence also causes incompleteness (Satir, 1967). Consider the following: "I really wanted that...Oh shoot, I forgot to make the phone call. Well now you see it's impossible to do anything. See, what did I tell you!" Even a very close friend of the sender of this message would have difficulty figuring it out. Finally, Satir noted that we can act as if we have sent a message when we really have not. Sometimes this results from a wish that the other person act in a certain way. Frequently, either spouse will expect the other to "know" something without this "something" being said out loud. Maybe the wife wants to be taken out to dinner. This is partly a "wish" and partly the idea that, obviously, if nothing is planned for dinner, he would "know" she wanted to dine out. This assumption can lead to some dysfunctional communications between the couple.

Satir (1967) also talked about contradictory and incongruent messages causing dysfunction in message generation. Contradictory messages are two or more opposing messages in sequence sent on the same communication level. "You're really smart. No, actually you're dumb," is a contradictory message sent on the content level. A smile and then a frown are two nonverbal contradictory metacommunications. We may even have a verbal metacommunication contradict a nonverbal metacommunication; *e.g.,* "That wasn't an apology," with a hug following. Incongruent messages are two or more messages sent on different levels that oppose or contradict one another. "That was only a request. I'll never ask you for anything," is a verbal metacommunication contradicted by a content message. "I love you," followed by a slap on the face is a content message contradicted by a nonverbal metacommunication.

The context in which a message is sent may also cause some incongruency. If a classroom teacher who is having difficulty controlling an unruly class suddenly jumps up on a desk, screams, and shouts obscenities, no one will know how to interpret the teacher's message. The setting and past role behaviors or expected roles of a teacher are contradicted by these new behaviors. Likewise, if I choose to ignore a close friend, I am contradicting the context of our relationship, and my message is incongruent.

——— Theoretical Applications To Group Practice ———

The Group as an Interactional System

The theory that describes interactional systems has application for nurses doing groups with clients and their significant others. Many of the groups which nurses lead or colead involve the families of clients meeting together without the client present. For example, supportive groups for parents of handicapped children or for significant others of terminally ill clients have members who are a part of the client's system as well as the group's system. Although the ill client is not directly participating in an intervention, his or her family or support system is. When the parents of the handicapped child are able to talk about their sadness and disappointment in a group of other parents, some of the grief work that would normally have to be done in the child's presence can be accomplished in the group instead. This frees up emotional energy for other kinds of work or interactions with the child once the parents are back in the family system. A similar process can occur with family members of the terminally ill. If the significant others are able to work through some of their denial, anger, and depression in a group, they can then return to the interactional system with the client armed with more awareness and understanding of how their feelings impact on the client.

The interactional system of the group may, at times, be at odds with some of the other interactional systems to which the client belongs. In an assertiveness training group, for example, members often work on changing either a nonassertive or an aggressive style of interacting (see Chapter Four). If the client succeeds in becoming more assertive in his or her relationships, the new style of interacting will be felt by the client's other interactional systems. If a spouse is comfortable with his wife's nonassertive way of behaving, her more assertive interactions may be difficult for him to handle. The client who attends a diabetic teaching group, learning to give his own insulin and regulate his diet while receiving support for these independent behaviors from the other group members and the leader, may have difficulty if the client's family members are uncomfortable allowing the client that much control. The nurse group leader needs to assess the membership of such a group from a system's point of view. Perhaps a teaching/support group for the client and his family would be appropriate. Remembering that the client is a member of many interactional systems is an important consideration for nursing care.

Nursing Care Planning as a Group Process

The process of nursing care planning most often occurs between the client, the nursing staff and, if possible, the client's significant others. A number of options are usually discussed, and the choice of interventions depends on how the systems of the client, the staff, and the family finally choose to interact. The nurse needs to remember the characteristic of equifinality which applies to all living systems. What the nursing staff envisions as steps towards the client's particular goal of wellness may not be the same path as that envisioned by the client or a significant other. If our earlier example of weight loss is applied to nursing care planning, the following illustrates the options available. Perhaps a goal of weight loss cannot be met through a low-calorie diet because the client's family is not interested in preparing low-calorie meals. However, the family might be enthused about an increased activity program in which the client and significant others can participate together. The client's goal has a good start in this systems's approach to nursing care planning.

The Family as an Interactional System

The family is a social system. As with all social systems, the family has a set of roles, behaviors, and practices developed to maintain the value structure, organization, and decision-making power of the family (King, 1981).

In family therapy, the family system is the client. The therapist is concerned with the relationships between individual family members rather than with individual intrapsychic processes (Foley, 1979). The outcome of a systems approach to family therapy is to change the family's rigidity to one where members may be free to express their individuality within the system. The therapist becomes "a model of communication" and a "teacher of individuation" (Foley, 1979, p.476). Nurses who have preparation at the graduate level (masters or doctorate) may function as family therapists after specialized training in family therapy.

Satir (1967) identified three goals for the family in therapy.

1(Each member is able to be congruent and complete with observations, feelings and thoughts about oneself and others.

2) Decisions in the family are made through exploration and negotiation rather than power plays.

3) Differentness is openly acknowledged and used for growth.

The family system as a functioning whole must be balanced by each member's need for individuality as he or she interacts with other systems. Techniques that family therapists use to realize this goal focus on the family's interactions, problem-solving methods, and role behaviors.

The following verbalizations by the therapist help clarify communications, roles, behaviors, boundaries, and the uniqueness of each family member within the power of the family system:

"Germane, I'd like you to tell Stan what kinds of things you expect from him as a husband." (roles).

"I don't know if John heard you when you complimented him just now. Maybe you should talk to him directly rather than telling me how you feel about him." (communications).

"When you leave the house each time your parents shout at each other, what are you wanting to happen with your mom and dad?" (behaviors).

"How do people in your family know when you're hurt? I've noticed that in our meetings you never tell us how you're reacting to what happens in here." (behaviors, individuality).

"Try telling Kathy what you want her to do to give you more space." (boundaries). The therapist might give the family homework to do, such as asking each member to give the others ten minutes of uninterrupted listening time once a day. The family would then report how this went at the next session. If one family member demonstrated control of the system by sabotaging the homework, this would give the therapist an excellent opportunity to examine the family's power structure using data from the interactions that had occurred at home. The therapist is constantly assessing the family system and will ask family members to give their perceptions of how the system is working. Therapy is designed to stir up the family system while promoting adaptive change.

A Family Assessment Data Form

Nurses will most often see a family or an individual member in crisis during times of illness. All nurses need to have basic assessment skills to help them recognize the characteristics of the family system in crisis and to determine when to involve other social systems for the client's or family's well-being. Table 1.1 is a composite of the observations and needed actions that will help the nurse working with families to assess a possible crisis and take appropriate actions. The nurse's knowledge of systems theory and communications will serve as the basis for appropriate actions with the family.

——— Fair-Fighting Techniques With Couples: ——— A Study in the Communication of Two Interactional Systems

A Brief Overview

Bach and Wyden (1969) and Engel (1975) have contributed a unique approach to helping couples deal with anger that is based, in part, on some of the principles of communication theory and, specifically, on the feedback cycle. Bach identified two types of aggression that couples may express to one another. Hostile aggression is the desire to hurt the other. It is present in an intimate relationship where the couple is vulnerable to the pain of each other's words. Impact aggression, however, is a specific demand for change in a relationship to promote growth for the couple and each partner individually. In order to facilitate the discharge of both types of aggression, specific exercises called hostile aggression rituals and impact aggression rituals are practiced by couples until such a structure is no longer necessary to allow the healthy expression of anger. Each partner must always have the spouse's permission to engage the other in a ritual (Engel, 1975; Bach and Goldberg, 1975). This means asking one's spouse if he or she will participate in a particular exercise that will involve expressions of aggression. When aggressive communications are planned, they lose some of their forbidding power. The nurse with a masters degree and specialized training in couples therapy might choose to teach a couple hostile and impact aggression rituals. A thorough assessment of the couple's communication pattern is necessary before any fair fighting techniques should be used.

Feedback is an important concept in both sets of rituals. Bach and Wyden (1969) used the concept of feedback specifically to prohibit one partner from responding to the other until he or she has fed back the exact content of what the other has just said. This takes good listening skills to paraphrase the other's words and assures the sender that the partner has heard the message and will respond to the meaning of what has been said. Finally, the feedback process slows down the couple's interactions, thus controlling the buildup of anger, encouraging a rational exchange, and reinforcing the positive experience of being listened to by the other.

Briefly, hostility rituals allow the individual to blow off steam while signaling the partner that this is what is going to happen. The person venting the anger does not have to worry about being rational in what he says, and the partner may just listen as the audience and applaud or say, "thank you." Hostility rituals prepare the couple to fight for change and have such interesting names as "haircut," "Vesuvius," and "Virginia Wolfe fight," all verbal exercises, and "bataca fight," which is a physical encounter using bats made out of foam rubber (Engel, 1975; Bach and Goldberg, 1975).

An Impact Ritual

The "fight for change" is an impact ritual that is the major vehicle for asking for a specific behavioral change by one partner to the other (Bach and Wyden, 1969; Engel, 1975; Bach and Goldberg, 1975). Engel compared this ritual to a labor-management negotiation. The couple must decide on a mutually agreeable time to have the fight for change, thereby allowing both partners a chance to meet at a time that will ensure the most willingness and respect for one another. The "beef" is a clear, behavioral description of what the spouse does not like in the other's actions and how those actions affect him or her emotionally (Bach and Goldberg, 1975). The beef might be compared to an assertive statement (see Chapter Four):

"I don't like it that you throw your clothes on the floor and will only pick them up after I've asked you repeatedly. I get irritated having to bug you about it. I feel sometimes like your mother and resent having to take on that role."

Unlike the assertive statement, the beef does not include a demand for a different behavior from the spouse. This is done in a "demand" statement after the other partner has repeated back to the sender what he heard her say. If he is correct, the spouse making the beef should reward the partner for good listening skills. This may be done verbally, nonverbally, or both. Hugs, kisses, and other touching is encouraged (Engel, 1975).

The demand statement must be clear, specific, and something the partner can manage to fulfill, if he so chooses (Bach and Goldberg, 1975; Engel, 1975). Going back to our original example, a demand statement might be:

"I would like you to not leave clothes around when we're going to have someone over. I'll remind you once on the day we're having company. If you don't choose to put them away, I guess our friends will see how sloppy we are."

Possible responses by the partner are unconditional acceptance, conditional acceptance, or complete unacceptance. The process of negotiation continues until agreement is reached. Each time the partners must feedback exactly what they heard from the other. A solution reached may end up not working, and either party has the right to request further negotiations (Engel, 1975). It seems that the value of the fight for change is that the couple knows they are in the process of working out a solution and are really talking and listening to one another. The opening of communications in the system allows for new input and, hopefully, growth. Ensuring that the feedback circuit is working successfully is an important step.

The communication principles for couples, presented by Bach and Engel, may be applied to interactions that occur with other groups. The nurse involved in any group work with clients can use some of the basic principles of listening and feedback, so important for fair fighting, with group members. This facilitates the communication process in a group.

REFERENCES

Bach, G. and H. Goldberg. *Creative Aggression.* New York: Aron Books, 1975.

Back, G. and P. Wyden. *The Intimate Enemy: How to Fight Fair in Love and Marriage.* New York: William Morrow and Co., Inc., 1969.

Bateson, G. "The Biosocial Integration of Behavior in the Schizophrenic Family," *Exploring the Base for Family Therapy,* eds. N. Ackerman, F. Beatman, and S. Sherman: New York: Family Service Association of America, 1961.

Engel, L. Written notes obtained on "Fair Fight Training," originated by Engel in a workshop given on the Family Study Unit, U.S. V.A. Hospital, Palo Alto, CA, 1975.

Foley, V. "Family Therapy," in *Current Psychotherapies* (2nd ed.), ed. R. Corsini. Itasca, IL: F.E. Peacock Publishers, Inc., 1979.

Haley, J. *Strategies of Psychotherapy.* New York: Grune and Stratton, 1963.

Haley, J. *Leaving Home: The Therapy of Disturbed Young People.* New York: McGraw-Hill Book Co., 1980.

Jones, S. *Family Therapy: A Comparison of Approaches.* Bowie, MD: Robert J. Brady Co., 1980.

King, I. *A Theory of Nursing: Systems, Concepts, Process.* New York: John Wiley & Sons, 1981.

Kinseth, L. "Spontaneous Nonverbal Intervention in Group Psychotherapy," *International Journal of Group Psychotherapy,* 32, no. 3 (July, 1982), 327-338.

Roy, Sr. C. and S. Roberts. *Theory Construction in Nursing: An Adaptation Model.* Englewood Cliffs, NJ: Prentice-Hall, Inc., 1981.

Ruesch, J. *Disturbed Communications.* New York: W.W. Norton and Co., Inc., 1972.

Satir, V. *Conjoint Family Therapy* (revised ed.). Palo Alto, CA: Science and Behavior Books Inc., 1967.

Sullivan, H.S. *The Interpersonal Theory of Psychiatry.* New York: W.W. Norton and Co., Inc., 1953.

von Bertalanffy, L. "The History and Status of General Systems Theory," in *Trends in General Systems Theory,* ed. G. Klir. New York: John Wiley & Sons, Inc., 1972.

von Bertalanffy, L. "General Systems Theory and Psychiatry," in *The American Handbook of Psychiatry Vol. I* (2nd ed.), ed. S. Arieti. New York: Basic Books, 1974.

Watzlawick, P., J. Beavin, and D. Jackson. *Pragmatics of Human Communication.* New York: W.W. Norton and Co., Inc., 1967.

Wilson, H. and C. Kneisl. *Psychiatric Nursing.* Menlo Park, CA: Addison-Wesley Publishing Co., 1979.

Yalom, I. *The Theory and Practice of Group Psychotherapy* (2nd ed.). New York: Basic Books, Inc., 1975.

TABLE 1.1 BEHAVIORIAL ASSESSMENT OF FAMILIES IN CRISIS

Assessment Dimensions[1]	Client Behaviors		Nursing Actions
	Verbal	Nonverbal	
A. Individual Subsystems			
1. Self-Concept	Statements of confusion re: self.[2] Asks for reassurance from others (especially strangers)[3]	May show less attention to self re: dress, hygiene, etc.	For individual client in family showing signs of being in a crisis: 1. Ask questions to supplement data collection; *i.e.*, "I notice you really want to talk a lot about your illness. How is it affecting you?"
2. Role Performance	Identifies problems in own role or roles of family members[2]	May take on one or more new roles in family. Readily accepts suggestions from others about roles to take[2]	"You seem to need a lot of reassurance from me. How come?" "How has your illness affected your relationship with family members?"
3. Interpersonal Relationships (Support Systems)	Increased tendency to self-disclose to strangers.[2] Decrease in normal interactional patterns with family members and others[2]	Prolonged eye contact with strangers[2]	2. Plan a nursing care conference with staff involved in client's care. Use collective data plus input from multidisciplinary staff to assess degree of crisis
4. Signaling Behaviors[2] (notifying others of distress)	Asks for help, protection.[2] Wants to talk about crisis.[2] Avoids interactions not crisis-related[2]	Narrowed attention span[2]	
5. Coping Styles	Exaggeration of verbal coping behaviors	Exaggeration of nonverbal coping behaviors	

TABLE 1.1 BEHAVIORIAL ASSESSMENT OF FAMILIES IN CRISIS (Continued)

Assessment Dimensions[1]	Client Behaviors		Nursing Actions
	Verbal	Nonverbal	
B. Family Interaction Patterns	Verbalizations with other family members by member in crisis may decrease[2]	Decrease in expressions of intimacy by member in crisis.[2] Other family members may increase intimacy between them	3. Discuss assessment with client. Hold a family meeting with client, family, other health professionals, and support persons (clergy, social worker, etc.) as further intervention to focus on helping client and family deal with crisis.
C. Characteristics of Family as a Whole			For the family showing signs of being in a crisis: 1. Ask questions directed at family members re: their perceptions of the family's coping, *e.g.*, "How have things been going for you as a family since Ted's illness?"
1. Problem-Solving Style	Verbalizes frustration and confusion over lack of success with normal coping style	Increase in normal problem-solving actions and in new trial-and-error methods	
2. System Boundaries	Decrease in interactions with systems outside the family. Less verbalizations re: uniqueness of individual members	Decrease in independent actions of family members	"I've missed you stopping by to chat. When Ted was first hospitalized you seemed to want to talk more about it. What's changed?"
3. Signaling Behaviors	May ask outside agency for help	One member becomes ill (illness may precipitate a family crisis or be the result of a family in crisis)	

TABLE 1.1 BEHAVIORIAL ASSESSMENT OF FAMILIES IN CRISIS (Continued)

Assessment Dimensions[1]	Client Behaviors		Nursing Actions
	Verbal	Nonverbal	
D. Environmental Field			2. Consult with multidisciplinary staff for input re: observations of family, further interventions by nursing staff, or possible referrals to social service agency for a home visit, crisis intervention, etc.
1. Community Value System	Verbalized difference in beliefs, attitudes, etc., with the community[1] (e.g., open marriage, religious preference, socio-economic background)	Behavior of family is incongruent with community (e.g., seclusiveness, purchase of many luxury items, etc.)	Referral to social service agency with needs for housing relocation, etc., in a more compatible community
2. Requirements of Community and Family	Interactions with individuals in community are difficult due to differences in language and culture or to sparse or overpopulation.	Problem with lack of schools, daycare centers, churches, employment, etc.[1]	Referral to social service agency for help locating needed services

SOURCES

1. Ann Whall, "Nursing Theory and the Assessment of Families," *Journal of Psychiatric Nursing and Mental Health Services*, 19 (January, 1981), 30-36.
2. Roseann Umana, Steven Gross, and Marcia McConville, *Crisis in the Family* (New York: Gardner Press, Inc., 1980), 62-68.
3. Martha Hill, "When the Patient is the Family," *American Journal of Nursing*, 81 (March, 1981), 536-538.

Psychoanalytical Theory and Group Practice

2

Introduction

Originally, psychoanalytical theory was associated with individual therapy and, more specifically, with the intrapsychic workings of the client. This meant that the behaviors and feelings of the individual had their source in the unconscious part of the mind where early childhood experiences influenced the client's current actions. It would seem, therefore, that present interactions between the client and others are greatly influenced by the client's past experiences. This sounds contradictory to the theory presented in Chapter One. Interactional units within systems engaged in communications with one another are constantly in the process of defining and redefining their relationship. However, what the individual brings to a relationship and how this person responds to the communications of another is affected by unconscious feelings and conflicts. Both theories have something to say about how people interact. I like to think of psychoanalytical theory as being the source of the covert rehearsal that precedes the generation of a message. When we multiply a two-person interaction with the number of interactions that a group of people would generate, the covert rehearsal part of each message becomes more important to the resultant communications within the group. Each communicant is exposed to the effect of multiple internal processes with which he or she has no awareness. If the covert processes can be made overt to the extent that communications remain functional for the group, the group may become a place where individuals gain more understanding of themselves and how they are affected by others. Clients gain more control over their intrapsychic processes and can use that in a way that facilitates their relationships with others.

This chapter describes both the individual's psyche and the group's psyche. Recall that a system made up of a group of interacting parts is an entity in itself and may be looked at as a whole. The primary group, the family, or any other group functions with both internal processes and observable behaviors. Psychoanalytical theory can explain the internal processes that occur in a group. Transactional Analysis (TA) is a therapeutic modality that has its origin in psychoanalytical theory. Whereas psychoanalysis creates a dependent relationship for the client with the therapist, TA invites the client into a partnership with the group leader to work towards observable changes in behavior and an understanding of the internal processes that can make further life-long changes possible. This chapter presents an outline of TA theory and its use in a group and in everyday communications with others. It is a helpful tool in many types of patient interactions.

Basic Ego Psychology

The Structures of the Mind

In an attempt to explain man's psyche, Sigmund Freud developed a theoretical construct of the topography of the mind and its functions. Brenner's (1957) description of basic psychoanalytical theory forms the basis of our discussion on Freud.

The mind is divided into three structures: the *id,* the *ego,* and the *super ego.* The infant is born with an id which responds only to instinctual demands, and desires immediate gratification of needs. Energy stored in the id, known as psychic energy, allows the internal processes of pain and pleasure to govern the infant's responses. Observing a newborn's behaviors, we can see the reality of this construct. If the newborn is in pain (*i.e.,* internal discomfort due to hunger, cold, wetness, or other stimuli), crying signals the desire for immediate relief. The infant will not stop crying until someone removes the source of the discomfort. Pleasure or the absence of discomfort allows the newborn to sleep peacefully. Bonding by the mothering figure adds to the infant's pleasure, although the newborn is not aware of "mother" as an entity separate from the self. The id does not distinguish any boundaries outside itself.

The remnants of the id can be illustrated by the primary-process thinking which persons engage in when they dream, play "mind" games with one another, respond to jokes, and so forth. Primary process characterizes the id's immature yet, paradoxically, complex form of thinking. Paradoxes are a part of primary-process thinking since contradictory ideas, condensation, and timelessness all may exist together. Condensation refers to the inclusion of many ideas into one symbol. It is much the same as the concept of connotation that was discussed in Chapter One. Recall that "mother" may have many emotional ideas attached to it. However, one symbol, the word "mother," represents warmth, love, security, and so forth. Poets frequently use symbolism to express a number of ideas with one word or phrase. Jokes would not be funny if the punch line were not a condensation of several different ideas or double meanings. Most people have experienced timelessness in dreams where friends from the past show up in present-day scenes and time seems to be very distorted or to stand still. Although the id is the most immature part of the mind, it has many functions in adult life. Freud said the id was the source of all sexual and aggressive impulses. Translating that into more workable terminology, the id allows us to respond at a feeling level without thinking. Our ego then tempers the strong, impulsive feelings from the id into more acceptable expressions of emotion.

The ego is the bridge from the spontaneous, impetuous actions of the id to the controlled and logical responses of a mature mind. Actually, the ego begins to form sometime during the first year of life when the infant begins to understand the breast or bottle and other mothering actions as being distinct from itself. Now the more mature infant will delay gratification of immediate needs as long as mother makes her presence known frequently and responds consistently to the infant's signals. The ego has many functions. It allows us to reality-test, to develop relationships with people, to defend against overwhelming danger or anxiety, to determine where our boundaries end and others' begin, and to do all those adult things that keep us surviving in the world of multiple living systems. The ego is a mediator between internal instincts and the demands of the environment. Our ego is our conscious concept of ourself. Since the ego is such a mature construct, its thinking process, secondary process, is more logical and sophisticated. Secondary process includes concept formation, problem-solving, concentration, memory, and the higher skills of synthesis and integration. Generally, it is not until after adolescence that the individual masters the latter two skills. It is interesting that the ego is smart enough to allow itself to regress or to let out more id in the interest of creativity. Artists, poets, playwrights, and others must be able to do some of those id primary-process activities to produce works that stir up one's fantasies. The ego may also regress to protect itself from overwhelming anxiety. This is a pathological response, the discussion of which lies outside the scope of this book. If the ego is not regressed, it is responding according to the laws of syntax that characterize secondary-process thinking. Comparing this to Sullivan's (1953) syntaxic mode of experience, the importance of secondary process in everyday communications with others is evident. The words we use in secondary process have universal consensual validation which allow us to be understood by others.

The last structure of the mind to develop in the individual is the super ego. Like the id, its functions are largely unconscious. Its development is a result of the child incorporating the mores, values, attitudes, and norms of the parenting persons with whom the child has interacted for four to five years. Thus, it is not until preschool age that the super ego even begins to develop. Notice the behavior of a toddler. She needs constant reminders from adults to keep out of trouble. Her only controls are external and do not serve her as a code of conduct based on a particular value system. Toddlers do not understand the meaning of right or wrong behavior. The preschooler, however, will begin to think morally about her actions, *i.e.,* "It is not right to hit my brother when he takes my toy." Freudians call the process of incorporating external events into one's psyche and making them one's own, introjection. Perhaps a prime example of introjection is a husband feeling sympathetic pains when his wife is in labor. Brenner (1957) noted that identification is another term often used in place of introjection. In communications with others, one may empathize by saying, "I can identify with that feeling." Identification and introjection will both be explored in greater detail later. Introjection of parental ideals is a slow process and occurs over a number of years until the child is ten or eleven. The super ego is the source of one's guilt, self-approval or disapproval, and even self-praise. Because of the super ego's functions, many problems related to the "OK-ness" of the individual have their source in such messages.

Repression

One of the ways the ego protects the individual from the pain of unpleasant memories or emotions is through the mechanism of repression. Repression bars from one's consciousness thoughts which would cause pain or unpleasantness (Brenner, 1957). A lot of energy goes into keeping things out of conscious awareness and may take away from the ego's energy to perform other functions.

Occasionally, some of the conflicts that a person has repressed will slip out subtly through the individual's behaviors. The meaning of such actions remains out of the person's awareness. This is called acting-out (Wilson and Kneisl, 1979). Suicide may be considered the ultimate expression of acting-out. Less serious forms of this would be getting intoxicated, having an affair, lying, "ditching" school, and so forth. It is important to note that a person is not considered to be acting-out unless his or her behavior is an expression of some repressed pain or conflict. Acting-up behaviors may look the same, but the origin is not repressed material. If a person steals to get money or because of a conscious decision to not obey the law, this is acting-up behavior. Stealing becomes an acting-out behavior when the person cannot identify any conscious reason for doing it. Acting-out sometimes occurs in a group setting. See the discussion of latent content for an understanding of how acting-out affects a group.

Acting-out is actually a form of resistance to letting out repressed material. Although something is slipping through to consciousness in the form of an observable behavior, what is observed is not the feelings or thoughts that would bring the individual pain. Any phenomena that keep the client from producing material from the unconscious are labeled by psychoanalysts as resistance (Wilson and Kneisl, 1979). Resistance may take many forms. Keeping silent, withdrawing, making superficial conversation, changing the subject, and being late for a group meeting are all forms of resistance. Resistance in a group is a clue to the leader that some unconscious pain is causing a member or members to use a lot of energy to defend against awareness of this pain. Support groups created to help members deal with emotionally and, often, physically painful occurrences in their lives will frequently see resistant behaviors occurring.

Psychic Determinism

Another phenomenon that has its origin in the unconscious is psychic determinism. Psychic determinism expresses the idea that no human behavior is a random act isolated from previous behaviors by the person. Actions do not happen by chance but are determined by events preceding them (Wilson and Kneisl, 1979; Arlow, 1979). An accident or a slip of the tongue has its origin in the unconscious intent of the individual (Brenner, 1957). This concept is useful when exploring resistance with a client manifested by repetitious behaviors for which the client is unwilling to take responsibility. Yalom (1975) noted that a behavior is not significant unless it is repeated at least three times. If a member is often late for group, this is probably an intentional behavior, although the client may not be consciously aware of the reasons for the behavior. The staff nurse might confront his supervisor when she keeps misplacing his request for attendance at various conferences. Her intent is probably not a conscious one but may signify the existence of some conflictual feelings towards the nurse. If he can get her to talk with him about their relationship, she may eventually become aware of her negative feelings. The ego, remember, helps to keep anxiety at a manageable level by repressing what the individual cannot handle. If the nurse in the previous example makes it less threatening or anxiety-producing for his supervisor to express negative feelings to him, he may break through some of this resistance.

Transference

Transference may occur between a client and the group leader. In a traditional psychoanalytical group, transference is important to the success of the group. It is purposely nurtured by the group leader(s) (Yalom, 1975a). Transference is a "very unique, highly emotional attitude" that the client develops towards the analyst which represents the feelings and wishes towards significant others in the client's past that are now projected onto the therapist (Arlow, 1979, p.17). Often, the most common feelings to be projected are those the client had towards mother or father. The analyst uses transference for diagnostic purposes as well as to promote a corrective emotional response within the client as the analyst responds with healthy mother or father transactions (Yalom, 1975a).

Parataxic Distortion

A term similar to transference but with more encompassing meaning is parataxic distortion. Parataxic distortion refers to those wishes and feelings an individual had for significant others in her past which are projected onto any number of current relationships. Sullivan (1954) noted that, in parataxic distortion, the characteristics of a person whose relationship with another is being distorted by the latter are of negligible importance to the interpersonal situation. If a client is projecting feelings of hostility onto another group member because his mannerisms remind the client of the way her husband acts when she argues with him, she is not seeing this person's real characteristics. Obviously, parataxic distortion causes problems in communications. Recall the discussion in Chapter One about the parataxic mode of experience. The individual relating in this way views the world from a very personal stance. No consensual validation can occur between persons if one is relating from the parataxic mode. Parataxic distortion is often "the basis for the really astonishing misunderstandings and misconceptions which characterize all human relations" (Sullivan, 1954, p.26). Parataxic distortion is a more inclusive concept than transference to use in work with clients. I sometimes catch myself relating with an unusual amount of emotion to what a client is telling me. This signals me to be alert to some subjectiveness within the client or myself. If I am reacting subjectively, I may be bringing into our relationship some past feelings I experienced in an interaction with some significant person in my life. Role appropriate feelings are the expected response in a particular situation; whereas, subjective feelings come from a very personal reaction to the same occurrence. Subjective feelings stand out because they are generally not congruent to the situation, *e.g.*, they are overly emotive, understated, or totally inappropriate. If a client screams at the nurse when she tries to help her out of bed, she is probably experiencing some personal stimuli of which the nurse is not aware. She may be feeling very depressed about her incapacitation; she may be in physical pain, or she may be recalling a time when someone else made her feel very helpless and dependent. The latter is parataxic distortion. Parataxic distortion is a phenomenon that has a significant impact on the interactions between people.

Anxiety and Self-Esteem

Sullivan added an interpersonal level to psychoanalytical theory with his concept of anxiety. Although he talked about the internal processes a person experiences, he stressed the importance the effect one's interactions with others had on one's psyche. His theories help us to understand resistances that occur in a group setting. According to psychoanalytical theory, resistance is anything that inhibits the client from allowing painful material to be made conscious. Sullivan said that resistance is a function of a threat to one's self-esteem (Sullivan, 1954). Anxiety is the signal that one's self-respect is in danger. An individual's need for interpersonal security leads to an attempt to rid oneself of the anxiety that is so threatening to the self-system (Sullivan, 1953). Sullivan suggested that responses to anxiety vary from anger to selective inattention where the individual overlooks whatever interpersonal interaction is provoking the anxiety and shifts to another topic. If all fails, severe anxiety sets in, and the person is incapable of any constructive communication (Sullivan, 1954). This is a more conscious process than the forms of resistance discussed previously. Although the act of resisting the feeling of anxiety is conscious, the individual may not make the connection between the resultant behaviors, *e.g.,* anger, selective inattention, and the original painful stimulus.

It follows that manifestations of anxiety in a group most likely have their origin with the interpersonal interactions that occur there or with the person's perception of a possible interpersonal transaction that might occur. A group member may anticipate a threat to the self by fantasizing about the nature of a relationship between herself and another member. It is also possible that an interaction within the group will cause someone to remember a significant past relationship that triggers anxiety (parataxic distortion).

The Group Psyche

In Chapter One, the group was identified as a system or entity of its own having certain properties. In psychoanalytical terms, the group has a psyche. Just as the individual responds to and acts upon internal stimuli, the group, collectively, may do this also. The internal stimuli for the group are the fantasies, wishes, anxieties, and other subjective phenomena that govern responses that are made by group members as a collective body. In future chapters, stages of group movement, the group emotion, group resistance, and other collective group phenomena will be explored in detail. It is the purpose of this chapter to introduce psychoanalytical terminology and theory that are applicable to the study of groups.

In a group setting, some of the individual distortions that occur because of a person's response to internal stimuli have a better chance of being corrected because of the presence of many "egos" to perform the function of reality-testing and feedback to the individual information that has been consensually validated. Yalom (1975, p.26) commented on this when comparing individual to group psychotherapy, "...the group setting offers far more opportunities for the generation of corrective emotional experiences." Recall that consensual validation is a term used by Sullivan to describe the process of correcting parataxic distortions by comparing one's evaluation of an interpersonal interaction with those of others. In a group, the existence of rules that require "honesty of expression offers ample opportunity for consensual validation." (Yalom, 1975, p.26). Reality-testing may be performed in the absence of an interaction with another. The mature ego is able to distinguish between one's own internal stimuli and actual phenomena in the outside world through a collection of experiences with one's environment over a period of time. Adults reality-test better than small children because they have had more experiences with the outside world. Santa Claus would not exist if children had the same ability to reality-test as adults do. In a group, individual reality testing is complemented with consensual validation by other group members and the leader. The leader performs many functions within the group. To the extent that the leader models reality testing and promotes consensual validation within the group, the leader is acting as an ego for the group psyche. Subsequent chapters will describe the process the leader uses to do this and will discuss other leadership functions in detail. Persons other than the leader may facilitate consensual validation within the group. Anytime consensual validation occurs, functional communication is enhanced.

Manifest Vs. Latent Content

In Chapter One, communication was defined as occurring on two levels, the denotative level and the metacommunication level. A similar concept taken from psychoanalytical theory describes the elements of a group session as existing on two levels: the manifest and the covert. The material expressed at each level is called the content. Manifest material consists of that which can be readily observed, *i.e.,* the verbal content expressed as well as verbal and nonverbal metacommunications that are obvious to the observer. Latent material is not expressed overtly, is most likely not within the group members' awareness, and is hardest to detect in groups where the manifest content is consistent and coherent, *i.e.,* in functional communications (Whitaker and Lieberman, 1964). Notice that the two levels of communication and the two levels of group content cannot be described as synonymous. Metacommunications may be part of the observable level of group content or part of the covert/latent level. A smile directed towards the group leader by a member may be considered a manifest expression of greeting or positive regard towards the leader. On the latent level, the smile may be a statement of a fantasized intimate relationship with the leader which the member may eventually act-out. The statement, "I'm going to apologize to the group by reading to you all from the Bible," is a verbal metacommunication sent on the manifest level. Covertly, the message may be, "I'm playing God in this group."

Manifest and latent content is expressed individually or by the group as a whole. A group verbalizes wanting an atmosphere where every member feels comfortable sharing painful feelings. However, behaviors of group members indicate the presence of latent content. Members may talk superficially, intellectualize, and rescue each other by changing the subject when any threatening topic begins to surface. The verbal acting-out is a covert collective group message, "We don't know if it's safe to self-disclose here," or, put another way, "We don't know if the leader can keep things under control." The latent content will vary according to the current stage of group development. These messages would be indicative of a group in the initial stage or the first part of the middle stage (See Chapter Six). The group psyche expresses the latent material of the group. Latent content reflecting an individual member's internal conflicts and fantasies certainly affects the other group members. Parataxic distortion, transference phenomena, resistance in the form of acting-out behaviors, and other individual internal dynamics all contribute to dysfunctional communications within a group. This, in turn, affects how future interactions will occur among members and how individuals perceive themselves and others within the group.

Transactional Analysis

The application of psychoanalytical theory to practice found in Transactional Analysis comes from Eric Berne. Berne was a student of classical psychoanalysis but broke away to develop more rapid methods to cure clients. Because he felt so strongly about this, he willingly shared his expertise with any professional that wanted training in TA (Dusay and Dusay, 1979). Thomas Harris, in the preface to his book, *I'm OK—You're OK*, talked about the difficulty the client has in understanding psychoanalytical jargon and applying it to his everyday practical problems, such as getting along with others (Harris, 1973). The language of Transactional Analysis eliminates this problem.

"The vocabulary of Transactional Analysis is the precision tool of treatment because, in a language anyone can understand, it identifies things that really are, the reality of experiences that really happened in the lives of people who really existed." (Harris, 1973, p.15).

The basic concepts of Transactional Analysis are found on the following pages. I use TA both with individuals and with groups and am still very much a novice in its applications. Because the terminology is relatively simple to understand, particularly the core concepts, the temptation to become a TA expert is great. As I read more about TA, I am convinced of its sophistication and complexity. When used by a therapist properly trained in its applications, it has universal effectiveness in helping people change. The therapeutic modalities discussed in the first four chapters are for the purpose of introducing the reader to the application of theory in a variety of group situations. Many require the facilitator to have graduate-level preparation and certification to practice. The reader is invited to read more on the various modalities and to obtain the appropriate training if this is desired.

The Ego States

Berne (1961) used this term to denote a person's "states of mind and their related patterns of behavior" (p.30). The ego states have some similarities to Freud's structures of the mind in that they roughly correspond in function to the id, ego, and super ego. However, they are more personal than the latter and can be applied directly to interpersonal interactions and current relationships. Berne named the ego states after the role figure to which their characteristics related. The Parent, Adult, and Child are capitalized to distinguish them from actual persons taking on these roles. They will be discussed in order of their development within the individual. Like the id, ego, and super ego, the ego states develop at different times as one's ego matures. Observations of the individual's verbal and nonverbal behaviors are cues to the ego state from which the person is currently relating. The ego states may be analyzed according to their structure and their function. The structure refers to the historical components leading to their development; whereas, the function describes how the ego states are used (Woollams and Brown, 1979).

The Child. Berne (1961) described the Child as those feelings, attitudes, and behavior patterns that originated from the individual's own childhood. The Child is the first ego state to develop. Its structure is made up of three smaller ego states as described by Woollams and Brown (1979) and discussed in the following paragraphs. The Child in the Child (C1) is the primary motivator of behaviors, expressing the uncensored feelings and needs that exist in all of us. C1 also contains tapes or memories of past feeling responses to events that were particularly intense, such as strong fear or expressions of love, frequently from significant persons in one's life. Since C1 is related to internal processing and often functions outside of our awareness, it is probably the closest ego state comparison to the id. C1 tapes may be played back to allow one to experience once again the feelings from one's childhood.

The Adult in the Child (A1), also known as the Little Professor, is, like C1, primarily operating outside of our awareness. The intuitive, creative preverbal infant is a Little

Professor trying to figure out how to get along with mother and other parts of a newly found environment. Adults are using the Little Professor when they comment on how they "feel" about something. They are making an intuitive, subjective statement that involves a hunch. Artists, writers, inventors, and other creative people must have a lot of A1 in their Child. Woollams and Brown (1979) make the point that a "freed-up Little Professor makes for a better therapist, as well as for a more interesting and exciting life." (p.13).

The Parent in the Child (P1) develops in response to a need for the child to gain the approval of the parenting persons. Spontaneous C1 expressions are frowned upon at times by parents. This gets the Little Professor working on figuring out what responses might be most acceptable to Mom or Dad. The automatic, conditioned feelings and behaviors resulting from the Little Professor's work, P1 responses, are used to deal with people perceived by the child as authority figures. P1 seems to be the most controlling part of the Child, and could be responsible for such behaviors as suicide or insanity if the person perceives that he or she has failed to live up to others' expectations (Woollams and Brown, 1979). Most of us have a set of responses to certain authority figures in our lives. One may observe individuals responding in a diffident manner to law enforcement officers even though the particular situation does not require such behavior. Some people never move beyond a Child-to-Parent interactional pattern with their own parents, although Adult-to-Adult interactions would be more appropriate.

In discussing the functions of the Child ego state, Berne (1961) described the Adapted Child as behaving under the dominance of parental influence in a compliant way that is acceptable to parent figures. Woollams and Brown (1979) added to this description by noting that the Adaptive Child behaves in ways that discount one's natural, spontaneous feelings, *i.e.,* responding with the feeling state that will be most acceptable in the situation, even though one is actually feeling something else. Rebelliousness is an Adaptive Child response because its motivation comes from meeting others' expectations. Generally, the covert message to a child behind a manifest request to "not get dirty" is "I don't expect you to stay neat and clean." If this is accompanied by a smile from the parent, the child has gotten an incongruent message and will most likely respond to the most powerful part of this message, the nonverbal. Even a stern look, making the same message congruent, might evoke a rebellious response if the child's Adaptive Child senses that getting dirty is the response the parents expect.

The Natural or Free Child responds autonomously and spontaneously without any concern for how others will react to the behavior (Berne, 1961; Woollams and Brown, 1979). Frequently, such Free-Child behaviors not motivated by a need to adapt to others are labeled by parents as rebelliousness (Woollams and Brown, 1979). The label depends on the motivation behind the behavior. It is possible that the Adaptive Child will decide that an expected behavior is "to be spontaneous." A shy person attending a party may be operating from her Adaptive Child when she becomes "wild and crazy" after drinking enough alcohol to become impulsive and let out C1 feelings. The fact that her motivation was to do what she thought was expected of her is Adaptive, although C1 responses most commonly would be associated with Free-Child activities. Woollams and Brown (1979) noted that negative Free-Child behaviors, such as driving a car at very high rates of speed, may hurt oneself or others while the Free

Child is expressing itself and having fun. "[M]ost behaviors which at first appear to be negative Free Child are actually self-destructive Adapted Child actions" (p.23).

Finally, Berne (1966) noted the difference between the id and the Child ego state. The Child is organized and has a will of its own as contrasted with the unorganized biological drives of the id.

The Parent (P2). At about ten months, the infant starts recording in the Parent events by significant others that are powerful people in the infant's life. Parenting figures get the most coverage, followed by older siblings, other relatives and adults living in the home, and teachers and others outside the home and influential in the child's development. Adults continue to make Parent tapes, but these tapes become more selective and might include messages from a mentor, a political or religious leader, a spouse, or boss. The Parent ego state contains judgments, opinions, values, and attitudes that attempt to define for the Child ego state how one should perceive and deal with the world (Woollams and Brown, 1979).

Examples from the Parent are best understood within the framework of a functional analysis. The function of the Parent is to reduce anxiety and conserve energy for the individual by making it possible for the person to come by certain decisions automatically (Berne, 1961). The Nurturing Parent is warm, protective, concerned, forgiving, permissive, and sympathetic (Woollams and Brown, 1979; Berne, 1961):

"I came over to see that you get some rest. Now go lie down."

"You'd better put your coat on or you'll catch cold."

"It's OK that you forgot my birthday. I know you love me."

"Go ahead and buy it. You've worked hard on that book."
Woollams and Brown (1979) made a distinction between the positive Nurturing Parent who cares for another when the person wants or needs this care and the negative Nurturing Parent who gives out this care when it is not needed or requested. The first two examples would be from a negative Nurturing Parent if the help and advice were not solicited.

The Prejudicial, Controlling, or Critical Parent is arbitrary, opinionated, powerful, punitive, principled, and demanding (Berne, 1961; Woollams and Brown, 1979):

"I said no and I mean it. You don't need a reason."

"That was really stupid. You go back and start all over again, and do it right this time."

"I'm in charge of this project, and I'm going to see that things are done correctly."

"We expect you to apologize to your teacher and give him the respect I know you can."
The first two statements come from a negative Controlling Parent, since they may negatively influence the other person's self-esteem level. Positive Controlling Parent statements, like the latter two, stand up for one's own and other's rights without putting others down (Woollams and Brown, 1979).

In comparing the Parent ego state to the function of the super ego, Berne (1961) noted that both constructs modify behavior on the basis of past experience with authority figures. However, the Parent deals with the individual's transactions with real parental figures and offers permission and encouragement which the super ego does not do.

The Adult (A2). Towards the end of the first year of life, the Adult begins to develop as the infant becomes more verbal. The Adult is called the Computer because it processes data in an objective, unfeeling manner. Its relationship with the external environment is based on autonomous reality-testing (Woollams and Brown, 1979; Berne, 1961). As a fully functioning adult, the individual will use both the creativity and intuition of A1 and the logic of A2. The Adult does not function independently of the other two ego states but responds to the Child's need for information to help with decision-making and maximizing fun and to the Parent's need for data to prove the correctness of its statements (Woollams and Brown, 1979). Both the ego and the Adult perform reality testing for accuracy of responses and to prevent distortion of the environment. Freud's concept of a weak ego was that it caused pathological distortion because it ignored data. According to TA theory, the Adult is never weak but may be handicapped by lack of available data. Pathologically, the Adult contaminated by the Child could be considered as synonymous to a weak ego (Berne, 1966). Discussion of pathological responses go beyond the scope of this book.

Transactions

One's ego states are the structure for interactions that define relationships with others. Woollams and Brown (1979) described transactions in two ways: an exchange of strokes between persons, and the stimulus and response between ego states. A stroke is a unit of attention that provides stimulation to the individual either in a positive or negative manner. Other than internal stimulation when we recall old tapes from our Parent or Child (*i.e.,* a memory that is either pleasant or painful), stroking is an interactional process. Strokes may be given through physical stimulation or by verbal or nonverbal messages. Even though negative strokes are unpleasant, they are a message that the person is being recognized. Often the misbehaviors of children are unconsciously motivated by recognition hunger or a need for attention (Berne, 1972). The opposite to being stroked is receiving a discount, the act of not being recognized (Woollams and Brown, 1979). The following are examples of strokes and discounts:

"I really liked the way you handled that situation today." (positive stroke).

"You've really been bad today. Go to your room until you decide to apologize." (negative stroke).

"Oh, have I met you before? I'm afraid I don't remember your name." (discount).

Nonverbally: a hug (positive), a spanking (negative), and a purposeful lack of eye contact (discount).

Complementary Transactions. In a complementary transaction, the response comes from the same ego state to which it was directed and goes to the same ego state that initiated the stimulus. In other words, the stimulus and response vectors are parallel (Woollams and Brown, 1979). A common occurrence in the nurse-client relationship is a complementary transaction with the nurse coming from the Parent ego state and the client coming from the Child. It is inherent in the nurse's role to be nurturing and critical at times, thus facilitating a Parent-Child relationship with a dependent client. If the client is a health care consumer, the complementary relationship most appropriate for transactions between the nurse and client would be Adult-Adult. The client makes decisions about his care in collaboration with the nurse. Certainly, there are times when the Parent-Child transaction between the nurse and the client is appropriate (*e.g.,* when the client is dependent on the nurse for basic need fulfillment during critical-care situations and immediately postoperatively). Some clients desire the more traditional Parent-Child transactions with the nurse. The nurse needs to assess the relationship status with the client to determine the type of complementary transaction most appropriate to the client's adaptation. See Figure 2.1 for examples of complementary transactions as they occur in nurse-client relationships.

Berne (1966) suggested that, as long as the vectors are parallel, communication may continue indefinitely. However, complementary transactions may become boring, frustrating, and so forth. Communication continues, but the relationship between the communicants might deteriorate because of the feelings one or both communicants

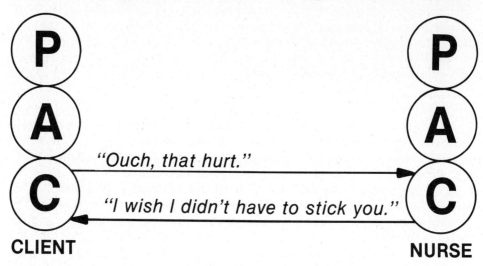

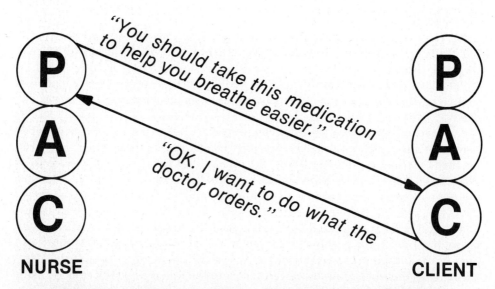

COMPLEMENTARY TRANSACTIONS

Figure 2.1

has about the transactions. Probably the most common example of this phenomenon is the Parent-Child transactions that many couples find themselves pursuing. If the husband becomes bored with his wife's wishes to be parented all the time, he may find himself looking for other relationships that would give him more strokes. Perhaps he wants more recognition for his Child or Adult ego states. His options with his wife are to continue to elicit her Child with his Parent or to cross the transaction by responding from the Adult, for example.

Crossed Transactions. Once one person responds from an ego state not intended by the stimulus of the transaction, a crossed transaction occurs. The vectors between the transactions are no longer parallel. If the vectors are crossed, communication stops, at least for a time, and the relationship as previously defined by the communicants is in danger (Berne, 1966). Figure 2.2 applies the theory about crossed transactions to nurse-client communications.

Recall the discussion on transference and countertransference reactions. Berne (1961; 1966) explained these phenomena in terms of transactional analysis. The classical transference reaction is an Adult stimulus from the therapist directed towards the client's Adult which elicits, instead, a response from the Child of the client to the Parent of the therapist. A countertransference reaction is just the opposite. The client attempts to elicit an Adult response to an Adult stimulus but gets a Parent-to-Child response from the therapist. Berne noted that transference/countertransference reactions were very accessible to analysis using transactional data. He saw this as a more efficient method than the difficult process of self-analysis which the psychoanalyst needed to use.

Ulterior Transactions. Although it takes a series of ulterior transactions plus what Berne (1966) called a "payoff" to make a game, ulterior transactions, because of their duplicity, have a game-like quality. Ulterior transactions contain both a social message (an overt or manifest message) and a psychological message (the covert, latent message). Ulterior transactions may be either angular or duplex. An angular transaction is a message sent from one ego state of the initiator to two ego states of the respondent. The initiator is trying to psychologically "hook" a second ego state without the respondent being aware of this. Salespersons will frequently initiate an Adult-to-Adult message to a prospective buyer while hoping part of the Adult's information will appeal to the Child. If the message to the Child were overt, it would probably not be as effective. A duplex transaction involves four ego states with two sets of complementary transactions sent simultaneously, one on the social level and one on the psychological level. The psychological level is always the most meaningful level, thus determining the outcome of the transaction. Very often, the nonverbal modes are used to send the psychological message (Berne, 1966; Woollams and Brown, 1979). Figure 2.3 illustrates the angular and the duplex transactions as they might occur in nurse-client interactions.

In Chapter One, the sending of dysfunctional messages was discussed. One may create a dysfunctional message by engaging in ulterior transactions. If the respondent does not pick up on the overt message level, the message is incomplete in regard to the initiator's goals. Because the respondent is frequently unaware of the psychological level or the initiator's intentions, ulterior transactions, even if successful, tend to encourage dysfunctional communications.

When ulterior transactions result in a predictable payoff called a game, participants

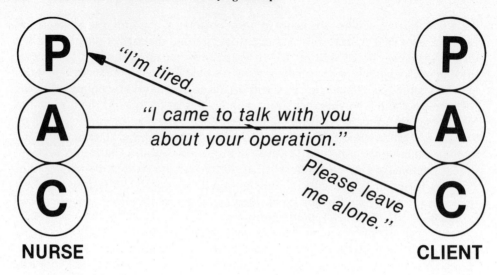

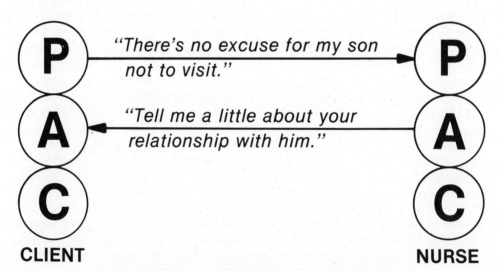

CROSSED TRANSACTIONS

Figure 2.2

end up with racket feelings. Racket feelings are not Free-Child feelings but learned responses by the Adapted Child which help the individual deal with "not OK" messages or discounts from others (Woollams and Brown, 1979). If a person is feeling hurt but finds it is more acceptable to feel angry, the anger becomes a racket feeling (genuine anger from the Free Child is not a racket feeling because it is not an adaptation to someone else's expectations).

Racket feelings may be cashed in with what Berne (1966, 1972) called "trading stamps." Berne was referring to an individual's tendency to save up racket feelings and cash them in to justify certain behaviors. Brown stamps are accumulated for bad feelings. If a colleague consistently allows herself to be yelled at or embarrassed by others and never says anything to acknowledge her hurt, she may be saving up brown stamps in the form of a racket feeling, such as self-pity, to be cashed in later. One day, she may leave the unit early saying she is too overworked and has a bad headache. Perhaps she "forgets" to carry out an important nursing order and blames this on "stress." More serious "cash-ins" of one's brown stamps include drinking alcohol, taking other drugs, or making a suicide attempt. Collecting brown

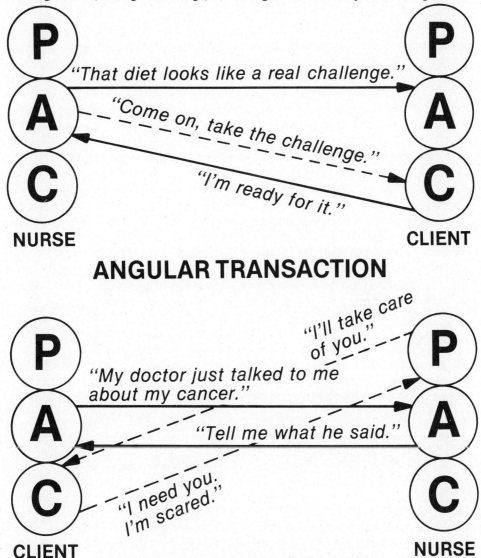

ANGULAR TRANSACTION

DUPLEX TRANSACTION

Figure 2.3

stamps precludes the individual from expressing feelings when they occur, thus preventing the communicants involved from clarifying their relationship through feedback with each other. For further discussion of specific games, racket feelings, and trading stamps, the reader is directed to Berne (1964) and other TA therapists who have written on this subject.

Scripting

A script is an ongoing personal life plan developed in early childhood through a set of decisions influenced by one's parents and in reaction to what is perceived as occurring in one's world (Berne, 1972; Woollams and Brown, 1979). Scripting begins with the infant's encounter with the parenting person, and the P1 tapes which the infant records in reaction to parental messages are the beginnings of the script. Messages for scripts are sent verbally or nonverbally by the powerful authority figures in the child's life. For example, always forgetting a child's name says, "You're not important," or "You're not an individual." Parents often sound like they are labeling a child when they may only mean to label a behavior, "You're a bad boy," or "That was stupid." As the child grows, the label may become real and believable. It is more difficult, then, for this individual to see him or herself as not "bad" or "stupid."

I use the scripting concept when I work with clients whom I see struggling with Parent messages that are keeping them from making a decision that would be adaptive for them. Perhaps a common problem nurses encounter with clients is compliance with doctor's orders or nursing actions. A client may not be staying on a prescribed weight loss diet. In talking with the client, the nurse discovers that the client's mother always gave her "be fat" messages (e.g., "You're my cute little chubby girl...I just love fat babies...I'm insulted if people don't clean their plates up for me...Heavy women don't get taken advantage of."). Most likely, the nurse will not be able to help the client deal with all these messages in a way that would free her to make her own decision about being fat, but the nurse does have more data about the client's lack of compliance. It is important to give clients the message that they may take the power to make their own decision if they wish to do so. It also important for nurses to empathize with those persons who cannot seem to free themselves from Parent tapes. The nurse may support a client's decision to look for psychotherapeutic help in making some script changes.

Applying TA to Work with Groups

Thomas Harris (1973) offered some comments on the uses for TA. "A central reason why Transactional Analysis offers such promise for filling the gap between the need for and supply of treatment is that it works at its best in groups...Anybody can use it. People do not have to be "sick" to benefit from it." (p.17). The traditional TA group is led by a trained TA professional. Each group member has a contract which is shared with the group. Berne (1966) noted the following as appropriate goals for members: reorganizing one's personality, achieving a symptomatic remission or cure, increasing control of feelings and behaviors, abandoning stereotyped relationship patterns, and increasing one's satisfaction with socialization.

As with all therapeutic modalities, judgment must be used by the health professional in applying such techniques. With TA, there is the danger that one can become so caught up in the terminology that the ultimate goal is lost. Labeling one's messages as Parent, Adult, or Child does not necessarily help someone to change dysfunctional ego states or transactions. Extensive work with a TA therapist is usually necessary before change can take place. I have found some principles of TA helpful, however, in work with both individual clients and with groups.

Hooking One Ego State: The Adult. The Adult makes change possible because it is free of the contamination of past messages and needs only to deal with the facts. Recall the discussion of psychic determinism in which all of one's present behaviors had their cause in past events and relationships. Harris (1967) noted that the cause-and-effect nature of the universe need not be the only way of explaining one's current actions. The Adult may contemplate the future and estimate probabilities in order to make a decision about an action to take. If I can get a client to respond from the Adult, perhaps this person will make a more adaptive decision with regard to behaviors. If the client is trying to get me to Parent her, I would choose, instead, to cross the transaction and come back in my Adult hoping to hook hers:

Client: "I don't know what to do. I'm so stupid when it comes to finances." (Adapted Child).

Nurse: "Well, how about looking at some of your options." (Adult).

The Child. If I want the client to get to some bottled-up feelings, I would try and hook the Free Child by coming across in my Child (C1): "Wow I get really angry when I hear you say that." Frequently, a group experiential exercise (see Chapter Nine), such as one to increase trust or promote expression of feelings, is best done when the group members can get into their child. Having the members sit on the floor or do a warm-up "play" exercise, such as tossing balloons, brings out the child.

Identifying Script Messages. We have talked briefly about looking at the client's script. If I get the sense that a client is operating from a Parent tape (*e.g.,* the person seems inflexible or in conflict about making decisions to act), I might ask the client what he is telling me about the decision he is making or what is influencing his decision-making. The individual may not be able to give me an answer, but I have probably started him thinking about his script or at least about his conflict.

Group members will often carry out a script in group, since the multitude of transactions may hook the client's script message. A client who has a script, "I don't belong," or "I'm the odd one," will tend to interpret other members' actions toward her as rejection or messages that she is different. Consensual validation by the group of what the actions or messages actually mean is very important for the client to hear. The group can be a powerful force in influencing a client to change a losing script.

Analyzing Transactions. It may be helpful in a group to point out crossed transactions when they occur, since this will have an effect on the communication process within the group. Likewise, a group member who complains about others in the group always giving him advice may need to look at what ego state he is in when he interacts with others. Perhaps his Child invites a Nurturing or Controlling Parent response. Teaching clients basic TA terminology makes it easier to talk about transactions between group members. It also dispels the power around some of the interventions the leader makes in a group, since the members also have a tool for looking at their communications with others. There is the danger that clients will want to intellectualize about their ego states instead of changing less adaptive transactions. If TA terminology is used in a non-TA group, it should be kept simple and applicable to the transactions occurring at the moment. Transactional Analysis is a very helpful tool for nurse/client interactions; however, it requires that the group leader understand the concepts of TA before attempting to use them with clients.

REFERENCES

Arlow, J. "Psychoanalysis," *Current Psychotherapies* (2nd ed.), ed. R. Corsini. Itasca, IL: F.E. Peacock Publishers, Inc., 1979

Berne, E. *Transactional Analysis in Psychotherapy.* New York: Grove Press, Inc., 1961.

Berne, E. *Games People Play.* New York: Grove Press, Inc., 1964.

Berne, E. *Principles of Group Treatment.* New York: Grove Press, Inc., 1966.

Berne, E. *What Do You Say After You Say Hello?* New York: Grove Press, Inc. 1972

Brenner, C. *An Elementary Textbook of Psychoanalysis* (Anchor Books ed.). New York: Doubleday and Co., Inc., 1957.

Dusay, J. and K. Dusay. "Transactional Analysis," in *Current Psychotherapies* (2nd ed.), ed. R. Corsini. Itasca, IL: F.E. Peacock Publishers, Inc., 1979.

Harris, T. *I'm OK—You're OK* (Avon Books ed.). New York: The Hearst Corp., 1973.

Sullivan, H.S. *The Interpersonal Theory of Psychiatry.* New York: W.W. Norton and Co., Inc., 1953.

Sullivan, H.S. *The Psychiatric Interview.* New York: W.W. Norton and Co., Inc., 1954.

Whitaker, D. and M. Lieberman. *Psychotherapy Through the Group Process.* New York: Atherton Press, 1964.

Wilson, H. and C. Kneisl. *Psychiatric Nursing.* Menlo Park, CA: Addison-Wesley Publishing Co., 1979.

Woollams, S. and M. Brown. *TA: The Total Handbook of Transactional Analysis.* Englewood Cliffs, N.J.: Prentice-Hall, Inc., 1979.

Yalom, I. *The Theory and Practice of Group Psychotherapy* (2nd ed.). New York: Basic Books, Inc., 1975.

Yalom, I. Observations of Dr. I. Yalom's outpatient group at Stanford University, Stanford, CA, 1975a.

The Existential Influence on Group Behaviors 3

---------------- Introduction ----------------

The existentialist views humans as being free to exercise their will, to make choices, and to assume responsibility for the choices they make. May (1967) described the existential approach as an emphasis on knowing by doing. Notice the autonomy inherent in the role of the person who embraces an existential philosophy. The individual who is actively engaged in making life work cannot really blame others for his failures. Implied in the autonomy of making choices is a chance to change the way one's life is going to make it better.

In comparing the existential movement to the psychoanalytical view, one is struck by the seeming dichotomy of the two perspectives. Psychoanalytical theory explains present actions by looking for their origin in the past. Unless the person resolves past conflicts, his or her actions will continue to demonstrate the effect of such conflicts on current behaviors. Thus, the person is always acting out the past. Existentialism gives the individual the freedom to make a decision for the present and to take some action. This action may be similar or different from actions taken in the past, and the outcome might also be the same or different depending on how the person reacts to current stimuli. Past unresolved conflicts are still present, but the individual does not have to act on them in the same way. Consider the following example.

Bill, a staff nurse, has always had difficulty dealing with women who are very aggressive in their interactions with men. Generally, he responds to aggressive females with the same interactional pattern he learned as a child in relating to his mother. His mother made him feel very inadequate when she jumped in to rescue him from losing an argument with a peer and then continued to "rescue" him from girlfriends and others whom she thought might take advantage of him. Bill patched up his relationships by explaining her behavior as "meaning well," but he never confronted his mother directly about the hurt he felt with her interference in his life. Instead, his legitimate feeling of hurt became the racket feeling of anger. His anger was displaced on less aggressive women in his life with whom he could exercise some control.

When Bill's head nurse confronted him about some medications he had failed to order, Bill's Child responded to the anger in her voice and replayed the tapes that had recorded his mother's anger at having to rescue him from his "messes" with others. Bill's Adapted Child again responded by walking away and storing up racket feelings of anger and resentment instead of directly expressing the hurt he felt. That evening, he was furious with his girlfriend for being five minutes late for their dinner date.

Psychoanalytical Interpretation

Bill will continue to behave this way as long as the original conflict with his mother is not resolved. Bill is paradoxically distorting current relationships with aggressive, confrontive females. The source of this distortion is the unresolved feelings around his mother's need to aggressively interfere in Bill's life. Since TA theory actualizes past conflicts by describing the present activities of one's ego states, Bill might understand his behavior if he examines his Adapted Child tapes. As long as his Adaptive Child is in control of his feelings, Bill will continue to respond in the same way.

Existential Interpretation

Bill's response to his head nurse originates in the choice he made at the time of the interaction when he became aware he was feeling hurt. He chose to deal with his hurt by walking away. When Bill's girlfriend was late, he reacted to this situation by becoming furious with her. He may have been feeling hurt again, but this time he responded with anger. Both times Bill blocked the direct expression of his hurt although he was aware of feeling some discomfort in the interactions. He may not be aware of the source of his pain but has chosen to respond in the way that makes him least uncomfortable. Bill does not deal directly with his pain and must take the consequences for this; *i.e.,* his expressed feelings are not authentic and will, therefore, interfere with his ability to be real or genuine with others, especially women.

Although the interpretations of Bill's problem seem very different, there are some significant similarities. Both interpretations identify conflict or pain around Bill's actions. The psychoanalyst says that the conflict existed in Bill's inability as a child to directly deal with the hurt that resulted from interactions with his mother. The existentialist identifies present pain connected with the awareness and expression of hurt. Both agree that Bill's inability to deal with the conflict, or to prevent the blocking of his pain, result in Bill's difficulty with current relationships. In this chapter, existential theory, expressed in clinical terms as Gestalt therapy, will be developed.

Existential Theory

Some of the basic tenets of existentialism, partly identified in the introduction, include the courage to be, to be authentic, and to be free to make choices. With choice comes responsibility.

Being or participating in life involves taking risks. The opposite of this is nonbeing and can be seen when one inhibits expression of the self or loses one's identity by molding the self to the expectations of others (May, 1967). Bill indicates his position of nonbeing by inhibiting the expression of painful feelings. His choice to become angry and hide his hurt may be considered by some to be a more "legitimate" way for a male to react. If Bill was attempting to respond according to the expectations of others, this would also be an expression of nonbeing or a loss of identity.

Being oneself is being authentic. Carl Rogers (1980) discussed authenticity when he described the realness or genuineness of a person. Realness involves congruency within oneself. For a therapist to be real, Rogers said there needed to be congruence between what the therapist experienced at the gut level, what he was aware of, and what he expressed to the client. If a person understands himself, that is, if he can relate awareness to expression of feelings and the two are congruent, then he is a more genuine person. Rogers noted that these characteristics led to the possibility of more growth for oneself and for others. May (1967) also talked about growth for the individual:

"Capacities emerge in the developing person which render him a new gestalt...the maturing person continually develops new capacities out of the old, new symbols, values in a new form.'' (p.74).

For the existentialist, the concepts of awareness, authenticity, and the result of this, growth, are inextricably bound. Part of one's awareness is a consciousness of the ''deterministic forces'' in one's life (May, 1967, p.175). May was referring to those childhood experiences and other past events that the psychoanalysts say determine one's present behaviors and interactions. But May felt that the individual had a choice about how such past events influenced current actions. He defined freedom as ''the individual's capacity to know that he is the determined one...and thus to throw his weight, however slight it may be, on the side of one particular response among several possible ones.'' (p.175). Bill would attain freedom for his person if he not only became aware of how his mother's interactions with him in the past were determining his current responses but if he also decided what he wanted to do with that. He may choose to do something, or he may not, but whatever he does is now under his control.

May (1967) talked about responsibility as one's response to and involvement in the world. He saw freedom being limited by the fact that man exists in the world and, therefore, has a relationship to it. The critical care nurse must constantly interact with persons who are in the midst of life-threatening crises. How the nurse deals with this painful situation is a function of the freedom of the self. If the nurse allows herself to feel the pain and take care of it from day to day, she will probably avoid the burnout that a less aware, less authentic nurse may experience. To take care of the pain, she may need to talk with other staff. A staff person not directly involved with clients or a special mental health professional may help the nurse to understand reactions of anger, powerlessness, sadness, and other feelings. Asking for a day off, a change of assignments, or other measures that would provide some relief are other ways of dealing with the pressures of critical care nursing. The nurse's ability to deal effectively with the situation makes her a responsive person to the clients in her care. The nurse less able to respond to the pain of working in the critical care setting is not a less caring person but may have less understanding of the self and may, therefore, be less congruent in dealing with feelings.

Gestalt Theory

Relationship to Existentialism

Gestalt theory is the basis for the interventions known as Gestalt therapy, a technique which views the client in an existential mode of being. The German psychologists who gave us the word, gestalt, talked about man's need to perceive things not as unrelated isolates but as parts of a meaningful whole. Human nature, according to gestaltists, is organized into patterns or wholes and can only be understood as a function of the wholes of which it is made (Simkin, 1979). Gestalt therapy allows the individual to be aware of his own existence and to work through disjointed parts of himself to become an authentic whole being. The client is encouraged to take responsibility for himself or to be ''response-able'' for his own decisions (Simkin, 1979, p.284). The individual in Gestalt therapy starts with the obvious, that existence is an actuality, an awareness of the self. For therapy to be called successful, the person must achieve integration. The client becomes aware of previously alienated parts of the self and assimilates these parts into the whole self if they seem to fit. If they do not fit, the client is free to discard them and move on to new experiences for the self (Simkin, 1979). Awareness of the alienated parts is preceded by some discomfort. Going back to Bill's example, we could label his difficulty with current relationships and the resultant painful feelings as the alienated part of his self. Bill resists understanding this alienation when he avoids total awareness of his pain. Gestalt therapy is designed to help the client deal with such resistance.

Resistance to Being

When a person, such as Bill, avoids complete awareness of the pain, which, if acknowledged and expressed, could lead to more freedom and authenticity of the self, the individual is said to be resisting. Freud talked about resistance as an unconscious process. The Gestaltists defined resistance as a process that keeps one from fully experiencing one's being (Perls, Hefferline, and Goodman, 1951). Resistance can take on several forms:

1) Introjection. Introjection is the process of "swallowing" whole ways of acting, feeling, or thinking. One passively incorporates the psychological "food" the environment provides without bothering to analyze and assimilate that which is good and to discard that which is not helpful (Perls, *et al.,* 1951; Perls, 1973). Recall the function of introjection as the process occurring when the child incorporates the attitudes and values of significant adults to form the super ego. This is a passive process and an unconscious one. The child does not make a value judgment on what to incorporate. Perls (1973) noted that the child assimilates the parents' good habits when he translates them into terms he can understand. This implies a more active process and occurs because the child observes that some of the values of the parents and other adults yield satisfying behaviors. The child attempts to understand the origin of these behaviors by putting their value structure into terms he can assimilate and use for himself. Bad attitudes, however, must be introjected rather than taken apart and assimilated, because the child does not know how to cope with or relate to the negative behaviors such attitudes produce (Perls, 1973). Our Parent tapes are where our introjects are stored. If our Adult takes a Parent message and submits it to scrutiny with hard facts or data from the real world, then the message may or may not get Adult sanction to be used again. If it is a "should" that will serve our purposes for living, then we hold onto it. Otherwise, we can discard it. The problem comes when the Child decides that there is too much discomfort or negativity to go through the Adult process of assimilation. The Adaptive Child just wants to "swallow" the "whole thing."

Bill may have introjected the belief that anger is a legitimate way to deal with hurts. If Bill had allowed his Adult to operate during the time he was learning this behavior from his mother, his Adult would have pointed out the reality that being angry did not necessarily make mother feel better. Anger can serve a very useful purpose at times, particularly if it is in an assertive form (see Chapter Four). However, anger can also be destructive. Assimilation of all the facts about anger will help a person to decide when and when not to use it. Introjection and assimilation are mutually exclusive. Introjection robs the person of some knowledge or awareness of the self, and assimilation brings together many separate pieces of information about the self.

2) Projection. This is the reverse of introjection. In projection, one makes the environment responsible for what originated in oneself. An attitude, feeling, or behavior belonging to an individual's personality is attributed, instead, to another object or person in the environment and is experienced by the individual as coming towards him from the environment. Generally, the person will disown parts of the personality that are unattractive or offensive (Perls, *et al.,* 1951; Perls, 1973).

Resistance to those parts of oneself which are uncomfortable to own certainly makes sense. A client in a group I led was frequently accusing other group members of not being open and honest about their feelings with him. In reality, the overwhelming characteristic he displayed was a very intellectualized interactional pattern with others. He would couch his feelings in intellectual jargon in order not to feel them so intensely, but he accused everyone else in the group of doing to him what he did so well to others. Not only was he projecting, but he was also avoiding awareness through intellectualization, another form of resistance to be discussed in more detail later.

3) Retroflection. Retroflection helps the individual resist awareness of powerful yet frightening impulses that the person originally wanted to act on towards another. Instead, the individual turns such impulses back on the self and becomes the target of behaviors originally intended for someone else. Frequently, these are destructive impulses (Perls, *et al.,* 1951; Perls, 1973). A child may bang her head against a hard object instead of striking her mother. The child has not made a conscious decision in her Adult that to hit oneself or others is destructive and not reasonable to do. Instead, the Parent tape tells her she should not hit others, but her Child wants to get rid of the bottled-up anger. Recall that the Adult is called into act when the other two ego states need some help. The Adult might advise throwing something or playing really hard rather than hitting oneself, but her Child apparently is not wanting this advice right now. Thus, retroflection becomes the means for handling some painful feelings.

4) Confluence. Confluence opposes the central principle of the Gestalt view of the world. The individual using confluence blurs the boundaries between the self and others. The parts and the whole are indistinguishable. Reducing the differences between oneself and others may be a way of not "rocking the boat." Society sometimes frowns on difference as being deviant and to be feared. One is reminded of the newborn who is born with only the id to define his state of being. At first, even mother is not distinguishable as a separate entity. In confluence, one's needs, emotions, and activities blend together (Perls, *et al.,* 1951; Perls, 1973). For example, a woman may not be able to pinpoint a particular feeling that causes her to burst into tears. She may just have a vague sense of discomfort. Her automatic response fits society's norm that crying is an acceptable and rather frequent behavior of females. Crying is safe and relieves some of the discomfort. The woman may also have discovered the secondary gain from this behavior, *i.e.,* that crying is a way to hook another's Nurturing Parent to get what one wants. Crying does not represent an authentic emotion for this woman but is a confluent response to several different situations.

5) Intellectualization. Gestalt therapists call intellectualization "being in one's head." Trying to explain "why" one is or feels a certain way does not give the individual an immediate awareness of the behavior to be modified. Perls (1973) said that the person needed to learn the "how" of what was happening to him. He said that trying to figure out the reason for transference kept the client from really experiencing the therapist as a person. In looking for the "why," the client was stuck on what he construed the therapist to be. This blocked the actual awareness of their relationship and prevented the client from working on it in the "here-and-now" (Perls, 1973). Intellectualization allows a person to talk about past experiences and avoid the pain of making them real again. Nurses may use intellectualization in talking about the death of a client or other experiences of pain that they have been through with clients or their families. Consider how much easier it is to talk about the death of a close friend if the dialogue is phrased in storytelling fashion:

"She was so thin I hardly recognized her. It was hard, but I'm glad I got to see her again. We talked about high school, some really special friends, and how much fun her parents used to let us have. Her children didn't even bother to say anything to me when I left. They didn't deserve such a wonderful mother!"

The Gestaltist would insist on the client talking about any past experiences in the "here-and-now." The above dialogue would sound like this:

"I'm sitting on the edge of the bed looking at her. I notice her cheek bones, how thin they are. I really don't want to keep staring at her. I'd rather look away, but I'm afraid that will upset her. She looks so different than I remember her. I feel like crying. I don't want her to die. I'm trying to think of something to say. Maybe we can talk about our high school days." (The client would then talk in first person with an empty chair or pillow that represents her friend: "Do you remember, Amy, the time we double-dated. . ." She would move into the empty chair or to the pillow to respond back to herself as her friend would. This technique will be explained in more detail later.) ". . . Here I am going out the door, and her children aren't even speaking to me. They don't deserve her."

The Gestaltist requires that the client "experience himself as fully as he can in the here and now" (Perls, 1973, p.63). Perls (1973) insisted that a client psychodramatically act out past incidents to make them a present experience. In the present, assimilation may take place. The client then has put a past event into perspective with the rest of the current self and is more integrated. Intellectualization prevents integration because it does not allow the person to be aware of present parts of the self as they react to a past event.

Owning Responsibility

The existential influence shows itself in the Gestalt concept that the client must take responsibility for any new awareness and must decide what to do with this new part of the self (Perls, *et al.,* 1951). If the individual decides that the new, unintegrated part of the self does not fit with the rest of her being, she takes responsibility for not integrating or assimilating that into her personality. To help clients with this process, the Gestaltists insist that "I" replace "it" in verbal expressions where "it" is the subject and "I" is the object. "The aim is to come to realize again that you are creative in your environment and are responsible for your reality." (Perls, *et al.,* 1951, p.216). This process would work as follows:

"My throat (it) is choking me," vs. "I am choking myself," (Note: this might might also be an example of retroflection, *i.e.,* doing to the self, choking, rather than doing this to someone else).

"It's really hard (for me) to talk about it." vs "I keep myself from talking."

"It's not my fault you were late." vs. "I'm not taking responsibility for your lateness."

Another bit of terminology which keeps the person responsible for his or her own awareness and actions is the use of the word "won't" vs. "can't" (Pappas, 1981). "I can't cry" is very different from "I won't cry." Using "can't" implies a passive approach to one's behavior in which the individual is saying, "I am not in control of my own being." If I "won't" do something, I take responsibility for the consequences and am being more authentic or honest with myself. For example, a psychiatrist who works with regressed, chronic mental health clients uses this principle of Gestalt to instill some sense of responsibility within the client for his own destiny. Instead of structuring the interview around a set of specific questions, he asks the client to tell him what he wants to have happen in their interaction. He insists the client begin with the premise that he is in the hospital because of actions he, himself, has taken. No one may use "can't" as an excuse for being "crazy." Many clients are unwilling to take such responsibility because they have to work, then, on getting well. The nurse counseling a client about hygiene, diet, and medications for diabetes needs to have the client see his or her responsibility in the outcome of the disease process.

The Figure-Ground Concept

In the process of Gestalt therapy, the concept of figure-ground is the primary unit of experience for the client. It forms the basis for the work the client does to increase awareness of a part of the self that is not yet integrated with the whole person. The individual's total self may be considered the ground, whereas, the particular prominant part of the self that is standing out and clamoring for attention is the figure. Perls described it in this way: "The context in which an element appears is called in Gestalt psychology the 'ground' against which the 'figure' stands out" (Perls, *et al.,* 1951, p.*ix*). I find it helpful for my understanding of this concept to use an example from the arts. In looking at a painting, one has a choice of viewing the work either as a whole (the ground) or in little parts that catch one's fancy (the figure). If one looks at the painting as a whole, then one may experience abstractness, realism, or whatever theme the artist was trying to convey in the work in its completeness. However, if one chooses to just experience the colors in the painting, or the way the lines of the brush flow, or other parts of the work separately, then one may have many different impressions and emotions in response to the particular field of attention. Too much attention to the painting's details will prevent the person from seeing the whole picture or getting the whole message from the artist. However, time spent focusing on a small part of the painting may then change the individual's perceptions of the painting as a whole.

After the individual has worked with the figure separately and then allowed it to become part of the ground once more, a new insight about one's self may occur. Gestalt psychologists call this the "aha" experience (Perls, *et al.,* 1951). This new awareness of the self means that the person will now present himself a little differently to others. What he does with this new understanding of himself is his choice. The process of examining the figure in detail and coming to closure with the realization of the "aha" will be discussed in the following paragraphs.

—————————— **Gestalt Therapy** ——————————

Sharpening the Figure: Contact

Contact is a word that personifies energy and activity for the Gestalt therapist. Contact means "in touch with" and describes the sensory awareness and motor behavior of the individual (Perls, *et al.,* 1951, p.227). Contact is more meaningful to our previous discussion of the figure-ground with this definition: "Contact, the work that results in assimilation and growth, is the forming of a figure of interest against a ground or context of the organism/environment field." (Perls, *et al.,* 1951, p.231). Contact, then, may be considered the opposite of resistance. Resistance certainly involves the use of energy, but it is the goal of the individual to avoid awareness through various behaviors that keep one's figure hidden within the whole or ground of one's being. Paradoxically, it is the client's resistance that signals the therapist that this person is in need of making contact. Something must be so disturbing to the client that all the energy this person has is going towards hiding that discomfort from the self and others.

The process of contact begins with either the therapist's observation of the client's discomfort and resulting resistance or the client's identification of a need "to work" on an area of pain. The therapist's goal for the client during contact is to have this individual accentuate that area of the self that is causing the discomfort. The figure is being sharpened against the ground. Following are examples of how the therapist might do this.

1) If the therapist notices a specific nonverbal behavior which is expending a lot of the client's energy, such as hand wringing, leg swinging, choking, or swallowing hard, she would ask the individual to exaggerate that movement (sharpening the figure). As the client did this, she would ask him to talk out loud about what he was experiencing/feeling (*e.g.,* "I feel silly waving my hands so fast...I'm afraid they're going to fall off. They feel so heavy"). This will heighten the person's awareness. The therapist might then ask the client to give his hands a voice and have them dialogue with each other ("I feel really aimless flopping around like this. Sometimes I feel like John wants to get rid of us. Maybe we're a handicap for him. I don't think he always knows what to do with us. He doesn't like us to touch other people. Maybe John's afraid to touch"). At this point the client, John, might be coming to some insight about his discomfort with touch. Right now, this is an incomplete Gestalt because there is more, most likely, to his discomfort with this. John will need to explore more specific incidents of discomfort with touch, perhaps with a particular person or set of relationships. In discussing some of the special techniques of Gestalt later, I will continue with this example.

2) The therapist may notice that the client is trying to restrict a particular nonverbal behavior or set of behaviors. The energy devoted to this resistance calls attention to the possible need for the client to make contact with these nonverbals. To help the client look at these behaviors, the therapist may ask a question (*e.g.,* "What are you swallowing so hard?" The client may be attempting not to cry or not to argue with someone. This would be confluence.). If the client is reluctant to work with the therapist on looking at her swallowing behavior, the therapist may then take the

resistance and work with that to bring about contact (*e.g.,* "What aren't you willing to give yourself permission to do?" If that does not get a response from the client, another question might be, "If you could make your discomfort an object, what would it look like?" Generally, the client sees this as a less-threatening question and can come up with some specific object. The client might then have a dialogue with the object. Dialoguing will be discussed later.). If the person is willing to work on the nonverbal the therapist identifies, the therapist will then determine what techniques might enhance the figure. Giving the throat a voice or exaggerating the swallowing might help.

3) A verbalization may be a way of asking for contact. The client may start talking about a present awareness, *e.g.,* "I am aware of my heart beating really fast." The therapist would ask the client to concentrate on the heartbeats, thus enhancing the figure. Sometimes verbalizations are resistances to feeling. The woman who tells another group member that he is always too loud and aggressive may actually be afraid of owning her own aggressiveness. Usually, a projection is occurring when the characteristic attributed to the other person is not totally accurate or is exaggerated. For example, the statement, "You always talk so loud, I'm sick of you trying to take control," might be a projection. The therapist could ask the client to "play the projection" by saying, "Try shouting as loud as you can and see how this feels. See if you can take control of this group." The client may contact some of her own need for power and control through expression of her restricted aggressive feelings.

Assimilating the Figure into the Ground: Withdrawal

Once the figure has been explored and worked with to the point that the client has some new information about the self, the client makes a decision about how to use this information. This process leads to closure of the gestalt and withdrawal of the energy used in contact. Withdrawal does not necessarily mean that the individual has come to closure with new behaviors or feelings to cause a change in his or her personality. The individual will have experienced an awareness of part of the self that had not been as prominent in the past. Perhaps the client does not want to accept the fact that she is withholding anger as a way of being controlling (see previous example). She has seen something new in herself but does not wish to risk being more direct with her anger and need to control. Although her behavior will not change because of her decision not to work further on this problem, she will be different after having had this contact with a new part of herself. She will be more aware of her controlling behaviors and may watch the outcome of her actions to see if her behaviors are getting her what she wants.

Recall that the Gestaltist subscribes to the existential belief that man takes responsibility for being a certain way. It is a choice the person makes. The Gestalt therapist is only helping the client to see what choices he or she may make. With new awarenesses of the self, the choices multiply. If the client decides to go for a change in the self, the therapist can help facilitate this change. Simkin (1979) noted Perls' description of the personality as being multilayered with the most genuine part of the personality being stripped of all phony ways of being. It is the therapist who may help a client get to this layer where the person then has an option to rebuild the self as he or she wishes.

The client, John, described in the previous section, had only begun to explore the significance of touch for himself and probably needed to do more work in this area before the gestalt would have closure. The gestalt is closed when the cathected object (the energy put into sharpening the figure) is dealt with in some way satisfactory to the individual. The figure and its detail are no longer needed and may disappear into the ground (Perls, 1973). Generally, the "aha" experience signifies closure. For John, his "aha" gave him a new insight about touch. Although the therapist may feel that this insight re touch is not complete, *i.e.,* that there are more "aha's" to come, the client may be happy to close at this point. The therapist's determination of closure always yields to the client's. The therapist may think a client has more work to do, but if the client does not think so or want to, then the therapist cannot make him work. If John decided it was too scary for him to explore the situations in which he was uncomfortable with touch, then the therapist would need to respect this decision. It seems to me that this is a "given" for any health professional working with a client. One cannot force someone to change or get well because the health practitioner wishes this to happen. A nurse may tell the client how she feels about his decision not to take care of his health, and I often do that. The client who makes a decision not to change must take the responsibility for this decision.

This basic principle of freedom and responsibility which the existentialists gave us is equally as important in group interactions between the leader and members as it is in a dyad between the nurse and client. If a group member is passing up an opportunity to "work" by withdrawing in some way from the group, I need to allow that person to be withdrawn. I make sure that, if other group members have not commented on the member's withdrawal, I do so since I feel both the group and the member need to be aware of what he or she is choosing to do. Withdrawal is a process that expends energy but which may or may not give the client comfort. If withdrawal comes after the member has worked, it is a natural process. If it is to keep from working, the member may eventually decide that the pain is not going away and will make a decision to work. In Gestalt terms, withdrawal of energy from the figure may take place without closure, but the incomplete gestalt may lead to some discomfort for the individual.

Unfinished Business: An Incomplete Gestalt

If, in Example 1, John begins to feel some anxiety around his new knowledge about his fear of touch, he is experiencing unfinished business. An incomplete gestalt may cause stagnation and regression rather than growth and development for the individual. Pain is a warning signal for unfinished business and indicates that something needs attention (Perls, *et al.,* 1951). Emotional pain may manifest itself in many ways. The person may find himself more anxious, more easily upset, more prone to getting angry and to being angry at the wrong people, and so forth. I rely on the client to tell me when his discomfort is bad enough to push him to want to work on those things that are bothering him. The best time to take care of unfinished business is when the client, himself, senses his discomfort. Since the client must produce the energy for another contact, I wait for him to identify when he is ready to expend this energy. The point of contact for unfinished business begins at the area of discomfort. The therapist must begin with the "here-and-now" awareness rather than trying to recapture a feeling the client had the last time he worked.

In Example 1, John might start by describing his discomfort as an object and having a dialogue with it. This allows him to ease into the really painful area of touch more gradually. The discomfort John has been feeling is probably resistance to the more painful feelings around touch. In Perls' description of the layers of the personality, he talked about the impasse layer as the feeling one has when being confronted with unfinished business. The impasse layer gives one a sense of emptiness or of being without a role to play (Simkin, 1979).

Unfinished business is a hazard in all relationships. Sometimes it is a function of not communicating what one really feels to the other person because of insecurities in one's self esteem. Recall the discussion in Chapter One on the covert rehearsal phase of message generation. The individual frequently ruminates about what her response should be according to how she perceives the other communicant to be reacting to her. Casual relationships are more subject to this tendency to not risk honest communications because of the uncertainty of acceptance by one or both communicants. Translated into TA terms, the more one feels "OK" about oneself, the more one is able to risk sharing and completing any unfinished business between others. The person is able to recognize the signals of unfinished business (*i.e.,* the discomfort and fear of encounter or emptiness) and looks for an opportunity to do something about it. If a person is not disturbed about an unfinished relationship, she may have decided that the relationship is not important to her, or she may be using resistance to avoid any pain. For one individual, a completed gestalt may be the realization that an unfinished relationship will stay unfinished. One or both communicants in an incomplete relationship may want the relationship structured this way. Unfinished business may also occur because one communicant wants the relationship on a different level than the other. The incomplete gestalt rests with the person who is not able to deal with this situation.

In close relationships, unfinished business is less likely to occur because of the way the communicants have defined their relationship. However, an abrupt end to the relationship due to death, or to the decision by one communicant to change the terms of the relationship, will often result in unfinished business for either communicant.

Most of the time, the individual with the incomplete gestalt around a relationship will not be able to finish communications with the other communicant because of unavailability of the other person. One of the most frequently used Gestalt techniques allows the individual to finish his or her end of the relationship regardless of whether another communication would ever take place. The dialogue for unfinished business using an empty chair or a pillow to represent the other communicant serves this purpose. The individual working will start in her own chair and then move to the space occupied in fantasy by the absent communicant. In this chair, the person will speak as she feels the other would have, but she must respond to the "here-and-now" communication just made from her own chair. The Gestalt therapist coaches the individual with dialogue as necessary as the therapist perceives areas of discomfort which need to be talked about. The person working switches back and forth with help from the therapist and identifies for the therapist when she feels finished. In the following dialogue, Jane is talking to her mother who recently died:

Therapist: "Tell your mother what you're feeling right now about her leaving you."

Jane: "I feel really alone like you deserted me. I never felt like you gave me enough of your time anyway."

Therapist: "Tell her how come this is so."

Jane: "Well you always paid more attention to Brad. I could see that you liked him better. It's like I wasn't as good at things as he was."

Therapist: "Change places and respond to Jane's comments as mother when you're ready."

Jane (to therapist): "I feel really stilted saying this. I'd never talk that way to my mother."

Therapist: "Tell your mother that." (Going with the "here-and-now" resistance)

Jane: (repeats, to the empty chair, the above statement that she made to the therapist and then changes chairs and speaks as mother.) "I'm not sure what to say to you. You certainly haven't talked to me like this before. How come you never told me this?"

Jane: (as herself back in the other chair): "I guess I didn't think you'd understand."

Therapist: "How come your mother wouldn't understand you?"

Jane: (hesitating a little) "I don't know. It doesn't really matter."

Therapist: "Try substituting I for IT."

Jane: "I don't really matter...to myself." (The last two words are spoken as an "aha" indicating that Jane has just learned something new about herself.)

This is not a completed gestalt yet, but the therapist would switch the focus to Jane's need to treat herself as a nonperson or a "not OK" person. The therapist might have Jane continue the dialogue with herself by having her decide what part of herself she cares about the least and then putting that part on the other chair. This technique is called "top-dog" vs. under-dog." Perls (1971) talked about the top-dog vs. under-dog as being part of the roleplaying layer of the personality that masks genuineness. He described the top-dog as righteous and the under-dog as being the very unsure part of the self. This technique is especially helpful for the person who is trying to accomplish a goal but is not succeeding. Chances are that the two parts of the personality, the top-dog and the under-dog, are vying for control and neither is winning. Someone who is trying to lose weight can split the two sides of the self, the part that says one must be thin and the part that does not have the willpower to diet. A client I worked with did this exercise. It soon became evident that the part that did not have the willpower to diet was winning. The technique did not help the client to lose weight, but it helped her understand that a part of her was successfully sabotaging her goal. She was then free to make a decision about whether she wanted to try and strengthen her willpower or give up dieting.

Switching to the top-dog/under-dog technique with Jane takes the focus off completing a dialogue with mother. However, the therapist and Jane have discovered that Jane's unfinished business was really with herself rather than with her mother. If Jane is successful in closing the gestalt on herself around the issue of liking herself, she will probably not feel any more discomfort about her relationship with her mother. She may also be more successful in future relationships with others.

The Gestalt Group

This chapter is not designed to prepare anyone to conduct a Gestalt group or use Gestalt with individual clients. However, some of the principles used in Gestalt are transferable to work in other groups. A Gestalt therapist, like the TA therapist, must take special training in Gestalt which involves both theory and clinical practice. In the following paragraphs, some of the features of a Gestalt group and the principles that are taken from Gestalt/existential theory that may be applicable to other groups will be discussed.

Member Roles

The lines of communication in a Gestalt group show more member-to-leader and leader-to-member interactions than member-to-member communications. Simkin (1979) described a Gestalt group as one in which individual therapy is done in a group setting. The therapist, traditionally, does not emphasize group dynamics or focus on group cohesiveness. Some therapists, however, see group process (the relationships between the leader and members) as important as the individual's work on personal issues (Simkin, 1979). I find that the more trust members have with one another or the more experience they have in taking risks with one another and sharing perceptions of each other's work, the more the growth experience is enhanced for the entire group.

Some of the primary roles members have are observing each other work and sharing the feelings they experience while each is working. As one person works to sharpen a figure for more awareness of the self, others experience vicariously some of the feelings related to the individual's situation. These feelings should be shared in the first person "here-and-now" mode. For example, while Jane is talking to her mother via the empty chair, Carl may be recalling an experience with a significant other in his life. It is not important that the two experiences be similar but only that Carl has some awareness of a feeling in himself that was triggered by what Jane was doing. Carl might share the following:

"I really feel my breathing getting heavy. Right now it seems like all I can remember about my father is that he always told me I was important to him. I never acknowledged that. I feel like I let him down. I'm really excited about what you just learned about yourself. Maybe I should appreciate more his caring for me."

By Carl's sharing his awareness with Jane, either Jane or Carl, or both of them, may gain some new insight for the self. Even if they do not, this sharing promotes feelings of caring and authenticity among members of the group and may be the catalyst for someone else working whose feeling level has been stimulated by the feedback in the group. As members sit quietly and observe (silence is important while a member is working), the other members are generally very much involved with the emotions generated in the group.

Often someone else working will get another member involved in contacting his or her unfinished business. Carl may not be ready to work on anything with the limited awareness he gained from what Jane did. However, the therapist may begin talking to Carl to help him explore if he, indeed, has any unfinished business with his father or with his relationship with himself.

Therapist's Roles

The therapist is constantly observing members for any anxiety, pain, or resistance (*e.g.,* any verbal and nonverbal behaviors which might signify some readiness to work). Notice the previous examples in this chapter where the therapist has changed the direction of a dialogue or asked a specific question related to a probable area of resistance or discomfort for the client. If the therapist asks a question related to some possible resistance and the response from the client indicates that there is no resistance at that point, the work or process of the group may proceed without the therapist needing to feel badly about not being on track with the correct perception. We will talk in later chapters about interventions the leader makes which may not do what the leader has in mind. No matter what happens to an intervention, it adds to the "here-and-now" quality of the group and may stir up some process much later.

Obviously, the primary role of the therapist is to guide members through the figure-ground process. Several illustrations have already been given of this process. We have discussed the importance of closure with any work the client does and have stressed that the client decides when a gestalt is closed or when there is still more work to do. The therapist never tells the client what he or she should feel or learn from the awareness of a gestalt experience. The client decides what goals he or she has reached. It is the process of the work the client engages in with the therapist's guidance that is important (Simkin, 1979). Whatever conclusions the client reaches about the self are only significant in their usefulness to the individual. Of more significance is one learning how to be aware of parts of the self that one has not been in touch with before and learning to recognize discomfort as a sign that one has more work to do in dealing with unfinished business.

Frequently, leadership in a Gestalt group is shared by two therapists. Because the work is often very intense, having a second person to share the responsibility of facilitating the group is helpful. There are specific balancing functions that coleaders perform. These will be discussed in detail in Chapter Thirteen. One of those balancing functions is the ability of one coleader to be an observer of the process in the group while the other coleader is working with a client. This is especially important in a Gestalt group, because the therapist working with a client must concentrate so intently on the client's verbal and nonverbal behaviors that attention to other members' processes is impossible. The other leader is free to observe other members' responses to the process going on in the group. A coleader is available to provide objectivity to a therapist-client interaction in which the other coleader has lost the ability to be objective. This happened to me when I was working with a client in a Gestalt group. As I interacted with the client, he became very upset with me, screamed at me, and then stormed out of the room. I reacted very subjectively, letting my personal feelings overwhelm me, and began to cry. At the time, I blamed my response on my being "with child." My coleader did an excellent job of helping me talk out loud about my "here-and-now" feelings and resolve my distress. This turned out to be a good experience for the whole group, since I modeled the working-through process and demonstrated my realness or authentic humanness for the members. Durald and Hanks (1980) make another point about coleadership in a Gestalt group. They suggest that two leaders make it easier for clients to work because a member may choose either leader to work with in the group: "(D)ual leadership offers a far richer spectrum of therapeutic resources to which the client can creatively respond." (Durald and Hanks, 1980, p.23). They also suggest that the coleaders be of opposite sexes. A member would probably choose that therapist with whom he felt the most rapport, thereby perhaps taking a greater risk to explore the unknown parts of the self because of the safety he felt.

Norms Applicable to Non-Gestalt Groups

The following are major points that we have talked about in relationship to existentialism and Gestalt theory that seem to me to be universal principles that may become part of the belief structure in any supportive group: 1) owning responsibility for one's behaviors and feelings; 2) maintaining a "here-and-now" orientation to the process of the group; 3) valuing feedback between members and the leader; and 4) taking responsibility for one's own growth.

These specific principles of conducting oneself in group will be developed in relation to the dynamics of the supportive group beginning in Chapter Five.

REFERENCES

Durald, M. and D. Hanks. "The Evaluation of Co-Leading a Gestalt Group," *Journal of Psychiatric Nursing and Mental Health Services,* 18, no. 12 (Dec. 1980), 19–23.

May, R. *Psychology and the Human Dilemma.* Princeton, NJ: D. Van Nostrand Co., Inc., 1967.

Pappas, S. "Gestalt Therapy," an inservice given at County Mental Health, Hillcrest, San Diego, CA, 1981.

Perls, F. "Four Lectures," in *Gestalt Therapy Now* (Harper Colophon ed.), eds. J. Fagan and I. Shepherd. New York: Harper and Row, 1971.

Perls, F. *The Gestalt Approach and Eyewitness to Therapy.* Ben Lomond, CA: Science and Behavior Books, Inc., 1973.

Perls, F., R. Hefferline, and P. Goodman. *Gestalt Therapy: Excitement and Growth in the Human Personality* (Delta Book ed.). New York: Dell Publishing Co., Inc., 1951.

Rogers, C. *A Way of Being.* Boston: Houghton Mifflin Co., 1980.

Simkin, J. "Gestalt Therapy," in *Current Psychotherapies* (2nd ed.), ed. R. Corsini. Itasca, IL: F.E. Peacock Publishers, Inc., 1979.

Behavioral Theory as a Basis for Group Interaction 4

Introduction

A basic assumption of the behaviorists is that a person acts a certain way because of learned behaviors (Chambless and Goldstein, 1979). B.F. Skinner (1971) expanded on this in his discussion of the individual's relationship to his environment:

"Man's struggle for freedom is not due to a will to be free, but to certain behavioral processes characteristic of the human organism, the chief effect of which is the avoidance of or escape from so-called "aversive" features of the environment" (p.42).

Up until now, we have talked about the importance of intrapsychic phenomena or one's internal processes upon one's actions and the effect of interactional processes on one's view of the self and the environment (specifically, other systems). The behaviorists place more emphasis on how man reacts to his environment and attempt to teach the individual to unlearn some behaviors which are causing problems and to relearn other, more adaptive behaviors that allow the individual to survive better in the environment (Chambless and Goldstein, 1979). Skinner was referring to the individual's desire to avoid unpleasant stimuli and escape. The desire one has to feel comfortable and not in pain has been a universal thread running throughout our discussions of how man views himself and his environment. Internal stimuli signal the individual that there are areas of anxiety or discomfort. In Gestalt, discomfort results in unfinished business; in psychoanalysis, repression; as viewed by systems theorists, a closed system and crisis behaviors. All of the above theoretical frameworks agree that the individual deals with discomfort initially by escaping or withdrawing in some way. The behaviorists see the person as having an automatic response to discomfort. A person's actions are dependent on an immediate result that either eliminates pain or increases his or her pleasure. Basically, a person learns to escape discomfort, and each time the behavior that is associated with relief works, it has more of a likelihood of being repeated.

This chapter will present the basic concepts of behavior modification, their ethical implications, and their use in a group setting with various client populations. Assertiveness training has become an important modality to help individuals have more satisfying interactions with others. Because assertiveness training is based on principles of behavior modification and is most often taught in a group, it is discussed in detail in this chapter. Assertiveness has application in both nurse-client and nurse-colleague interactions. Behavioral rehearsal is a basic technique used to teach assertiveness. It has a variety of uses in many different types of groups in which nurses are involved. A section on behavioral rehearsal and other behavioral techniques is included.

Principles of Behavior Modification

Behaviorists look at behavior modification as a method of helping the client substitute more adaptive behaviors for others which are causing the client some difficulty. An identifiable goal is to teach the individual some general strategies for behavioral change which can be applied to both current and future problems (Chambless and Goldstein, 1979). An important aspect of this goal, then, is to work with the client to make sure that any modification in his or her behavior generalizes to the client's natural environment. Those aspects of the treatment environment that have resulted in behavioral changes for the client must be present not only in the therapy setting but also in the client's daily environment (Baldwin and Baldwin, 1981).

Terminology

Operant Conditioning. Operant conditioning is a term used by Skinner to describe the process whereby the frequency of one's overt behaviors may be increased or decreased by consequences operating in the immediate environment to affect the individual's response. Consequences that cause behavior to increase are called reinforcers. Those that cause behavior to decrease are called punishers (Skinner, 1971; Chambless and Goldstein, 1979; Baldwin and Baldwin, 1981). The toddler's behaviors are very much a function of operant conditioning. Recall that the toddler has not developed the internal controls that make actions the result of the toddler's value system or super ego. Instead, the two-year-old responds to mother's praise or punishment. The toddler who is put in her room after breaking a dish begins to learn that an unpleasant consequence occurs as a result of her behavior. To avoid the unpleasant result in the future, she may modify her behavior; *i.e.,* she will decrease the number of times she breaks dishes. Specific terms used in operant conditioning include the following.

1) Positive Reinforcers. As stated earlier, a reinforcer increases the frequency of a behavior. Reinforcers are highly individualized. What will increase the frequency of a behavior with one person may not have any effect on another individual. The reinforcer's value lies in its importance for the person being affected by the reinforcement. For example, a nurse may think praise is a positive reinforcer. However, the client may feel he is not worthy of praise and will avoid behaviors that result in praise by the nurse. Skinner (1971, 1974) noted that a reinforcer strengthens any behavior that it follows. A behavior change that occurs immediately or shortly after a particular response or event has most likely been caused by that response. The greatest change in behavior occurs when the reinforcer follows immediately after the behavior (Baldwin and Baldwin, 1981).

Positive reinforcers may be tangible objects such as food, toys, money, tokens, flowers, a hug, or a multitude of other things present in the environment. Less tangible but equally as powerful are such reinforcers as recognition by one's boss, a compliment, or a smile. Recall that stroking is a way of recognizing an individual and is, therefore, a powerful reinforcer. Even negative strokes may be positive reinforcers. For example, children whose parents seem to have little time for them may discover that some acting-up will result in a response by the parent in the form of a negative stroke, such as a spanking or a verbal rebuke. If children with recognition hunger find that acting-up gets the parents' attention, then these children will increase their acting-up behaviors. The negative stroking is a positive reinforcer for the acting-up behavior.

Nurses frequently use positive reinforcement with clients to increase compliance. Praising a client who is on a reducing diet for losing two pounds between weigh-ins is a reinforcer if this praise causes the individual to increase those behaviors which will help the client lose more weight next week. Sometimes a client will hook the nurse into reinforcing a negative behavior. A nurse who responds each time a client asks for help with some treatment he should be doing for himself is reinforcing the client's dependency. It would be important for the nurse to discover what independent behaviors she could positively reinforce with her attention to the client since her presence is a desirable occurrence for him. Looking at this in another way, the client's help-seeking behaviors are positively reinforcing for the nurse's action in keeping the client in a dependent relationship. The nurse must discover ways of meeting a need to be helpful in a situation that does not compromise the client's move towards more independent functioning. A nurse who constantly finds herself responding to help-seeking behaviors to the detriment of the client's well-being may benefit from some personal work in this area.

In groups, positive reinforcers have many uses. In Chapter Five, we will talk about the development of group norms. The group leader has the primary responsibility for seeing that the norms, or ways of operating in the group, are adaptive and are understood by the group members. One way of facilitating member participation in the formation and compliance with norms is to positively reinforce behaviors occurring in the group that would lead to these goals. For example, if the leader believes that self-disclosure is an important process for group members to experience for self-growth as well as for the growth of the group, the leader will stroke members who appropriately self-disclose. Other uses of positive reinforcement in a group include promoting behavioral change or acquisition of new skills for individual members. A member may have difficulty speaking loud enough to be heard in a group. An adolescent group member may have a hard time allowing others in the group to speak or in sharing the leader's attention with other members. All of these situations are appropriate ones for the use of positive reinforcement. In our discussion of assertiveness techniques, we will look at how the group structure positively reinforces assertive behaviors.

2) Negative Reinforcers. A negative reinforcer strengthens those behaviors or responses that reduce or terminate it (Skinner, 1974; Baldwin and Baldwin, 1981). The reinforced response is capable of terminating an aversive or punishing stimulus (Chambless and Goldstein, 1979). Nurses frequently encounter the results of negative reinforcement if they give pain medication upon the client's request, and it is effective. Whenever the client asks for medication and receives relief from discomfort or pain (the aversive stimuli), the action of requesting medication for pain is reinforced and will probably increase in frequency. Because pain increased a response which ultimately caused its termination, pain is considered a negative reinforcer in this example. In an attempt to discourage a client from using too much pain medication, the nurse might search for another behavior that can be reinforced. Relaxation exercises and guided imagery might be an alternative to medication for some types of pain. Sometimes a supportive group experience will help clients deal with chronic pain. Attending the group then becomes a negatively reinforced behavior to reduce pain. Because negative reinforcers are unpleasant and tend to be avoided, if possible, any behavior that prevents them will be reinforced. This makes it more difficult to control what behaviors the client learns. Cold, hunger, embarrassment, and anxiety are also negative reinforcers. Anxiety over a particular surgical procedure is a negative reinforcer for such behaviors as requesting an excessive amount of the nurse's attention or asking pertinent questions about the procedure. Of course, the latter is a more desirable behavior for the client to exhibit.

Positive and negative reinforcers may work together to ensure compliance by a client. For example, the nurse who wants a new adolescent diabetic client to be responsible in giving his own insulin may positively reinforce this by setting up a family meeting where the adolescent can show his parents how he has mastered this skill and can teach them what he knows about insulin and its precautions. If the adolescent's family is not supportive, another reinforcer may work. Perhaps the adolescent has a positive attachment to the nurse as an adult he admires. A few extra minutes spent talking with the adolescent after the regular clinic appointment would, therefore, be a positive reinforcer. A group for new adolescent diabetics might be positively reinforcing if peer support is prominent. Recall that a positive reinforcer must be highly valued by the client. Initially, minor skin irritation at the injection site may discourage the adolescent from continuing. However, the physical effects of a diabetic coma, when discussed with the adolescent, may be so devastating that this negative reinforcer will promote compliance with insulin administration. The nurse controls the positive reinforcers, and the negative reinforcers are a deterrent to noncompliance.

3) Aversive Stimuli. Punishment or aversive stimuli serve as negative reinforcers, as noted above, when they are reduced or terminated. Punishment may be thought of as the reverse of reinforcement, since its goal is to reduce the occurrence of a particular behavior or response (Skinner, 1974; Chambless and Goldstein, 1979; Baldwin and Baldwin, 1981). Punishment is the least effective means of teaching a client new behaviors, since aversive techniques serve to decrease undesirable behaviors but do not help the individual know what acceptable behavior to substitute in its place.

An example of applying aversive techniques in a group setting illustrates its ineffectiveness in promoting adaptive behaviors. If Debbie is consistently disruptive in a group because she talks out of turn and monopolizes the conversation, the group leader may decide to punish her by asking her to leave the meeting. Excluding Debbie from the group does not help her to deal with her inappropriate behaviors. She may just seek another way to satisfy whatever need the monopolizing and interrupting meets. If it is a need for attention, Debbie might start calling the group leader at home. It could be that Debbie is merely demonstrating her stress by these behaviors and could benefit from some problem-solving around the source of her stress. Being able to talk with someone individually might help. Excluding Debbie from the group may take care of the initial disturbance, but it will probably not help Debbie deal with the problem. The group members may fear that they cannot exhibit any behaviors out of the ordinary or they, too, will be asked to leave. In a support group, expressing stress is inevitable, since it is one of the problems that brings members together. The group leader needs to be prepared with interventions that lead to more adaptive coping behaviors.

4) Extinction. As with punishment, extinction causes a behavioral response to become less frequent. Although the outcome is the same, punishment and extinction are different in process. Discontinuing the use of the reinforcer that has maintained the behavior eventually causes extinction. Punishment is a more rapid and complete way of extinguishing a response, because it is an active process of applying aversive stimuli. Punishment must be continued, however, or without the threat of aversive stimuli, the undesired behavior will again increase in frequency (Baldwin and Baldwin, 1981; Chambless and Goldstein, 1979).

Sometimes it appears that extinction is not working because the nonreinforced response continues on for a time and may even increase in intensity (Chambless and Goldstein, 1979). Children's behaviors seem to support this statement. A child demonstrates much faith in the continuing reinforcement of behaviors that have been reinforced in the past. Notice how a toddler will continue to bring an adult a toy for play even after the adult is no longer reinforcing this behavior by engaging in the interaction with the toddler. The two-year-old may even try harder to get the adult's attention by throwing the toy or using some other forceful behavior.

It is especially difficult to extinguish behaviors that are reinforced by attention. Frequently, the members of a group want attention from the leader. This, then, becomes positively reinforcing. However, the leader does not want to give attention to those behaviors that disrupt the group or prevent the growth of the group or its members. Someone who tends to monopolize the group's time by excessive talking, interruptions, and so forth, calls attention to herself because of her behaviors. If the leader pays attention to the member, even if it is with a negative stroke in an attempt to discourage the behavior, the leader ends up reinforcing what he would like to see stopped. Generally, monopolizing behaviors and others that disrupt a group provide the actor/member not only with the group's attention, but with some more basic needs such as those related to self-esteem. Behavioral techniques such as extinction are not usually effective with the underlying problematic dynamics.

5) Shaping. When the client's desired behavioral goal is quite complicated or complex, it is often not possible to reach the terminal behavior immediately. One may notice that the client is able to learn intermediate behaviors that will eventually lead to the goal behavior. If these intermediate actions are reinforced, the client will continue to move towards the goal. The process of reinforcing closer approximations to the goal until the terminal behavior is achieved is called shaping (Steckel, 1980; Chambless and Goldstein, 1979).

Walking is a complicated skill for the child to learn. Anytime the toddler pulls himself up, stands holding on to an object, or takes a step while holding on, he is reinforced by the parent for these behaviors. He is not walking yet, but the parent knows that these are preliminary steps to walking and wants to positively reinforce their continuing. Thus, he is shaping the child's behaviors.

In a group, the leader might shape actions that are preliminary to self-disclosure, which is a heavy risk-taking behavior. If a group member is willing to share demographic data, this is a precursor to sharing more intimate data about oneself. Giving feedback to other members is not sharing information directly about oneself but is another step towards self-disclosure if the feedback is in the form of "I" statements in response to another member's communication. The leader needs to positively reinforce these two steps as actions that are leading the member towards personal self-disclosure.

6) Token Economy. Although token economy programs are only a small part of the total realm of possible behavioral therapies, their use is widespread with many different populations. Many elementary school teachers use a form of token economy in their school classrooms. Paper money or points for completing homework on time, doing extra credit projects, and having appropriate classroom behavior are "tokens" paid to the children. With paper dollars or points, they may then purchase items such as pencils or small books, or exchange points or money for special privileges at the end of the week. Groups of clients who frequently participate in token economy programs include chronic mental health clients, alcoholics and drug addicts, adolescents struggling with emotional problems who express their distress through maladaptive behaviors, the developmentally disabled, and children with mental health problems.

Token economy programs apply operant conditioning to individuals and groups in a standardized manner. Target behaviors that are considered most desirable are reinforced with tokens that are then exchanged for concrete items or privileges. These items, called back-up reinforcers, are such a variety of different goods that the client should never lose interest in obtaining them, thereby ensuring the viability of the program. The token is a secondary reinforcer that gives the client immediate feedback for appropriate behavior. Tokens serve to bridge the gap between the client's performance of target behaviors and the privileges or goods the client will receive later (Craighead, *et al.*, 1981). Tokens are often more powerful reinforcers than praise or a verbal stroke for the client populations that participate in token economy programs. Shaping may be used to increase the quality of the behaviors performed and to reach target goals that are not possible initially (Chambless and Goldstein, 1979).

Staff that administer token economy programs must be very familiar with the behaviors that are to be reinforced. Obviously, extinction may occur if consistent reinforcement of target behaviors does not take place. Clients who can handle a more sophisticated procedure than concrete tokens may be put on a point system for reinforcement. Receiving so many points for attending an activity does not offer the immediate reinforcement of tokens which may be spent as money. Generally, points must be accumulated over several days and then exchanged for weekend passes, extended hours of television, and so forth. Rewarding clients with tokens or points may be difficult for staff if a range of points or tokens is allowed rather than a set number. The staff members must then use their judgment, and consistency may be jeopardized if the range of behavioral possibilities is not specific according to a reinforcement schedule. Attempting to individualize the token economy program, therefore, may cause problems (Galle, 1979). The advantage of a clearly defined reinforcement schedule is that nonprofessional staff may quickly and easily learn to administer such a program (Chambless and Goldstein, 1979).

The greatest problem of token economy programs is the transfer and maintenance of learned behaviors to the client's natural environmental setting where some of the target behaviors may no longer be reinforced. The solution is to select behaviors that will be reinforced or to consider what environmental reinforcements are available and attempt to incorporate these into the program (Chambless and Goldstein, 1979). If attending group is a behavior that has been reinforced by tokens or points while the client is in the hospital, what might be reinforcement for continuing this behavior as an outpatient? The group leader would need to provide some in-group reinforcement that would increase the probability of future attendance. Clients that need very concrete, tangible rewards will continue to respond to these if they become part of the group experience. Sometimes providing refreshments immediately after group not only positively reinforces attendance but also encourages informal socialization between group members. If one of the goals for group is to increase the members' ease in interacting with others, after-group refreshment time might also help members accomplish this goal. Chapter Twelve will present in more detail the group techniques important for accomplishing goals with a chronic client population.

Contingency Contract. This term is used to describe the contractual agreement between a client and a health professional that provides a reinforcement schedule for specific health-seeking behaviors performed by the client over a period of time. The client is an active participant in choosing both the positive reinforcements desired and the target behaviors which the client agrees are priorities for his or her health needs. Shaping may be used to reinforce intermediate behaviors if the terminal behavioral goal is very complex. All items of the contract are explicitly written down, dated, and signed by both parties. Specifics of how the behaviors will be monitored, such as with weekly weigh-ins or daily diaries of activities, are included in the written contract (Steckel, 1980). The contingency contract is quite different from the token economy program described for chronic populations in which the client is an inpatient on a unit where token economy is the form of treatment provided. In this case, the client cannot actively participate in choosing behavioral priorities or specific personalized reinforcements. Certainly, an individualized program for a client is more desirable. Those persons who are motivated to increase their level of wellness do well with contingency contracts. The individual is able to see the results of specific health-seeking behaviors and to more easily connect certain health problems with those behaviors that will correct them. "...(T)he use of reinforcement contracts is increasingly being recognized as an effective means of increasing patient participation in health care and improving patient adherence." (Steckel, 1980, p. 1599).

Contingency contracts are a way of personalizing the work that clients may be doing in a behaviorally structured group. The assertiveness training group which will be discussed later in this chapter works well with the use of individualized reinforcement contracts. All members of the group have the goal of increasing their assertiveness level, but each member may be working on a different skill and responding to a different reinforcement for accomplishing that goal. Generally, assertiveness behaviors are graded in their complexity, and a client may have a terminal target goal that involves incremental behaviors that are smaller steps towards that goal. Rewards for accomplishing each step may come from the group, its members or leader, or from some outside source. However, group feedback, itself, serves as one means of reinforcement. The group is a supportive environment for the member participating in a contingency contract. Supportive weight loss groups, for example, may include individualized member contingency contracts for specific pounds lost. The interaction between members in the group serves as a support for meeting individualized goals.

Ethical Implications of Behavioral Techniques

1) Influence vs. Control. Szasz (1977) discussed the issue of control of involuntary clients and prisoners who found themselves the recipients of behavioral techniques, especially aversive controls. He noted that child molesters were forced to receive electric shock while being shown pictures of nude children. The doctrine of the least restrictive alternative is a court decision that speaks to the issue of involuntary confinement. It holds that the least restrictive condition of confinement that will achieve the purposes of therapy must be used. Persons hospitalized under the legal system against their will may have to participate in a token economy or other contingency management program. There is concern that this violates the doctrine of least restrictive treatment (Craighead, *et al.*, 1981). Professionals who support behavioral interventions note that the goal of behavior modification is to generate stimuli that the client, himself, controls. The process of applying behavioral interventions should be a collaborative one between the client and the therapist (Chambless and Goldstein, 1979). Involuntary clients may not always fit in this category. Chambless and Goldstein (1979) commented on their perceptions of this issue of control: "The application of behavioral principles has not resulted in the exertion of more control over institutionalized clients, but rather in clearer contingencies for such rewards and punishments." (p.232). One's set of values and ethics as a health professional determines how one might use behavioral techniques or any other therapeutic intervention. I am aware that, when I choose to point out one observation to a client and to withhold another, I am choosing to control what information the client receives. I am using my judgment as to how to influence the client at that point towards a new learning experience or an opportunity to try out a different behavior or perception of the self. It seems to me that the issue of influence or control is germane to more than just the field of behavioral interventions.

2) Desirable Behavioral Change vs. Necessary Life-Saving Sanctions. The issue of influence or control is closely related to the use of behavioral interventions when it may be necessary to save a life. For example, clients who are diagnosed as anorexic are struggling with a number of underlying dynamics. Among these is the issue of control over their lives. As long as the client with anorexia nervosa can feel some power and control by withholding nourishment to herself, she is meeting a need that has been lacking for her. Behavioral therapy is a common intervention for anorexia nervosa and frequently involves punishment, such as withdrawal of privileges, unless the client eats. This challenges the client's ability to control her food intake (Claggett, 1980). However, the client may die of malnourishment if control is not placed over what she eats. Helping the client gain control over other areas of her life besides food is an important long-term goal. Steps toward this goal may be supported by positive reinforcement. The use of behavioral controls to prevent injury or loss of life applies to individuals engaging in any self-destructive behavior. The courts have ruled that, in such cases of extraordinary circumstances, even the use of aversive techniques are acceptable if this prevents self-injury (Craighead, *et al.,* 1981).

3) Aversive Stimuli vs. Positive Reinforcement. The anorexic client who is being denied privileges is being punished. Should aversive treatment be used when positive reinforcers help persons to develop new, adaptive behaviors, whereas aversive stimuli simply decrease the occurrence of certain undesirable behaviors? If punishment is used by denying positive reinforcers to someone, reinforcers are considered privileges rather than rights. Some recent court decisions make it illegal to withhold privileges in order to modify behavior. Institutional programs must use as reinforcers items that are not readily available to clients. Isolation or keeping the client from having the opportunity to receive positive reinforcement may only be done for brief periods and only if the individual has been a danger to himself or others (Craighead, *et al.,* 1981). Chambless and Goldstein (1979) stated that electric shock is seldom justified, since viewing unpleasant images will produce the same results. Baldwin and Baldwin (1981) also noted some problems with the use of punishment. Punishment teaches one to be aggressive; *i.e.,* one learns that punishment is an effective coping mechanism to use on others. Punishment only provides for temporary suppression of the undesirable behavior and is, therefore, a temporary solution. Part of the learning that takes place with people who are punished is the desire to avoid both the punishment and the punisher. The socializing agent, then, is less able to exert control over the individual or to influence that person in a positive way. It should be noted that "(b)ehavior modification programs rely more heavily on positive reinforcement than on negative reinforcement and punishment." (Craighead, *et al.*, 1981, p.192). Since the behavioral experts see aversive stimuli as being less than desirable, it seems that, both therapeutically and ethically, punishment should be avoided if possible.

The Group and Behavior Modification

Client Populations

As with the token economy program, a variety of client populations participating in groups may benefit from behavioral techniques. Groups that focus on breaking a behavioral pattern, such as those dealing with smoking, overeating, or lack of assertiveness use many behavioral techniques including operant conditioning, modeling, and reciprocal inhibition. The latter two techniques will be discussed in the section on assertiveness training. Children and adolescents respond quite readily to positive reinforcement and to such active techniques as behavioral rehearsal, where they may practice behaviors that have been modeled for them by adults. Clients with organic mental syndromes who have difficulty with memory, concentration, and other cognitive skills practice these skills in groups where any efforts are rewarded with positive reinforcement, often in the form of concrete items as well as verbal and nonverbal strokes.

The clients selected for behaviorally focused group should be a homogeneous population with easily isolated behaviors for change for the purpose of applying behavioral techniques. Ten to twelve members make an appropriate-sized group. A smaller number of members is found in a group where the leader is less directive, and the members focus more on expression of feelings and their process with each other (Griffith, 1982).

Group Characteristics

Behavioral groups have more directive leadership with circumscribed, specific goals, simulations, explanations, and with most interaction leader-centered rather than member-centered. The group as a whole may participate in a reinforcement schedule, or such a program may be individualized for each member. It seems that the peer pressure within the group to earn reinforcers increases the motivational level of the members. Reinforcers may be adjusted as the group increases its level of functioning. Typical behaviors that may be reinforced in a group include the expression of positive feelings, meaningful conversation, and acceptance of the group leader's decisions and direction (Griffith, 1982).

The Assertiveness Training Group

Definitions

Assertive Behavior. Assertive behaviors are a group of actions which are self-enhancing to the individual and facilitate the honest expression of feelings (Alberti and Emmons, 1974). The nonverbal behaviors of an assertive person include an open and relaxed stance with an erect posture, natural and appropriate movements, direct eye contact, and a natural and confident voice tone. The individual who is assertive is in an "I'm OK" life position (Bowman and Spadoni, 1981). Alberti and Emmons (1974) described the assertive person as one who is "open and flexible, genuinely concerned with the rights of others, yet at the same time able to establish very well his own rights." (p.4). A person who is assertive would be likely to do what Jean demonstrates in the following incidents.

1) When the sales clerk asks, "Who's next?" Jean speaks up to identify herself as the person who has been waiting the longest.

2) Jean is comfortable saying "no" to someone when she does not want to do what the person is asking of her.

3) Jean does not hesitate to tell someone what she thinks even though it is not in agreement with the other's viewpoint.

4) When the smoker sitting next to her blows smoke in her face, Jean asks him to stop.

Nonassertive Behavior. In contrast to the assertive person, the nonassertive or passive individual is self-denying and is often unable to express how he or she feels, although this person typically feels inhibited and fearful (Alberti and Emmons, 1974). The body language of the nonassertive individual includes a slumped or cowering posture, avoidance of eye contact, a closed body position, and fidgeting behaviors. When this person speaks, it is usually in a soft, quivering tone, a high-pitched, nervous, or rambling and hesitant manner. Generally, the passive individual has low self-esteem and is in an "You're OK, I'm not OK" position (Bowman and Spadoni, 1981). Some examples of nonassertive behaviors include the following behaviors that Bill demonstrates.

1) A group of friends is trying to decide where to go for dinner, and the suggestion is made to try a new Mexican restaurant. Bill does not like Mexican food, but agrees to the decision when asked his preference.

2) Several people are pushing in front of Bill in line. He is really feeling angry about this but is afraid to say anything because he does not want to get anyone angry with him.

3) The supervisor asks Bill to work a double shift. This is not convenient, and he knows that several other nurses have not worked as much overtime as he has recently. Bill says "yes" but ends up "stewing" about this the whole shift and decides he will not go out of his way to help any of the other nurses out. (This example illustrates a passive-aggressive mode of behavior in which the anger one feels is not expressed directly but comes out in indirect negative behaviors, such as stubbornness, procrastination, and so forth.)

One may be generally or situationally nonassertive. Most people have at least one or two categories of responses in which they feel nonassertive. Such individuals are comfortable with their assertiveness in all other situations but would like to change their behaviors in those one or two key areas (Alberti and Emmons, 1974). For example, I am very reluctant to ask others to do favors for me, even though the requests I have are reasonable, and the other person has asked and received favors from me. I think I have a Parent tape that tells me I should not impose on others. In this area of interactions, I am situationally nonassertive. The situationally nonassertive person works on those areas that are giving him difficulty. Practicing responses to deal with authority figures or to disarm manipulators are examples of more specific, selected activities that would help the situationally nonassertive person.

The generally nonassertive person has a chronically low self-esteem and experiences anxiety in almost all social situations. Alberti and Emmons (1974) identified this individual as needing comprehensive assertive training from a trained therapist. The generally nonassertive person needs to start at a very basic level with assertiveness skills. This may mean practicing introducing himself to others, initiating a conversation, and so forth.

Aggressive Behavior. The aggressive individual gets his or her needs met at the expense of others. This person is self-enhancing and is able to express herself in a situation, but has little regard for the worth of others (Alberti and Emmons, 1974). Frequently, an individual who fears losing his or her sense of power or becoming vulnerable will become increasingly more aggressive. One who is aggressive shows impatience in her body language, boredom with others, aloofness, and a tendency to be demeaning. Sarcasm and loudness characterize one's tone of voice. This person's view of the world is that "I'm OK, You're not OK" (Bowman and Spadoni, 1981). Examples of aggressive behavior are the following demonstrated by Courtney.

1) Courtney lives in an apartment but feels okay about playing the stereo loud even though several neighbors have complained. She feels she has a right to live as she wants to even if it disturbs others.

2) The paperboy has missed delivering the paper two consecutive nights. Courtney is outside watching for him. As he drops the paper off, she starts screaming at him for missing her. He does not have a chance to explain because she cuts him off each time he tries to say something.

3) The seat Courtney is assigned on the plane is in the No Smoking section because the smoking area is all filled. Courtney feels it is OK to smoke, however, because she has no control over the airline's lack of accommodations for smokers. She decides to challenge the No Smoking rule by lighting up.

As with nonassertion, aggression can be expressed as a generalized behavior in almost every situation or as situational aggression. Alberti and Emmons (1974) described the characteristics of the individuals who fit these two groups. The generally aggressive person has difficulty getting along with most people. Although this individual may feel as much anxiety as the generally nonassertive person, the anxiety is expressed through volatile, aggressive outbursts out of proportion to the situation. Situational aggressiveness is a function of the individual's inability to handle the anxiety he or she feels in certain situations. This person has learned to handle the anxiety by being aggressive instead of nonassertive. Often, people find that, when they are first learning to be more assertive than passive in certain situations, they sometimes tip the scale towards aggressiveness in an effort to overcome any passivity.

Assertive Training

Kolotkin (1981) defined assertive training as a "multifaceted behavioral intervention designed to teach social skills, encourage appropriate and affective self-expression, increase personal awareness of maladaptive cognitions, and reduce anxiety in interpersonal situations" (pp.238–239). Assertive training is based on the behavioral theories of reciprocal inhibition and operant conditioning. Reciprocal inhibition is the pairing of an anxiety-provoking stimulus with another stronger stimulus that produces a feeling opposite to that of anxiety and is able to suppress it (Wilson and Kneisel, 1979). Wolpe (1973) found that a nonassertive person is often inhibited from being assertive because of anxiety. Anger is a stronger impulse than anxiety. Expressing anger is, therefore, a way of suppressing one's anxiety. Appropriate expressions of anger are assertive responses. The nonassertive person very often has difficulty expressing anger. For example, if a client in an outpatient clinic yells at a nurse because he has been waiting over an hour, the nonassertive nurse would most likely experience some uneasiness inside related to anxiety, and this would lead to a more inhibited response, such as an attempt to soothe the client. An assertive response most appropriate would facilitate the nurse's discharge of anger but prevent defensiveness with the client; *e.g.,* "I understand you are frustrated about waiting, but I don't appreciate being yelled at, and I would like you not to yell at me again. Perhaps it would help if you went to the canteen. I'll come find you when it's your turn." This is an appropriate expression of anger in a controlled manner.

Wolpe (1973) noted that nonassertion is sometimes a process of not having the correct motor habits to respond assertively. For those people who needed to change their motor responses, Wolpe found that assertiveness would increase if the correct motor responses were met with positive reinforcement (operant conditioning). For example, a member of a group who turns away from other, more verbal members and holds his head down, avoiding eye contact when speaking, may not have success at having other members pay attention to what he says. The group leader may work with him on more assertive motor responses outside of group (*e.g.,* open posture directed towards whom he is speaking, erect head, some eye contact). In changing his body language, this person will often find that the group members are more attentive and responsive to his comments. This positive reinforcement will tend to perpetuate the new body language he has learned.

Progress in assertion depends on success. Therefore, the group leader or therapist needs to help the client assess the most appropriate areas in which to try out assertive skills. If one area produces too much anxiety, an easier skill should be mastered first (Wolpe, 1973). Grading assertion skills is a process of isolating anxiety-producing stimuli and arranging them in a hierarchical order (Chambless and Goldstein, 1979). If a client has difficulty saying her name out loud to others, she would probably experience overwhelming anxiety if asked to introduce herself to the group. Therefore, the group leader would not have her work on talking in front of the whole group initially. The client might start by introducing herself to one person in the group first. Her partner could then introduce her to the group.

Preparation of the Group Leader

Bowman and Spadoni (1981) stressed the difference in the level of preparation and intervention of a group leader doing assertive training and one doing assertive therapy. The latter requires a broader knowledge base, including concepts of learning theory, a knowledge of the effects of anxiety on behavior, and an understanding of the cultural influences on assertion. "Assertion is a powerful tool that is potentially disastrous when initiated by the hands of the inadequately prepared." (Bowman and Spadoni, 1981, p.9). As with other therapeutic modalities discussed in this book that require both clinical preparation and theoretical understanding, assertive therapy should be done by a professional prepared at the graduate level. However, the communication or social skills that are often taught in specific assertive training exercises are techniques that one could learn as an assertiveness trainer (Bowman and Spadoni, 1981). The rest of this chapter will present a brief outline of the structure of an assertive training group and the basic behavioral techniques that facilitate learning. I believe it is important that the nurse leading a supportive group understand the theory of behavioral interventions and their application. The nurse may then make a more accurate assessment of client needs and interventions based on his knowledge of theory and the accompanying therapies. Specific behavioral techniques presented here are to acquaint the reader with their roots in theory. Chapter Nine will teach the process of behavioral rehearsal and other experiential activities that have a variety of uses in a group.

The Group

The assertiveness training group provides a laboratory where the client may practice confronting the anxiety that prevents assertive behaviors. People often share similar problems in assertiveness and find the group a supportive place to try out new assertive behaviors. Observing others acting assertively is helpful. Group feedback and reinforcement are powerful tools to facilitate change for individual members (Alberti and Emmons, 1974). Alberti and Emmons (1974) recommended that the size of the group be between five and twelve members with a balance of men and women if possible. This ensures a large enough group for feedback and observation of a variety of behavioral styles while giving members the opportunity to work out interactions with both sexes. Meeting twice a week is recommended. Frequent meetings to practice new behaviors are more helpful than one meeting. Repetition and positive feedback are reinforcing. As with other groups, coleadership adds to the growth potential for the members. Two leaders are available to model behaviors and offer group members two different personalities with which to interact. A male-female coleadership structure is very effective (Alberti and Emmons, 1974).

Members are screened to determine their assertiveness needs and appropriateness for a group experience. Frequently, the chronic mental health client is a candidate for assertiveness training. This person generally suffers from a low self-esteem and poor social skills. Bowman and Spadoni (1981) suggested that screening is important to assess the client's degree of reality orientation. A client who is poorly oriented to reality would probably not do well in an assertive training group where the structure demands compliance. The screening process for clients for assertiveness training includes a questionnaire or survey of their assertiveness level to determine their comfort with specific social situations (Wolpe, 1973; Alberti and Emmons, 1974; Bowman and Spadoni, 1981). Areas to look for would be the client's comfort with nonverbal behaviors, with saying "no," with interactions with authority figures, and with typical daily living activities, such as ordering a meal or exchanging an item at a store.

I always begin my assessment with a client by defining assertiveness, nonassertiveness, and aggressiveness. After I have asked specific questions to determine his or her assertivenss level, I suggest specific areas in which I feel the client needs to work. If the person is agreeable to my assessment, I write up a contract specifying the behavioral goals, the exercises the client will be working on in group, and homework assignments. This model of assertiveness training has been used with chronic mental health clients at the Veterans Administration Hospital in Palo Alto. Both inpatient and outpatient groups followed the same model. Contracts were written on 3 × 5 cards. Members referred to their cards in group as they performed the practice behaviors. Constructive feedback with positive reinforcement for improvement helped each client assess his progress. When the behavioral objectives of the contract had been met, the client would negotiate after group with the leader to formulate a new contract with a more challenging assertive skill to master. See Table 4.1 for some examples of assertive training contracts used in a group.

Specific Group Techniques

The facilitative components of assertive training include covert rehearsal, modeling, and behavioral rehearsal (Alberti and Emmons, 1974). Recall the discussion on covert rehearsal in Chapter One. The internal process of covert rehearsal helps the communicator to imagine the outcome of the message she is about to send. For persons who are struggling with their inability to make assertive statements, this internal process helps these individuals to picture themselves being assertive. Alberti and Emmons (1974) suggested two uses for covert rehearsal. If the group members have been asked to introduce themselves to each other, for example, each group member would initially imagine the exercise being completed using the interaction style the individual finds least anxiety-producing. The group leaders would then model the task for the group, demonstrating an assertive approach. Finally, after some discussion about this approach, each member would perform another covert rehearsal using the assertive skills modeled. The second covert rehearsal should help the member to see herself being an assertive person. The role response she anticipates receiving from others will become more positive as she learns how assertive responses affect others. Kolotkin (1981) suggested that cognitive restructuring, which is what the person does during covert rehearsal, helps an individual become aware of irrational thoughts that inhibit assertive responses. He stated that didactic lectures and reading assignments would teach rational thinking, a skill which the individual needed to become assertive.

It is important for the group leaders to prepare the members for a response not anticipated. Since being assertive precludes forcing another person to behave a certain way, the group should understand that they have no control over another person's willingness to meet or not meet their needs. Group leaders should teach members to assess a situation before deciding whether to be assertive or not. Since positive reinforcement comes from getting one's needs met, a leader needs to suggest practice situations for the client which will have the highest probability of success. However,

TABLE 4.1 ASSERTIVE TRAINING GROUP CONTRACTS

Group Member: J.D. (inpatient)   Contract 1   Date: 3/5

Assertiveness Level: Generally nonassertive with some situational aggressive outbursts when J.D. experiences frustration from not getting his needs met.
Speaks in a high-pitched voice. Has difficulty speaking without swinging his
knees in and out. Makes requests to others by pleading and repeating self.
Cannot sustain a conversation.

Strengths: Smiles frequently; initiates conversation; some eye contact.

Behavioral Goal: Introduce self to group using normal tone of voice and keeping knees still.

Homework: Twice a day initiates a conversation with a different staff member.
Asks staff member for feedback about voice level and nonverbal behaviors.
Reports back to group.

Group Member: J.D. (inpatient)   Contract 2   Date 3/26

Assertiveness Level: Change noticed in ability to maintain level voice and control knee movements. Otherwise, unchanged.

Behavioral Goals:
   1) Introduces self to each member of the group; shares *2* items of
      demographic data and asks each member *1* question to elicit data about
      the other person.
   2) Makes at least *1* statement of feedback for another member each group.
      Uses appropriate voice level and nonverbal as specified above.

Homework:
   1) Keeps a journal[1] of the times he elicits a response from another person
      and is able to offer a return response.
   2) Initiates a conversation with *1* staff member each day and attempts to
      sustain the conversation for *1* minute using appropriate voice level and
      nonverbal. Gets feedback from staff member.
   3) Notes in journal anytime he feels frustrated about not getting needs met.
      Describes situation: who was present, what he did to try to get his needs
      met, the outcome.
   4) Reports back to group.

Group Member: M.H. (outpatient)   Contract 1   Date: 3/5

Assertiveness Level: Situationally nonassertive. Unable to say "no" to a request
by a friend. Hesitates to ask friends for any favors. Feels this is imposing.
Feels uncomfortable receiving compliments; turns red, stammers, and
mumbles a "thank you." Does not get angry with friends even when she
has a legitimate reason to do so. Works to keep voice level at an even tone.
Appears stiff when holding in anger.

TABLE 4.1 ASSERTIVE TRAINING GROUP CONTRACTS (Continued)

Strengths: Eye contact and body language appropriate except when attempting to hide anger. Says "no" to strangers when she wants to do so. Responds to others' needs for contact by initiating and sustaining a conversation. Expresses feelings (except anger) in "I" statement form.

Behavioral Goals:
  1) Tells the group *2* things she likes about herself using a strong voice and good eye contact.
  2) Receives positive feedback from group members with a "thank you" said audibly, clearly, and with eye contact.

Homework:
  1) Keeps a journal[1]:
     a) Identifies times she is given compliments or positive feedback. Notes her response.
     b) Identifies situations where she is unable to say "no." Notes with whom this occurs and the feelings she has about it.
     c) Identifies situations where she feels angry. Notes with whom this occurs, the incident, and the outcome. Pays attention to her body language, voice level, and verbal responses.
  2) At least once between group meetings asks a friend to do something for her. Writes down her feelings about this in her journal.
  3) Reports back to group.

Group Member M.H. (outpatient)   Contract 2   Date 3/12

Assertiveness Level:
  1) Reports more ease at asking friends for favors. Feels anxious before asking them but feels good after she does this.
  2) Speaks in an audible voice with appropriate body language to acknowledge compliments/positive feedback from others. Good eye contact.
  3) Wants to practice making assertive statements when she feels anger towards friends. Admits to such feelings and is aware of her inappropriate body language.

Behavioral Goals:
  1) Assertively demonstrates the expression of anger in behavioral rehearsal of a particular situation with friends.
  2) Rehearses saying "no" assertively to friends.
  3) Demonstrates no. 1 and no. 2 responses in real situations with friends.

Homework:
  1) Practices no. 1 and no. 2 outside of group as the situation arises.
  2) Keeps a journal noting each situation, her response, and the outcome.
  3) Reports back to group.

---

[1]Source: Robert Alberti and Michael Emmons, *Your Perfect Right: A Guide to Assertive Behavior* (2nd ed.) (San Luis Obispo, CA: Impact Publishers, Inc., 1974), p.76.

part of being an assertive person is knowing when not to be. Alberti and Emmons (1974) noted several instances where not being assertive might be the "assertive" thing to do. Sometimes others are oversensitive, and being assertive with them will not work. There may be extenuating circumstances in which the individual may not be meeting another's needs, but he or she is unable to do so at the moment. I tend to ignore being overlooked by a salesperson who is appearing quite hassled from her work. Instead of making an assertive statement, I will usually just wait my turn and feel good about my patience. I believe it is caring to be assertive under most circumstances since I am honestly expressing my feelings and letting the other person know where I stand. Alberti and Emmons (1974) summed up the issue for or against assertiveness this way:

"Perhaps the key issue is whether or not the assertion, which one feels morally obligated to make, in actuality will make any difference. It might be better for all to accept the fact that some things are better left as they are." (p.52).

Modeling is done by an "expert" who displays a behavior that others are to observe and copy. Models may be real or symbolic (such as TV heroes). The observer initiates the modeled behavior because of positive regard towards the model or because the observer has noted the behavior results in positive reinforcement for the performer (Baldwin and Baldwin, 1981). It is important, then, for the group leaders to be seen as legitimate models by the members. I find that, if I am assertive with a group by being open and honest in my interactions, the members will more likely find me to be a credible person with whom to relate. Modeling takes on particular importance when the group leader is attempting to influence the members in appropriate norm development. The group leader must be seen as a credible model by the members in order that the behaviors the leader sees as important for the group's functioning are adopted by the members.

Behavioral rehearsal is a term that originated with psychodrama (Wolpe, 1973). In psychodrama, a scene is recreated by the client and several others who act out a past situation in the "here-and-now." The terminal goal for the client performing a psychodrama is an "aha" experience related to the resolution of internal conflicts. The psychodramatist comes with a psychodynamic background to facilitate an awareness for the actors that behavioral rehearsal alone cannot achieve (see Chapter Nine). Behaviorists describe behavioral rehearsal as practicing behaviors in a simulated setting that need to be learned for the person to function more adaptively (Wolpe, 1973). One may learn new behaviors without coming to any insight about internal processes. Behavioral rehearsal is an appropriate technique for the goals desired in assertive training. In an assertive training group, the leaders initiate behavioral rehearsal for teaching new behaviors to one or more clients. Members will frequently choose other members to help them try out new behaviors practiced initially with the leader. Specific assertive responses that group members may practice with behavioral rehearsal include the following: the "I" statement, the broken record, fogging, negative assertion, and disarming anger. Many of these are sophisticated responses that an already assertive person would learn in order to refine his interactional skills and avoid manipulation. The many assertive-training manuals available explain these exercises in detail. In order for these behaviors to be applicable for the client outside the group, the person practices using real-life situations he or she has encountered before in interactions with others.

Warm-up exercises are part of assertive-group sessions and may consist of a variety of experiential exercises which help the members become more comfortable with each other and with the leaders. Alberti and Emmons (1974) suggested that the group leaders participate in exercises to model assertiveness and other appropriate interactional process. Such exercises may be done at the beginning of a group meeting as well as for closure in the final group session. Chapter Nine presents a set of experiential exercises and discusses the process of using them effectively.

The behavioral techniques and principles of assertiveness that make up an assertive training group may be introduced in a supportive group. I try to be an ongoing model of assertiveness in any group I am leading or coleading. For example, if I notice a client using nonverbal behaviors that are distracting from his ability to express himself, I may use this process to introduce some assertiveness skills. As a responsible group leader, I feel that I need to offer the client all of the options I have available. The client may choose to not work on particular behaviors. As with other interventions, behavioral changes are negotiated with the client.

REFERENCES

Alberti, R. and M. Emmons. *Your Perfect Right: A Guide to Assertive Behavior* (2nd ed.). San Luis Obispo, CA: Impact Publishers, Inc., 1974.

Baldwin, J. and J. Baldwin. *Behavior Principles in Everyday Life.* Englewood Cliffs, NJ: Prentice-Hall, Inc., 1981.

Bowman, C. Sr., and A Spadoni. "Assertion Therapy: The Nurse and the Psychiatric Patient in an Acute, Short-Term Hospital Setting," *Journal of Psychiatric Nursing and Mental Health Services*, 19, no. 6 (June, 1981), 7–21.

Chambless, D. and A. Goldstein. "Behavioral Psychotherapy," in *Current Psychotherapies* (2nd ed.), ed. R. Corsini. Itasca, IL: F.E. Peacock Publishers, Inc., 1979.

Claggett, M. "Anorexia Nervosa: A Behavioral Approach," *American Journal of Nursing,* 80, no. 8 (Aug., 1980), 1471–1472.

Craighead, W., A. Kazdin, and M. Mahoney. *Behavior Modification: Principles, Issues, and Applications* (2nd ed.). Boston: Houghton Mifflin Co., 1981.

Galle, M. "Point System vs. Level System: Effects on Adolescent Psychiatric Nursing Staff," *Free Association*, 6, no. 6 (Nov.-Dec., 1979), 3–4.

Griffith, L. "Group Work with Children and Adolescents," in *Life Cycle Group Work in Nursing,* eds. E. Janosik and L. Phipps. Monterey, CA: Wadsworth Health Science Division, 1982.

Kolotkin, R. "Preventing Burn-Out and Reducing Stress in Terminal Care: The Role of Assertive Training," in *Behavior Therapy in Terminal Care: A Humanistic Approach*, ed. H. Sobel. Cambridge, MA: Ballinger Publishing Co., 1981.

Skinner, B.F. *Beyond Freedom and Dignity.* New York: Alfred A. Knopf, Inc., 1971.

Skinner, B.F. *About Behavioralism.* New York: Alfred A. Knopf, Inc., 1974.

Steckel, S. "Contracting with Patient-Selected Reinforcers," *American Journal of Nursing,* 80, no. 9 (Sept., 1980), 1596–1599.

Szasz, T. *The Theology of Medicine.* Baton Rouge, LA: State University Press, 1977.

Wilson, H. and C. Kneisl. *Psychiatric Nursing.* Menlo Park, CA: Addison-Wesley Publishing Co., 1979.

Wolpe, J. *The Practice of Behavior Therapy* (2nd ed.). New York: Pergamon Press, Inc., 1973.

Supplemental Learning Activities

1-4

1. Identify the reference groups that currently influence your beliefs and behavior. How does your frame of reference influence your interactions and activities in the primary group to which you belong? In what way does your frame of reference influence your interactions with clients?
2. Examine one of the interpersonal systems with which you interact. Good examples of an interpersonal system might be the staff with whom you work, your family, a set of friends, and so forth.

a) Describe the feedback loop operating between the two systems.
b) Describe the quality of the boundaries between you as a personal system and the interpersonal system.
c) If the boundaries seem rigid, to what do you attribute this? If the boundaries are fluid, what changes have occurred with either you or the interactional system as a result of the permeability between the two systems?

3. Using the nursing process, identify a client problem and include an assessment of the most important systems interacting with the client. Keeping in mind the principle of equifinality, identify several options for nursing interventions/nursing actions that might be appropriate to deal with the problem.
4. Recall an interaction you had with another person that resulted in a blocked communication (*e.g.,* game-playing, guardedness, unexpected anger). Analyze the interaction using either psychoanalytical or TA concepts, such as parataxic distortion, or crossed or ulterior transactions. How might you interact differently if you could repeat the communication now?
5 Identify moments in your interactions with others in which you do not own responsibility for your feelings. For example, notice when you use "one," "you," or "it" to talk about a feeling you are experiencing. If you take responsibility for how you feel, how does this change the way you might respond in the interaction? What effect does this have on your relationship with the person(s) you are interacting with at the moment?
6. Below are some problems the nurse might encounter in interactions with clients and other staff. Some are similar to experiences my students encountered. In each example, using the "I" statement, determine an assertive response the nurse might make to improve the situation. The "I" statement lets the other person know how his or her interaction or behavior has affected the speaker. The speaker may also include a request for the other person to do something about the behavior. Notice that the "I" statement has a particular form. For example: "I really feel angry when you blow smoke in my face. I get all choked up. I would like you to exhale in the other direction." The receiver of this message is not obligated to change his or her behavior. The speaker has been assertive and must now rely on the receiver to correct the behavior in question. Ob-

viously, assertiveness does not guarantee results. However, the assertive person has done what he can to make his needs known.

Using the process of covert rehearsal, carry the "I" statement through to imagine how the receiver might respond (*e.g.,* identify the receiver in each case; describe the role behavior of the nurse and the receiver; imagine the nurse's reaction to the receiver's role behavior).

The Situations

A. A seventeen-year-old Hispanic client has a diagnosis of lymphoma and respiratory distress. He speaks English, but his mother does not. The family has many questions about the diagnosis and chemotherapy. However, the mother is generally the person in the room when the nurse is giving care. She is constantly trying to communicate to whomever is in the room but only seems to end up upsetting her son and the care giver. How should the nurse handle this situation in an assertive manner to express legitimate frustration over the mother's intrusiveness while keeping in mind the needs of both the son and the mother?

B. In a mental health setting, a student observed a staff member reprimanding a client for putting her feet up on a chair during a meeting. The staff member always props up his legs on a special stool because of his varicose veins. However, the staff member has never explained this situation to the client. She does not understand why she has been singled out. The student wishes he had talked with the staff member about this. How would he do this in an assertive way?

C. A client in a prenatal clinic does not understand why her doctor is so abrupt with her. She has some questions about the various methods of birth control and is also considering a tubal ligation after the birth of her third child, which should be within the month. Your experience with the doctor is that he generally listens to clients. You have observed this woman being very hesitant about stating her needs to authority figures. How would you facilitate the woman's assertiveness with her doctor and for future encounters with authority figures? What role should you have in this situation?

Section Two

The Group:
Its Personality and Development

This section builds a structure for dissecting the movement of any group over a period of time looking at the way the members relate to one another and to the leader as the group works to accomplish its goals. Whether the member is seen as part of a system, as an individual with many unconscious motivations, as someone with the drive towards authenticity of "here-and-now" feelings, or as a person who is attempting to modify previously learned behaviors, he or she will be part of a group that has a predictable structure and process. These predictable characteristics of every group fall under the terminology of group dynamics. Dynamics refer to ongoing movements of energy between forces resulting in ever-changing circumstances. It is precisely this situation which occurs in any developing group. A group, therefore, may be described as a collection of people that, over time, creates a collective personality and moves in a particular direction. Chapters Five to Eight will look at the group's personality and the particular movement and goals which all groups share to varying degrees.

Structural Components of the Group

5

Although all groups have a certain predictable structure and process and some similar goals, it is in the latter characteristic that groups tend to vary the most. It is, therefore, valuable to classify groups according to their purpose for existing and desired goal attainment. Wilson and Kneisl (1979) presented a classification system for groups which may be used for a basic comparison of their differences in these two, similar areas. I have chosen to discuss those groups which I believe nurses are most likely to interact with as consultants, participate in as members, or lead, and have fit them under the broader categories that Wilson and Kneisl described.

The Task Group

Most of us have been members of various task groups. Beginning in childhood, as a member of a family, one might join in a project directed towards the accomplishment of a particular task or job. As a family group member, individuals tend to respond within the predictable role behaviors of an ongoing, established system. Once the family group becomes task-oriented, the predictable role behaviors will continue to occur, but the accomplishment of the task will be the overriding goal for the group. A task group, then, is a group formed to accomplish a specific job agreed upon by the group membership. The leader is usually called the chairperson and guides the group in task-oriented behaviors (Wilson and Kneisl, 1979).

Nurses are frequently members of task groups formed in the work setting to formulate nursing care policies and procedures, accomplish quality assurance tasks, develop training modules for auxiliary staff, and so forth. Such groups are not always voluntary but are required to fulfill the role of a professional nurse. The nurse member will find it helpful to have a knowledge of group dynamics as a way of understanding the movement and processes that a group goes through. Although the nurse member will not be in a position to facilitate the process in a staff group and may not always want to take on such a role, understanding why the group is experiencing conflict, and so forth, makes such a group experience less stressful. Chapter Ten will explore staff work/task groups in more detail.

The Self-Awareness or Growth Group

Wilson and Kneisl (1979) defined this type of group as one with broad objectives that address a variety of goals related to growth for the members. The growth group is designed to help members become more aware of their own process of relating, feeling, and behaving, and to increase their interpersonal strengths as a way of improving the functioning of the primary groups to which the members return. Growth groups focus on problem-solving, interactional processes, and specific issues that might be of interest to the members. There are several different categories of groups coming under the broad focus of the self-awareness or growth group.

1) The Self-Help Group. The health professional has an ancillary role in the workings of the self-help group. A nurse may be asked to be a resource person on questions of health which the group members could not adequately address, but he or she would not intervene in the process of the group. Goldberg (1979) suggested that the best position for a nurse in the self-help group would be as a member. In this role, the nurse could share health expertise as a peer rather than as a leader of the group. Goldberg described the members of a self-help group as being in a helper-therapy role. The member, who is the helper, aids another in dealing with the problem or issue around which the group is formed and also receives self-healing by learning more about how to deal with the issue herself. This function, central to self-help groups, would be negated if a professional health care worker stepped in to facilitate and teach in the role the members themselves cultivate.

The group's formation is identified by a focal issue or problem; the goal is to bring about social change and/or improved personal functioning and effectiveness. Through the group, the members attempt to meet a need not being met by currently existing agencies (Levy, 1982; Goldberg, 1979). The leader of a self-help group is most often someone who has experienced and conquered the problem with which the group members are dealing (Nix, 1980). Some well-known self-help groups include Weight Watchers, Alcoholics Anonymous, Make Today Count (a group for persons with a diagnosis of cancer), Recovery Incorporated (a group for rehabilitated mental health clients), Parents Without Partners, and Parents Anonymous.

2) The Consciousness-Raising Group. Closely related to the self-help group, the consciousness-raising group focuses on a problem issue that is shared by the members of the group. Generally, the issue is not of a personal nature, such as the abuse of alcohol, the state of single parenting, or the recovery of mental illness, but is an issue that involves a segment of society. Issues related to the women's movement, nuclear war, or the plight of the aging are all appropriate for exploration in a consciousness-raising group. Personal experiences are shared around the particular issue, and individual members might make personal contracts to assume roles in dealing more actively with a certain part of the issue that is most important to each of them. Commonalities of experiences and activities that facilitate the group members' cohesiveness and ability to work together further the chance that the members may make some impact on an issue. Often the leader, a member who is active in the particular issue, also has a background in group dynamics. This person can facilitate the process of self-awareness and provide for a safe atmosphere where constructive work might be done (Randolph and Ross-Valliere, 1979).

A consciousness-raising group is generally time-limited, lasting a minimum of ten to twelve weeks. Randolph and Ross-Valliere (1979) also suggested that the group be closed to new members after the third meeting in order to preserve the ongoing process of developing trust and cohesiveness among the members.

3) The Growth Group. The emphasis of the growth group is on self-understanding through increased awareness of one's feelings, values, attitudes, and the way the individual's own process prevents growth. Such groups may offer a variety of experiential exercises that facilitate self-awareness. The leaders or group facilitators may provide a balance of confrontation and support as a catalyst for increased awareness and the breakdown of resistance (Silbert, 1981). The "here-and-now" focus of the Gestalt group is also a part of the approach of the growth group. Often, an extended session of a half-day or as long as twenty-four hours (a marathon) of nonstop dialogue, encounters, and so forth, allow for deeper exploration of the self and a chance to take the risk of more self-disclosure. Frequently, mental health professionals join growth groups as a way of understanding their own process of interacting to be better prepared to help clients in that same endeavor. Students preparing for careers in the helping professions may be in a growth group as part of their class work. Such groups might include a focus such as death and dying, human sexuality, or general self-awareness. The groups out of the Esalen Institute in California and the T-groups of management training seminars are examples of growth groups. Exploration of issues, such as those relating to sexual values and intimacy as well as much less personal issues, such as one's use of power in the marketplace, are all topics for growth groups.

The great variation in the content and process of these groups makes them difficult to evaluate. As a mental health professional, I am concerned about a group facilitated by someone not trained in the appropriate use of experiential techniques. Such techniques promote the expression of a volume of highly emotional feelings, some of which can be very frightening. If the facilitator does not know how to help the individual deal with these feelings satisfactorily, this can be very detrimental to the person's mental health. A discussion about the use and misuse of experiential techniques can be found in Chapter Nine. My own experience as a member of several growth groups as part of my graduate education left me with positive feelings. Nursing curriculums, even at the undergraduate level, are including more experiences for students that may be labeled as growth groups.

The Support Group

Although Wilson and Kneisl (1979) do not include the support group within any of their categories, it is a very appropriate one for nurses to structure and lead for almost any client population experiencing a stress related to illness. A support group does just what the word implies; it is a place to gain an emotional boost by reinforcing one's consistent coping mechanisms, teaching new ones, and providing an atmosphere for sharing and acceptance. Support groups serve both the client and significant others. Often, particularly when a child is ill, the parents are the ones that need the most support. The nurse may combine teaching about the child's illness, the disease process, and the technical care involved with some ideas to help parents restore as normal an atmosphere as possible for the child's development. The group may also help the parents deal with those family stresses related to the illness (Johnson, 1982). In summary, a support group is the strengthening and reinforcement of the members' personal and environmental resources which help them alter or prevent maladaptive coping patterns and maintain healthy behaviors (Johnson, 1982).

As with self-help groups, support groups thrive on the members' sharing of their personal experiences. This becomes a more authentic and accepted process than guidance solely by health professionals. The support group is led by a professional, often a nurse, who facilitates the group members' interactions, but it is this interaction among members that actually leads the group towards its goals (Johnson, 1982). Because increased knowledge often helps allay anxiety, the nurse or other group leader who can offer some teaching to the members about their illness increases the effectiveness of the support process.

Johnson (1982) suggested that it is important for the leader to help significant others in the group to focus on those issues over which they have some control in changing, such as the way they interact with the client or structure the home environment. The disease process itself, which may be taught in the group, is not something that significant others can alter. As a group leader, the nurse needs to be comfortable with the expression of emotions, such as fear, anger, and anxiety. Since families or other significant others may not have had a group experience before, some nurse leaders doing a group for the families of burn patients found that it was helpful to begin with didactic teaching and then gradually ease in to more "here-and-now" expressions of emotions. Their last formal teaching focused on the response to tragedy as a way to move towards the group members' emotional needs (McHugh, *et al.,* 1979). Chapter Twelve will discuss the support group as it is used for several different client populations.

The Therapy Group

Although the therapy group certainly offers support to the client, it is primarily designed as a modality to further change towards more adaptive ways of behaving and feeling. To do this, the group must be not only supportive, but also probing and confrontive with clients. A support group helps members to allay their anxiety; a therapy group may cause members to feel more anxiety. McHugh, *et al.,* (1979) noted that, in a support group, one's defense mechanisms are not challenged. In fact, if denial, for example, is helping a client over a difficult period of illness, the group leader will not ask this member to give up that defense. In contrast, the psychotherapist would work with the client on the denial, helping the individual to gain insight into the need for the defense mechanism, and work towards substituting a more adaptive means of coping. Certainly, while the client is trying to give up the defense, she is feeling some anxiety, particularly since this person is now aware of the thoughts that she so successfully had denied before. Eventually, the client will feel much less anxious and will be handling anxiety much better because of a more adaptive coping style. It is important to tell a client, who is in pain because of the inability to deal in an emotionally healthy way with some aspect of his life, that therapy will probably make the pain even greater for awhile since he will need to deal directly with the hurt rather than denying it or repressing it. It is through this painful process called therapy that real adaptive changes can take place for the client. Wilson and Kneisl (1979) described a therapy group as helping the client work towards self-understanding and more satisfying relationships. The leader or therapist facilitates interactions between members and between himself and members to do therapy. The therapist helps the client gain insight into his or her own process. Much work is done by the therapist prior to beginning group meetings in holding individual group interviews to select those clients that would be most appropriate for the group. This protects members from being in a group with others that do not have the motivation to be in a therapy group and allows the therapist to select the most appropriate client population for the goals of the particular group. An individual interview also prepares each client for the group experience. Chapter Thirteen discusses the techniques for facilitating a process-oriented insight therapy group.

The crisis group is a special therapy group that includes a lot of elements of the supportive group and focuses on helping members learn a more adaptive coping style. As with individual crisis therapy, the goal is resolution of the immediate crisis and restoration of at least the client's previous level of coping. The leader is more directive than in a regular therapy group, and more focus is placed on content than on the interactions between members (Janosik, 1982). The group provides the therapy for the individual. Sessions are limited as with individual crisis therapy, and usually the group is open-ended, allowing members to join at any time. It is important for the client to have a pregroup interview just as he would in preparation for joining a non-crisis-oriented psychotherapy group. Clients who could benefit from some of the curative factors of a group, such as increased interpersonal relationships, would be better suited for the crisis group than for individual crisis therapy (Aguilera and Messick, 1974). Since the crisis group serves those who are experiencing a need for extra support, it might sound as if such a group fulfilled similar needs to that of a support group. Although the crisis group does provide support to the clients, it is primarily a group where a therapy commitment must be made by the member. Table 5.1 highlights the differences between a support group and a crisis group.

The Social Group

All of us are members of one or more social groups where the primary goal is recreation and mutual enjoyment of friends. Wilson and Kneisl (1979) recognized this as a group worthy of comment, probably since it is such a pervasive force in our culture. As a nurse, I see the value of the social group for clients that are hesitant to develop close interpersonal relationships. I might, therefore, provide a social group as part of a client's therapy schedule. Nurses should not forget that this group serves a legitimate function, especially for the elderly client who has experienced many interpersonal losses and for the chronic mental health client who needs some social contact to prevent withdrawal and who could benefit from an increased sense of self-worth. The social group, although more informal in structure, experiences some of the same stages of group development as do other groups. This is helpful for the nurse to understand, since clients often are confused by the interactions in social groups to which they belong. The nurse who understands group dynamics may help the client realistically evaluate his or her interactions and behaviors in groups.

The Normative Structure

All groups have an unwritten set of norms or rules of conduct that prescribe how the members and leader(s) of the group will behave. Although norms are unwritten ideas of the appropriate behavior for a specific setting, each group member has a sense that the others hold the same beliefs in the behavioral expectations for the group (Lieberman, *et al.*, 1973). It is precisely this belief in the existence of a universal set of rules that results in the norms being carried out in the group. Some norms are spoken out loud by the leader or group members. Some are just reinforced nonverbally by the leader when they occur. Everything that goes into the development and enforcement of these behaviors is part of the normative structure. Norms will differ according to the type of group and the goals for the group. In our discussion, we

TABLE 5.1 COMPARING A CRISIS GROUP AND A SUPPORT GROUP

	Crisis Group	Support Group
MEMBERSHIP	Homogeneous re: current experience with a crisis	Homogeneous re: life situation or illness
DESCRIPTION OF GROUP MEMBER	In crisis with one or more of the following: decreased attention span; narrowed focus; decreased problem-solving ability, etc.	May or may not be in a crisis. Frequently has potential for a crisis because of current life situation
GOALS OF GROUP	Resolution of immediate individual crisis and restoration of function to at least the previous level with prevention of future, similar crises[1,2]	Emotional support to prevent a crisis during a period of illness of self or significant other; a recent life situation causing emotional distress.
THERAPEUTIC MODALITIES	Crisis intervention with didactic instruction, problem-solving, and development of new coping skills. Focus on content with high task-orientation and directive leadership[1]	Problem-solving; didactic instruction on the course and treatment of the particular illness or the developmental course of the particular life situation. Focus on both content and the relationship between members
LENGTH OF GROUP	Usually limited to six sessions[2]	May vary in length from six to ten weeks to six to twelve months or more. Meetings may be scheduled weekly or at longer intervals, particularly if an illness is ongoing.[3]

SOURCES

1. Ellen Janosik and Lenore Phipps, *Life Cycle Group Work in Nursing* (Monterey, CA: Wadsworth Health Science Division, 1982), 67-70.
2. Donna Aguilera and Janice Messick, *Crisis Intervention Theory and Methodology* (2nd ed.) (St. Louis: C.V. Mosby Co., 1974), 30.
3. Mary Johnson, "Support Groups for Parents of Chronically Ill Children" *Pediatric Nursing*, 8 (May-June, 1982), 160-163.

will focus on the normative structure that would be appropriate for a supportive group and will spend some time discussing the normative structure of a therapy group. Our discussion of norms will focus on their characteristics, the difference between explicit and implicit norms, the process of developing the normative structure within the group, and the process of norm enforcement.

Characteristics of Norms

The above paragraph contained a cursory definition of norms that introduced the idea of the normative structure. Norms are an important part of any group and consist of four basic characteristics. They provide for the following.

1) Role Behavioral Patterns. Norms predict how a group of people will react at anytime in the future (Mackenzie, 1979). They are rules of conduct that maintain behavioral consistency and are derived from the common beliefs of the group members and leader about acceptable behaviors. Some norms will apply to specific members in specific roles (Callahan, *et al.,* 1980; Wilson and Kneisl, 1979). Thus, norms speak about the role behavioral patterns that are appropriate for the group.

A role is a set of behaviors expected when one occupies a position in a social system (King, 1981). The family, as a social system, has defined behaviors for the position of mother, father, and child. Both Roy (1981) and King (1981) talk about role function as being an important aspect of the client's identity as a system and as a member of other systems.

The role, labeled as mother, father, and so forth, exists as a necessary set of functions or behaviors that must be done to make the system work. However, the functions performed in that role change as the system and its members change. Nursing mothers provide milk for their child up to the time the child is ready to be weaned from the breast. When this particular function for the mother no longer exists, other functions take its place. A parent, usually the mother, with help from other family members, toilet-trains the child. The child gradually takes over this behavior also.

The roles in a group are established by the group's norms just as the family has norms to define its basic roles. The role behavioral patterns in a group also change as the group grows in its development as a system (see Chapter Six for a full discussion on the movement of the group through its stages). The roles of member and leader are the two basic roles whose behaviors are defined by the group. Norms of the group establish these behaviors in a general way, but both the members and the leader have as much flexibility in their roles as the group allows. A task group may set more rigid role behaviors. It is crucial that all members and the leader direct their energies towards a particular goal. If a member is allowed to take over some of the leader's functions and steer the group in a different direction, the task may be compromised. In a therapy group, a member who is helping another member understand a particular communication is performing a leader role behavior. This intervention is very appropriate in the group because of the individual growth possible when the members interact in this way. Various members may take over this behavior at different times because there is no norm prohibiting it, and it has, most likely, been established as an appropriate group norm.

Just as the members often perform leadership interventions, the leader sometimes responds as another participant in the group, rather than as a leader, to show members how to act in the group. There needs to be an understanding in the group of how the leader behaves to fulfill leadership functions and to what extent the members would supplement the leadership for there to be some predictability within the group. This norm is often established as the leader models appropriate member behaviors. For example, if the group leader decides she could facilitate self-disclosure more effectively by moving from her normal leadership role and imitating a member behavior, she would temporarily take on member role actions of sharing personal feelings with the group. She might do this by saying something such as:

"I'm feeling uncomfortable right now and need to share that with you. David, I appreciate what you just said because it reminded me of how I dealt with the death of my mother. That's still a painful subject for me, and I don't like to think about it. I realize that sometimes my reactions are a result of that pain. I almost cut you off just now, and I guess that was my pain wanting to make you be quiet."

The leader is responding as a member, although this response also performs a leadership intervention which is to facilitate self-disclosure. The members will recognize the leader's self-disclosure as a behavior that is expected of them and might be more likely to comply with this behavior, because the leader has just modeled the behavior and has not suffered any negative reactions from that. How do members know what role behaviors are expected of them? This has to do with norm development and will be discussed at that time, but it is obvious that modeling by the leader as well as statements by the leader are two ways members begin to understand what behaviors are expected of them. Members, likewise, have an influence on the type of leadership that develops. Members who are dissatisfied with the leader's behaviors will try and change those behaviors or take over the leadership role. It is not uncommon for group members to vie for control with the leader, particularly during the middle stage of the group's development. Chapter Six discusses this process in more detail.

Bion's (1959) work in developing the idea of the basic assumption group identified the member's influence in the role structure of the group. Bion's reference to the basic assumption group has to do with the members of a group behaving "as if such and such were the case," although this is usually outside the member's awareness (Rioch, 1972, p.21). Bion (1959; Rioch, 1972) cited three types of basic assumption groups and described the role of the members in influencing the leader's behavior in each case. The *dependency* group represents the members' need to attain security and be protected by an individual, primarily the leader. Members see the leader as omniscient and omnipotent and would behave towards the leader in this manner, shaping their own behaviors to conform to what would be described as a dependent role. Such behaviors as making safe comments, staying on safe subjects, and asking the leader to do all the problem-solving are examples of member role behaviors in those desiring a dependent role (Whitman, *et al.,* 1979). Bion's second basic assumption group behavior, *fight-flight,* occurs when members believe the group exists for self-preservation and that this can only be accomplished through fighting or fleeing. Whitman, *et al.* (1979) noted in their support group for cancer patients that the members saw cancer as the enemy and would often use anger as a defense against confronting their own inability to cope with the disease. The anger would be directed at staff, the insurance company, the drug manufacturers, and so forth. If flight were chosen as the role behavior, this would manifest itself in reinforcing those who wanted to present a totally optimistic picture of cancer and not consider the possibility of death. One might see a member interrupting or changing the subject when someone begins to talk about death. *Pairing,* the other basic assumption group behavior, was described by Bion (1959) as the formation of subgroups by two or more members who hoped to save the group somehow by creating a new leadership. Subgroups are an expected occurrence in the life of any group (Yalom, 1975). Subgroups will frequently derail the leader from the task at the moment by creating an opposing force. For example, two group members might begin chatting together and create a diversion to whatever is being discussed or occurring in the group. It is also possible to overwhelm the leader by joining forces as a twosome and trying to lead the group in a different direction. In a social group, Bion's description of pairing activities occurs when two individuals move away from the larger group to have a more intimate conversation (Hare, *et al.,* 1965). The fact that member behaviors can have a great deal of influence on what happens in a group speaks to the power the members hold. We will discuss this in more detail when we look at the leadership in a group.

Role behaviors are predictable because roles develop over time within any group and come to be very stable. A study of the family group, who stays together for many years, shows the importance of predictable roles in the functioning of the group. Although the actual behaviors performed within a role may change over time, even that is predictable as part of the characteristics of the role. As discussed previously, the behaviors performed by "mother" change over time, but in a predictable way as the children grow. In the family group, an implicit understanding exists about the appropriate hierarchy of roles for any situation, such as when the family must deal with an outside system as, for example, a health care facility (Robbins and Schacht, 1982). Robbins and Schacht described a system the nurse might use to infer the communication hierarchy in a particular family with which he needs to interact in order to treat the client. One needs to observe the interactions of family members to see who speaks first, most often, to whom and when; who acted as an agent for another family member; and who followed whose advice. Nursing interventions can then be carried out according to the family's communication hierarchy. The nurse may be trying to persuade a client that a certain medication is important for his treatment. If she is getting nowhere with the client, she might try to engage the support of other family members. Depending on whether the nurse addressed the most influential member would determine how successful she was in swaying the client towards compliance.

Making an analogy to a group situation, the group leader needs to know which members are most influential with their peers. He can then engage those members as helpers in facilitating specific therapeutic actions in the group. Although the leader has a great deal of influence in norm development, the members may become powerful forces in the actions that occur in the group, as seen with the theories of Bion and others.

Once norms have established expected role enactment for the leader and the members, if either deviates from those expectations, the group becomes confused and productivity declines. A deviant member who rejects the group's norms for role behavior becomes the subject of the group's attention and pressure towards conformity (Phipps, 1982). Eventually this deviant member may be rejected from the group (Yalom, 1975).

2) Standards of Action. The ideal group has a set of norms that allows for the accomplishment of the greatest number of tasks in the most effective way (Callahan, *et al.,* 1980). It is important to note that the function or goals of the group determine the standards of action for that particular group, and these will vary according to the type of group. The norms of a therapy group, for example, are very different from those of a social group. Members are expected to comment on their immediate feelings, whether they be positive or negative, and are, therefore, more honest and spontaneous in their expression than those at a social gathering (Yalom, 1975). One would not, for example, offend the hostess by telling her about the offensive odor of her dogs or that the dessert was bland and unappetizing. In a task group, there is a norm against dealing with interpersonal issues that come up while the task is being performed. Generally, these issues are ignored as much as possible; whereas, in a therapy group, such interpersonal conflicts become the fruit for growth for the client. Yalom (1975) noted that norms are "a prescription for as well as a proscription against certain types of behavior" (p.108). As norms or standards of action are established, the group's goal-directed behaviors are more likely to be accomplished.

3) Rewards and Punishments. Part of the norm structure are sanctions for deviation or violation of the group's norms (Lieberman, *et al.,* 1973). Wilson and Kneisl (1979) made some observations regarding the group's compliance with norms. Norms vary in the degree to which they are accepted by the members. It would seem then that those members less accepting of certain norms would tend to violate these norms more depending on the penalty for such action. If the group leader believed that group should start on time, but only one or two other members felt the same way, this norm might be violated quite frequently, especially if there were no punishments for its violation. Because the leader has a lot of the power for norm-setting, she may institute norms that are not acceptable to a majority of the group. It is then that behavior such as in the above example might occur. The extent to which the group may permissibly deviate from norms also varies. For example, norms regarding confidentiality would most likely have stiffer sanctions and, thus, would not be violated as readily. A member who violated confidentiality might find herself emotionally ostracized from the group. Norms also differ in the degree sanctions are applied for their violation. Of the two behaviors we have discussed, being late to group would probably not carry as great a punishment as violating confidentiality. It is interesting to note that anticipation of sanctions is often as effective in controlling deviancy from the norms as the actual use of the sanction (Lieberman, *et al.,* 1973).

The norms most highly valued vary with the type of group they serve, allowing the same norm violation to be treated quite differently in two separate groups. A task group whose leader highly values punctuality and attendance to the task would probably punish lateness more severely than the breach of a confidentiality in the group. Members sharing with others outside specific group content might not be a grave violation of norms for a task group. Likewise, a support group might be less concerned with confidentiality than a therapy group.

Some sanctions or punishments which I have used or observed being used in groups with a chronic mental health population include withdrawing attention from a member who is being inappropriate, talking out loud to the group members about another member's refusal to speak while "guessing" out loud what the silent member must be thinking and feeling inside, and insisting a particularly disruptive member make an individual contract regarding his behavior in the group before he is allowed to remain. The leader can use her position of power to enforce such sanctions; however, if the majority of the members is not in agreement about the value of certain norms, the leader's position alone might not be enough to make such enforcement work in furthering compliance.

Punishments are a negative way to enforce the normative structure. Recall that in Chapter Four we talked about positive reinforcement as being a much more effective tool to support behavioral change than aversive stimuli or punishment. Therefore, if following the group norms leads to positive reinforcement or rewards for the member, it is more likely that the normative structure will remain intact. Verbally stroking members that adhere to the norms is a form of positive reinforcement. Group members recognize their peers who are following the norms and often show their positive regard to a member who has begun to be more compliant with specific norm behaviors. Members receive internal strokes when they follow the norms and find that this leads to growth or success for themselves.

4) Identity for the Group. A norm is "a straight forward description of what happens in a given group" (Mackenzie, 1979, p.473). Wilson and Kneisl (1979) noted that norms develop around situations important to the group. The norms a group follows seem to identify the behaviors most important to the group in its goal attainment.

Explicit or Implicit Norms

Explicit norms are spoken out loud in the group, and everyone is aware of their existence. If the leader were to say: "I really feel it's important for this group to be a place where members can say what they feel without having to explain their feelings," he would be making a norm explicit. A norm often made explicit is one that forbids physical acting-up or acting-out within the group. Frequently, norms built around how a member begins or terminates the group will be made explicit; *e.g.,* members terminating must discuss this with the leader and the group first (in therapy groups, especially). However, most norms are formulated in an implicit manner with the group members not always being consciously aware that their actions are governed by prescriptions for behaviors (Yalom, 1975). Members act a certain way because they have modeled the leader's behaviors or because they have gotten reinforced for certain behaviors and not for others. They even may learn norms by avoiding behaviors that lead to sanctions. Some typical implicit norms would include: acknowledging the leader as the expert in group process, expecting all members to self-disclose personal data (most prevalent in a therapy group or support group), and avoiding issues that would cause conflict (most prevalent in a task group). As we look at how norms develop, we will discuss the reason most norms are implicit. Norms that have been in operation in an implicit form may be made explicit, especially if they are hampering the work of the group. It is then up to the group to decide if these norms ought to be changed (Yalom, 1975). In a support group, for example, members may feel that they must consistently make only positive statements to each other to maintain the idea of the group being "supportive." However, it is often very caring to give feedback to let someone know a statement is not helpful, does not make sense, and so forth. If the leader gets a sense that this is occurring, she may explicitly state the implicit norm, "It seems that the group feels it is important to always give positive statements as feedback. I'm a little uncomfortable with that because I don't know if everything I've said to each of you is really helpful or not. I wonder how others in the group feel?'' The leader's second statement is giving the group permission to talk about changing the norm, and she makes herself a target for the discussion, thus providing a fairly safe atmosphere for the rest of the group members. Now that the norm has become explicit, it may be more easily handled by the group.

The Development of Norms

The leader is the most powerful norm setter (Yalom, 1975; Callahan, *et al.,* 1980). The leader has several ways of influencing the development of norms, and Yalom (1975) noted that many of these are implicit actions, thus making the majority of norms implicit in origin. The leader's comments carry more weight than the members'. Just by speaking, then, the leader may emphasize a certain behavior that is taking place in the group. If the leader chooses to comment on some actions in the group and not on others, the nature of his comments determines how the actions will be seen by the group. Repeating comments made by members, stroking a member for a particular comment, or following up on a statement made by a member by expanding on it or asking for more information are all interventions by the leader that make certain behaviors norms for the group. If the leader makes relatively infrequent comments, these comments are probably seen as very important, because the leader does not speak just to be talking. Yalom (1975) indicated that what the group leader does not do is as important as what he does do in the process of norm setting. The leader models behaviors he feels are important norms, and his style of leadership becomes an implicit norm in itself. We will talk about how leadership styles influence the way the members behave in a group later in this chapter.

In the development of norms, members make value judgments about what behaviors ought to be performed in a particular role and what behaviors are not appropriate (Yalom, 1975). It is interesting to note that members sometimes influence the development of nontherapeutic norms, as in the previous example when members of a support group gave only positive feedback.

Most norms develop early in the group's existence, and it is sometimes difficult to change a norm that has been in operation from the beginning of the group (Yalom, 1975; Callahan, *et al.,* 1980). In a viable group that is meeting its goals, those norms that do not serve the group well are eventually made less important or eliminated as members learn to operate an adaptive group. A healthy group is not afraid to discard some norms and formulate others in the interest of making the group more functional. Since the group leader is the most powerful normsetter, he is most influential in determining what norms are changed.

The leadership role remains a powerful one for norm enforcement. However, it is not always the leader who is enforcing the norms. As the members learn more about appropriate role behaviors and become more invested in the group working, they may, at different times, take on a leadership role in construction and enforcement of norms. Those members who are most influential with the highest status in group facilitate this happening (Loomis, 1979; Lieberman, *et al.,* 1973).

As a group leader, one of my goals is to instill in the members a desire to help each other take some responsibility for what happens in the group. For example, if one member in a support group is uncomfortable using the group's time to talk about his stressors, I would ask the group how we might help Jim feel more comfortable. A group member in a task group might repeatedly come to group without her assignment completed. Although, as the leader, I could impose some sanction because of her violation of an important task group norm, I would rather have the group decide what to do about her behavior. The gain for group members who will work with this problem is not just more compliance by the member, perhaps, but a greater sense by the other members about how they can influence, as a group, another person's behavior. Yalom (1975) called this norm self-monitoring. If a member enforces a norm for the group, then the other deviant member or members are often more accepting of this intervention than if the leader were to make it.

Deviance from the established norms of the group is handled according to the "norm" for deviant behavior and varies greatly among groups as to the amount of deviance permitted (Wilson and Kneisl, 1979). Those members with higher status in the group, as well as the leader, are given more freedom to deviate temporarily from the norms without receiving any sanctions for their behavior. They are seen as "good" group members and earn the right to not always be compliant (Lieberman, *et al.,* 1973). Some group leaders may have established an implicit norm that deviance need not be discussed because it would take too much energy away from the group's work. Any deviant behavior is handled as it comes up; however, in some groups the leader does not expect deviance to be such a problem that it would cause disruption and would need to be addressed by the group. The staff task group is an example of a group that would not be particularly concerned with punishing deviance from the norms unless such behaviors greatly interfered with the group task. Most often, such a group meets for a time-limited period, and task functions are the primary focus. Those functions that would provide for conflict resolution, for developing an atmosphere conducive to the members working together, and so forth, are called maintenance functions (Phipps, 1982). These functions are less important in a task group. Therefore, the provision to deal with deviancy to the norms, which is most often a maintenance function, would not be as important in a task group. Probably, extreme deviance to the norms, such as not completing an assigned task, would be dealt with overtly by the group leader or members (recall the previous example).

In groups where more attention is paid to group interaction among members, and where such interaction is part of the group's growth or goal, deviance from the norms might cause more concern among members. Generally, deviance would create some conflicts and might interfere with the group's interactions. An option for dealing with norm deviance would be to exclude the member. However, I choose to use that option only when there are no others. Since part of the reason the member has joined a group that focuses on interpersonal interactions is because this process would be valuable for this person, to exclude the person would not help the member reach her goals. A task group has goals unrelated to interpersonal growth, whereas a support group or a therapy group exists for the emotional support and growth of the members. Some options for punishing norm deviance in an interpersonally focused group include censoring the member's behavior in the group meeting and suggesting alternate acceptable behaviors or talking with the individual outside of the group, particularly if the problem behavior deals with issues of confidentiality or out-of-the-group socializing between members (if there is a norm against this). Sometimes a comment by the leader is enough to correct the behavior if the deviant member values the leader's regard. The group as a whole may put pressure on the member to conform (Phipps, 1982). This is especially effective if the member values the relationships he has with other members.

Norms give one a sense that there is some conformity of behavior in a group (Mackenzie, 1979). Norms help create a cohesion or force to help members feel that they want to remain in the group (Callahan, *et al.* 1980). Therefore, as the cohesion within a group increases, which normally happens in the middle phase of a group's life, uniform behaviors are more likely, and agreement with the norms exist also.

The Executive System

The executive system of a group refers to the group's leadership, both the role and behaviors of the group leader and those functions which the leader and various members perform to influence the behaviors of the rest of the members. Leadership has been defined as the frequency with which a group member is identified as the person influencing or directing the behaviors of others in the group (Callahan, *et al.,* 1980; Calkin, 1980). Many authors noted that leadership functions may be part of each member's behavior at one time or another within the group (Cartwright and Zander, 1960; Callahan, *et al.,* 1980; Wilson and Kneisl, 1979). This is especially noticed in staff groups where the members are comfortable assuming a leadership role. Even though one person may be designated as the leader, a staff group where the leader and members relate as peers will have many members assuming the leadership. In groups made up of clients led by a health professional, the members will perform leadership interventions, while the staff person remains the identified leader of the group. Part of every group's development is a phase where the leader's role is challenged by one or more members. This, however, is a different process than that of the leadership being a shared function with the group members at various times. The former has to do with the identified role of leader which is assumed by one person or a set of coleaders. The shared function of the leadership process refers to behaviors which are shared by the identified leader and the group members when any of them attempt to influence the group.

Dynamics of the Individual Leader

The literature on management talks about two elements present in the leadership role: authority and power (Calkin, 1980). Authority is the influence that results from possessing a position within a hierarchical structure. Power is the ability to influence behavior or cause or prevent a change (May, 1972; Peterson, 1979; Calkin, 1980). May (1972) talked about the five kinds of power one might use.

1) *Exploitative Power.* This type of power is most often used by the person who feels very unsure of his own abilities to influence another and who feels little self-worth or acceptance by others. Exploitative power subjects others to being used by the person holding the power in whatever way this person chooses. It is destructive power by force. Anytime the hospital administration decides to close a patient unit and move staff to other areas of the hospital without consulting the staff affected

by the move, the administration is exercising exploitative power. Often, this happens because those in administration are unsure of their ability to positively influence the staff in their way of thinking.

2) *Manipulative Power.* May (1972) described manipulative power as the power one has over another through shrewdness as with the "con job." He noted Skinner's use of operant conditioning as a form of manipulative power and cited Hitler's behaviors as those of someone who was feeling desperate or anxious with his choice of this kind of power. Certainly, Hitler did not present himself to others as he really was, and apparently conned the German people into believing in the worthiness of his leadership. Manipulative power, like exploitative power, is used by those who do not think they can allow others to be a part of the change taking place, *i.e.,* to be participants in the decision-making process. Politicians frequently use manipulative power to convince others of the merits of their ideas. Recall the discussion in Chapter One on the connotative meaning of words and the emotions some of these words evoked. Politicians are skilled in using connotative meanings to influence others, certainly a manipulative behavior if done in a purposeful manner.

3) *Competitive Power.* In its destructive form, competitiveness often results in hurting another. If friendly rivalries allow the competitors to do their best and grow by the experience, this is a constructive use of power. Using politics again as an example, one can see the results of competition for elected positions in the character assassinations and implications of ineptness or wrongdoing one candidate makes of another. The competition of some sporting events, particularly children's events, probably comes closer to a constructive use of competitive power. Even the worst player on my son's soccer team is allowed to play in the game, and a win or loss is secondary to the fun of playing the game.

4) *Nutrient Power.* When one exerts oneself for the sake of others or uses one's power for another, this is nutrient power. A teacher or a parent frequently exercises nutrient power for the sake of the children for whom he or she is caring. A parent must be a child advocate with the school system, with the medical system, and with all the commercial systems that have products the child needs. Often a head nurse, supervisor, or clinical specialist will exercise nutrient power towards a new staff nurse who does not yet understand the health care system but must function within such a system to provide patient care.

5) *Integrative Power.* This kind of power comes from within the person when he or she stimulates another with constructive criticism to promote new insights and growth. May (1972) suggested Martin Luther King as an example of someone using integrative power. We think of mentors or role models as using this type of power when they gently confront or challenge their students. The person who is willing to take a risk to challenge another with constructive criticism, thus risking the relationship with this person, must feel comfortable with his or her own interpersonal relations. Recall that one's self-esteem is related to one's public esteem or how one is accepted in relationships with others. Someone with a high level of self-esteem may risk a relationship with another if he or she feels it may lead to growth for that person. Integrative power, then, is most likely exercised by one with a positive self-esteem level.

May (1972) described the same person as exercising all five types of power at one time or another. Most people do not feel equally as comfortable with themselves in all possible situations. Therefore, it is likely that even the most well-adjusted person might resort to a more controlling type of power if his or her self-esteem were threatened. As health care professionals, we need to keep this in mind when working with clients. The ill person experiences powerlessness in many situations in the health care delivery system. In an effort to regain some of this power and a sense of one's worth as a person, the client might resort to exercising manipulative or exploitative power with staff, family members, or friends. Being able to understand the client's need to do this and explaining this need to significant others are areas in which the nurse may be very helpful.

The use of power and authority occurs within the group by the person in the leadership position and by others who attempt to influence the group. The designated leader of the group begins with the influence inherent in the authority of his or her role. When the leader vetoes a suggested norm, *e.g.,* that group members may interact socially outside of the group, she is using her authority of her position to influence the group. Even if the other group members move into a position to influence the group, none of them will have the authority of the designated leader. However, one or more members may use various kinds of power to influence the group. Consider the following examples of member influence within a group.

Jim rescues Bob from having to deal with the painful subject of his mother's suicide by telling the leader that he feels Bob has a right to keep such a personal subject to himself (manipulative power, although it appears that Jim is using nutrient power. Jim is most likely conning the group into thinking he is really caring for Bob as he tries to influence the group against the leader, *i.e.,* the leader is uncaring, and take over that position himself).

Kim has had experience in writing behavioral objectives, which is one of the tasks in a nursing procedures task group. The group leader is less skilled in this as are most of the other members. Instead of using her experience to facilitate the rest of the group's learning by offering constructive criticism (integrative power), Kim chooses to withhold her knowledge until everyone gets so frustrated that they are willing to let her step in and tell the group what to do (competitive power).

Exploitative power is probably not used very often by group members, since influence by force is highly unusual in client groups where there are normally sanctions against such behavior. In informal social groups of school-aged children, the use of exploitative power occurs when one child begins to bully another and succeeds in taking over the group leadership in this way.

Leadership Styles

Much has been written about the leadership styles found in various groups. Style is usually closely tied to the intrapersonal dynamics of the person assuming leadership. In the previous section, we discussed low self-esteem, a sense or lack of relatedness with others, and the level of anxiety as being intrapersonal factors to affect one's use of different types of power. Generally, felt anxiety causes one to have a greater desire to exert control when in a leadership position (Smith, 1980). The following are the styles most widely discussed as occurring in group leadership. The first three discussed are data from a well-known study by Lippitt and White (1960).

1) Authoritarian Group. In the authoritarian group, all policies and procedures are determined by the leader. The group members are not privy to future goals or direction for the group and are not aware of what criteria the leader uses to dole out praise or criticism to members. The leader remains very aloof from active group participation. Getting attention from the leader becomes one of the few member satisfactions available in the group. In their study, Lippitt and White (1960) noted that two responses emerged in the authoritarian-led groups. Either the members became totally submissive and dependent on the leader, resulting in apathy and a lack of competition, or the members became very frustrated and developed a channeled aggression toward the leader, increasing the cohesion among members. Individuality is lost in the authoritarian group. An authoritarian approach is useful if a group is in danger of disbanding, and an immediate decision is needed to maintain the group's existence. It is also helpful when the group has a complicated task to perform and limited alternatives for action (Phipps, 1982).

2) Democratic Group. Policies in a democratic group are decided by the members through discussion with encouragement and assistance from the leader. The leader communicates what objectives he uses to evaluate group member performance. The group can be productive in the absence of the leader. However, when the leader is present, he is a participant-observer, interacting with group members but not forsaking his leadership position.

3) Laissez-Faire Group. In the *laissez-faire* group, the leader takes a passive role in any group decisions, leaving this totally up to the members. He does not participate in the group except to supply information when asked. Although the leader may be friendly, he is not socially interactive with the members, nor does he offer any praise or criticism. The group's achievements in tasks are very low, and this results in a feeling of dissatisfaction. Ideas seldom become realities, although there may be a number of ideas expressed throughout the life of the group. It is interesting to me that the lack of obvious overt leadership in the *laissez-faire* group actually results in a strong leadership influence with its nonstructure. The leader has a high degree of influence in the group's inability to function.

4) Distributive Group. In a distributive leadership, any member may become a leader by performing actions that fulfill the group's various functions. Different members fulfill these functions and may change roles several times during any group meeting (Wilson and Kneisl, 1979). Some members may be more skilled at conflict resolution, while others may have experience at promoting creative problem-solving.

"Distributive leadership is believed to be the most effective approach, because it teaches people the diagnostic skills and behaviors needed to accomplish the group task and maintain good interpersonal relationships." (Wilson and Kneisl, 1979, p.443.).

In a distributive approach, no one person holds a designated leadership role, but the group has leadership through its members assuming this role. Many staff groups with a collegial membership have a distributive leadership. Other terms associated with leadership styles include the following:

a) Directive. The leader exerts a lot of control over what is discussed in the group and is a highly verbal participant orchestrating the movement within the group towards its goals. The directive leader exerts more control than a democratic leader but less control than an authoritarian leader. A task group or a crisis group often has a directive leader.

b) Nondirective. The leader is often listening rather than talking and allows direction for the movement of the group to come from the members. However, the leader sees that the group remains on target to accomplish its goals and exerts more direct influence than does the *laissez-faire* leader. Many psychotherapy groups have nondirective leaders.

Selection of a Leader

The type of group is a factor in leadership selection. For example, an informal group with a small membership may not have an assigned leader. One person emerges as the leader as he or she offers ideas for group goals, and so forth (Phipps, 1982). The type of leader selected corresponds to the purpose or function of the group. Note the examples of leadership style as they relate to a particular type of group (discussed in the previous section).

It is also important to note that the needs of the members influence the selection of a leader. If the group membership is one of self-directed, knowledgeable staff, the leadership may rotate or exist only as needed for the group to function. Sometimes a group of autonomous staff has much difficulty working as a cohesive unit. In this case, a specific leadership assignment is necessary, probably with the leadership role going to someone who may not work daily with the rest of the group but whom the group members can respect. A leader who can allow peer-centered autonomy for growth of the members (*i.e.,* allowing them to discard unwanted goals and to handle as much intragroup conflict as they are able) is good for a psychotherapy group. In support groups, the leader should be someone knowledgeable on the illness or life situation that is occurring with the members. Staff groups will often select a leader from among their members unless a leader has already been appointed by those in power within the hierarchy. Client-centered groups get their leadership by staff making a decision to organize a particular group.

Covert leadership refers to the process of group members taking over some control or power from the designated overt leader. Members who perceive that they have influence through the exercise of one or more types of power tend to readily use this power to take over the group leadership, frequently in covert ways (Phipps, 1982; see the examples under the section on leadership styles.). Efforts by the members to covertly control the group leadership occur more often during the second stage of group development. We will discuss this more thoroughly in Chapter Six.

Task Functions

The task functions which help to structure a group towards its goal are an important part of the leadership role and may be performed by the leader or interested members (Cartwright and Zander, 1960). In task groups where the reason for the group's existence is to accomplish specific tasks, the leader needs to be skilled in task functions. These functions include facilitating and coordinating group actions in the selection, definition, and solution of group problems (Wilson and Kneisl, 1979). Tasks might include appointing specific members to work on a particular part of a project, assigning individual members to some homework outside of group time, scheduling future meetings to meet deadlines, appointing or electing a secretary to keep minutes, or structuring a brainstorming session (see Chapter Eight). Members skilled in delegating tasks can handle those duties that are not part of the leader's skilled functions. The executive function of how to divide the tasks might best be performed by the leader. In a group where there is more than one leader, one leader may handle task functions while the other is more concerned with maintenance functions or maintaining a working relationship among the members. Using two leaders to divide these functions is important if the group has only minimal commitment to task accomplishment, such as when the members have been assigned to the group without a say in their appointments (Phipps, 1982). It is obvious that structure within the group is necessary for the accomplishment of the group's tasks. In the next chapter, we will look further at the group's inner workings.

REFERENCES

Aguilera, D. and J. Messick, *Crisis Intervention: Theory and Methodology* (2nd ed.). St. Louis: C.V. Mosby Co., 1974.

Bion, W. *Experiences in Group*. New York: Basic Books, 1959.

Calkin, J. "Using Management Literature to Enhance New Leadership Roles," *Journal of Nursing Administration*, 10, no. 4 (April, 1980), 24–30.

Callahan, J., S. Fertig, P. O'Dell, and B. Marlowe. "Processing a Task Group: A Continuing Education Committee at Work Planning a Conference," *Journal of Continuing Education in Nursing*, 11, no. 5 (Sept.–Oct., 1980), 8–15.

Cartwright, D. and A. Zander, eds. *Group Dynamics: Research and Theory* (2nd ed.). Evanston, IL: Row Peterson and Co., 1960.

Goldberg, C. "The Health Self Help Groups as an Alternative Source of Health Care for Women," *International Journal of Nursing Studies*, 16, no. 3 (1979), 283–294.

Hare, P., E. Borgatta, and R. Bales. *Small Groups Studies in Social Interaction*. New York: Alfred A. Knopf, 1965.

Janosik, E. "Theoretical Frameworks: Interpersonal Groups," in *Life Cycle Group Work in Nursing*, eds. E. Janosik and L. Phipps. Monterey, CA: Wadsworth Health Sciences Division, 1982.

Johnson, M. "Support Groups for Parents of Chronically Ill Children," *Pediatric Nursing*, 8, no. 3 (May–June, 1982), 160–163.

King, I. *A Theory for Nursing: Systems, Concepts, Process*. New York: John Wiley & Sons, 1981.

Levy, L. "Mutual Support Groups in Great Britain: A Survey," *Social Science and Medicine*, 16, no. 13 (1982), 1265–1275.

Lieberman, M., I. Yalom, and M. Miles. *Encounter Groups: First Facts*. New York: Basic Books, Inc., 1973.

Lippitt, R. and R. White, "An Experimental Study of Leadership and Group Life," in *Human Development: Selected Readings*, eds. M. Haimowitz and N. Haimowitz. New York: Thomas Y. Crowell Co., 1960.

Loomis, M. *Group Process for Nurses*. St. Louis: C.V. Mosby Co., 1979.

Mackenzie, K. "Group Norms: Importance and Measurement," *International Journal of Group Psychotherapy*, 29, no. 4 (Oct., 1979), 471–480.

May, R. *Power and Innocence: A Search for the Sources of Violence*. New York: W.W. Norton and Co., Inc., 1972.

McHugh, M., K. Dimitroff, and N. Davis. "Family Support Group in a Burn Unit," *American Journal of Nursing*, 79, no. 12 (Dec., 1979), 2148–2150.

Nix, H. "Why Parents Anonymous?" *Journal of Psychiatric Nursing and Mental Health Services*, 18, no. 10 (Oct., 1980), 23-28.

Peterson, G. "Power: A Perspective for the Nurse Administrator," *Journal of Nursing Administration*, 9, no. 7 (July, 1979), 7-10.

Phipps, L. "Group Dynamics: Leadership Roles and Functions," in *Life Cycle Group Work in Nursing*, eds. E. Janosik and L. Phipps. Monterey, CA: Wadsworth Health Sciences Division, 1982.

Phipps, L. "Group Dynamics: Membership Role Enactment," in *Life Cycle Group Work in Nursing*, eds. E. Janosik and L. Phipps. Monterey, CA: Wadsworth Health Sciences Division, 1982.

Randolph, B. and C. Ross-Valliere. "Consciousness Raising Groups," *American Journal of Nursing*, 79, no. 5 (May, 1979), 922-924.

Rioch, M. "The Works of Wilfred Bion on Groups," in *Progress in Group and Family Therapy*, eds. C. Sager and H. Kaplan. New York: Brunner/Mazel, Inc., 1972.

Robbins, M. and T. Schacht. "Family Hierarchies," *American Journal of Nursing*, 82, no. 2 (Feb., 1982), 284-286.

Roy, C. Sr., and S. Roberts. *Theory Construction in Nursing: An Adaptation Model*. Engelwood Cliffs, NJ: Prentice-Hall, Inc., 1981.

Silber, D. "Human Sexuality Growth Groups," *Journal of Psychiatric Nursing and Mental Health Services*, 19, no. 2 (Feb., 1981), 31-34.

Smith, L. "Finding Your Leadership Style in Groups," *American Journal of Nursing*, 80, no. 7 (July, 1980), 1301-1303.

Whitman, H., J. Gustafson, and F. Coleman, "Group Approaches for Cancer Patients: Leaders and Members," *American Journal of Nursing*, 79, no. 5 (May, 1979), 910-913.

Wilson, H. and C. Kneisl. *Psychiatric Nursing*. Menlo Park, CA: Addison-Wesley Publishing Co., 1979.

Yalom, I. *The Theory and Practice of Group Psychotherapy* (2nd ed.). New York: Basic Books, Inc., 1975.

The Processes that Define Group Movement   6

Introduction

In this chapter and the next, we will look at the movement both of the group as an entity and of individual members within the group. The group's movement is usually referred to as group phases or stages. The individual movement or actions between group members as they develop a relationship with each other is called process. Sometimes the process between one or more group members overlaps with that of the movement of the group. This overlapping may be called a group theme. In Chapter Seven, we will discuss the development of group themes. The reader will recall a reference to group themes in Chapter Two in the discussion on latent content. In this chapter and the following one, some of the material in the first section of this book on the metacommunication level, the "here-and-now" process, and covert or latent content should become clearer as it is applied to the process of group movement.

The Group: A Dynamic Interactional Process

Throughout the movement of the group towards its goals, there is a dynamic flow between individual member needs and the group's need for growth as well as order and stability. Recall that in Chapter One, the group was described as a system with the family group as an example of a dynamic interactional system. The healthy family allows external systems with which it interacts to influence it, providing growth for its members and thereby causing a change in the characteristics of the family as its members change. All adaptive groups depend on the members, as individuals, to bring their experiences and ideas to the group. In the psychotherapy group, members are creating a social microcosm as they interact with each other and learn about their process, which they then try out in systems outside the group (Yalom, 1975). Thus, there is a constant interchange between a group and those outside systems with which the members identify. This movement creates the dynamic interactional process that influences group growth.

Part of that dynamic process is the group's desire to maintain some order within the change. A family in crisis often becomes more protective of its system and tries to maintain some status quo of roles, predictable behaviors, and so forth, within the family structure. A group that forms for a limited time (any group is short-term when compared with a family group) will not be quite as good at preventing the build-up of chaos and tension as members experience changes in themselves. One of the ways a group protects itself is through the development of some predictable rules of conduct or behaviors which we have already defined as the norms. The fact that the group is meeting for a designated purpose, whether it be for psychotherapy, a particular task, support through a difficult period, or other reasons, allows some predictability, and stability. Group goals help keep the group on its course. A task group, for example, does not allow a lot of time spent on developing the interpersonal relationships between members or the probing for resolution of conflicts. The purpose for the task group's existence precludes the luxury of individual interpersonal growth for the members. A crisis group does not allow a member to dwell on past dynamics related to childhood or other unfinished business but totally absorbs the member in immediate problem-solving of the crisis situation. Thus, the predictable group structure of norms, purpose, and goals contributes to the group's stability.

Another predictable mechanism is the group's movement in definable stages. We will talk about each stage in detail in this chapter, but as an example of the predictability of this process, one may consider the recurring dynamic of anger directed towards the leader. Generally, this occurs during the conflict stage or the working phase of the group's process. Although I know this will occur in each group I facilitate, I am never quite ready when it comes. It is not pleasant to be a "bad guy," and I cannot completely hide my subjective disappointment when the group becomes angry with me. If one is coleading, there is some support when this happens, especially if the other leader is spared some of the members' wrath. Since I know it is coming, I intellectually understand its presence and can deal with it on a scholarly level. In fact, as a clinician, I should be more concerned if the group never reaches the point of directing its anger towards me. That would tell me that the group was stuck and had not moved from the feeling that the group leader is infallible, a belief that is characteristic of the first stage of development. At this point, the group needs help in examining this process. If a group leader knows how to use the process unfolding in the group, it does not matter how long the group takes to go from stage to stage. By looking at what the group is doing at the moment, the leader can use that to help the group members become more aware of their process with each other. We will talk more about how to do this in Chapter Seven.

Balancing the predictable mechanisms within the group are the individual members' needs that also take on a dynamic interactional process. Schutz (1958) talked about the predictable phases the group members must go through in defining their relationship with each other. These phases parallel to a certain degree the group's developmental stages or phases of movement.

1) *Inclusion Phase.* "In or out" as Schutz labels it, is the inclusion phase. The initial anxiety of joining a group originates in the member's fear of not being accepted by the leader and his or her peers, and, at a more basic level, a fear of rejection from the group. Inclusion needs generally occur in the beginning phase of group development but may also be important to a particular member at anytime during the group's existence. Someone who has difficulty believing the "I'm OK" script will keep testing her acceptance in the group and will behave in ways to either promote this inclusion by others or will behave to carry out the script that she is "not OK." Behaviors to promote inclusion might include: agreeing with the group consensus regardless of one's personal preference; constantly checking out with the group leader if what she is saying is acceptable to the group; strict compliance with those norms the group feels are important. Behaviors that demonstrate a belief that one will be rejected include: taking the blame for other members feeling badly; consistently apologizing for taking up the group's time; and deferring to other members.

2) *Control Phase.* "Top or bottom" is Schutz's label for the control phase. The control needs of members begin to emerge towards the end of the initial stage of

group movement (Janosik, 1982). Yalom (1975) identified the second stage of group as the conflict stage in which dominance and control are the most prominent needs being expressed in the group. Schutz described the control phase as a need to have some say in one's future in the group and to define one's place in the midst of both an identified leader and an unspoken one. Schutz said the member experiences anxiety around the amount of responsibility taken on in the group. One may be anxious with too much responsibility or without enough. Behaviors that the group leader might observe in members expressing control needs to be on top include the following: 1) a demand to the leader that he or she share with the group what the members are supposed to be doing; 2) a member challenging the leader's credentials; 3) a member bringing a "buddy" to group without consulting with the leader or the rest of the group first; 4) repeated incidents where several members verbally support another member's power stand on a group issue that is contrary to the leader's position; and 5) expressed negativity over the amount of "work" the leader is demanding of the members when the leader does not appear to be working nearly as hard.

The member who is threatened by too much responsibility may ask the leader to intervene in situations that are best handled by other group members, tends to seek the leader's advice, and hesitates to make any decisions about his or her own movement within the group.

3) *Affection Phase.* "Near or far" is Schutz's phrase for what happens in this phase. Yalom (1975) saw affection developing in what he called the third stage where the group becomes very cohesive. This is also the time where more work is taking place in the group; *i.e.,* the group is highly productive in moving towards its goals. Janosik (1982) defined the middle stage as the period of the development of intimacy or needs for affection and a definite movement into a working phase. It is obvious that different authors have chosen to label the group's movement differently, although there is a commonality to the description of the behaviors occurring during this time. The concern of members in the affection phase is how to get close enough to each other for warmth and caring yet be able to avoid the hurt or pain of such closeness (Schutz, 1958). Members express this need by approach-avoidance behaviors or by taking a position at one end or the other. Some members withdraw from intimacy to protect themselves against hurt. Some plunge into intimacy with one or more members. Approach-avoidance behaviors demonstrate ambivalence and might be seen, for example, when a member self-discloses to the group and then retreats from the reciprocal disclosure by someone else. Members protect themselves from intimacy with others with such behaviors as limiting self-disclosure, engaging in superficial social interactions, and intellectualizing. Recall the discussion on subgrouping in Chapter Five as a way of gratifying intimacy needs, as well as serving many other purposes related to felt hostility towards the group leader and some issues around the need for control (Yalom, 1975). Examples of members pursuing affection show up in such group behaviors as a member suggesting a post group party to celebrate another's birthday or a member consistently going to the rescue of another in the group. As with subgrouping, many observable behaviors may have several underlying motivations. In the chapters to follow, we will discuss the process for making interpretations of such behaviors and determine when the meaning or motivation behind a behavior is important to examine.

Along with the individual's needs around inclusion, control, and affection, the group member also has personalized growth needs that have probably been an impetus for the person joining a particular group. Schutz found that inclusion, control, and affection were needs that everyone in the group exhibited in varying degrees. However, the individual's need for growth, although a predictable part of voluntary membership in a group, may vary greatly in the specific areas of change the person desires. In Chapter Five, we discussed a variety of groups that offered the member potential for growth: the self-help group, the growth group, the consciousness-raising group, the therapy group, and so forth. The self-help group may have a particular growth focus for all the members, although the motivation each member has for joining the group may be quite different. One member of a self-help group for weight control may want to develop life-long eating habits to stay slender and has never been successful at permanent weight loss before. Another very self-sufficient person may be looking for social support systems to make this behavior change (losing weight) a way of expanding his interdependence with others. A third person may just want to understand how a self-help group functions as data for a social research project. The therapy group has an even greater variety of possibilities for individual growth needs. Generally, each person in a therapy group makes a contract with the therapist prior to the beginning of the group sessions. It is much more enriching for the group if members come with a variety of skills and needs. For example, one member may problem-solve well and can model appropriate problem-solving to supplement the therapist's activities in this area. However, this person may have a fear of interpersonal closeness. Another member demonstrates excellent self-awareness but has difficulty with assertiveness. As more needs surface in the group, the group becomes more of a social microcosm of the everyday world of its members and can be a rich area for learning.

Balancing the individual's needs with the group's needs creates conflict and other processes that provide the group with a constantly changing character that can be used skillfully by the leader to allow a group of individuals to grow together. The rest of this chapter will be a description of the group's movement and the leadership activities that facilitate this movement. How the individual member's growth interfaces with the group's movement will be clearer in the next chapter.

The Initial Stage: Orientation

The initial stage may be broken down into one or more smaller phases, labeled differently by a variety of authors. What is most important is that the characteristics of this stage are clearly defined for the reader. Someone observing a group over time should be able to identify specific behaviors that indicate the group's stage of development.

Characteristics

The orientation period in a group is much like that in a new job or any new setting. The members are feeling unsure of their position with others and attempt to size each other up and to understand the behaviors requested of them by the leader (Yalom, 1975). Schutz talked about the individual's need for inclusion which occurs in the orientation phase of the group's development. Dependency on the leader for directions, for relief from the discomfort or anxiety of the newness of the group experience, and for assurance that their individual needs will indeed be met are all possible expressions by the group members (Yalom, 1975; Janosik, 1982). Both the group as an individual unit and each member as a distinct person behave in a dependent manner towards the leader.

The group deals with its anxiety by two distinct processes, one related to the content of communications between members and the other related to the nature of the therapeutic interactions that occur. Group discussions are superficial, characterized by mostly demographic self-disclosure related to topics such as occupation, daily activities, family data, and a sharing of the reason one has chosen membership in the group. Occasionally, members will discuss current events and other topics of universal concern, looking for some commonalities with which to identify. The therapeutic interactions that take place are the giving and receiving of advice and a superficial attempt at caring for one another (Yalom, 1975). Yalom noted that "the process of advice-giving rather than the content of advice may be beneficial, since it implies and conveys a mutual interest and caring" (p.12). Since advice is a personal opinion about what to do or how to handle a certain situation, it is generally not valuable in its content to the person receiving the advice. To grow, one must decide for oneself what to do based on self-awareness and self-understanding. What works for one person may be detrimental for someone else. Advice giving is a way for the group to express to the leader a need for structure or "advice" from him or her.

Leadership Functions

There are specific actions which the leader undertakes as part of her responsibility that are a result of her understanding of the dynamics of group behavior and its effect on accomplishing the purpose for the group's existence. The members do not come with this understanding, and they are often the recipients of the reason for the group's existence. Therefore, only the leader can perform these actions or functions. Lieberman, *et al.* (1973) listed the following as leadership functions: caring, emotional stimulation, executive functions, and meaning attribution.

Caring relates to the leader's concern, genuineness, acceptance, and empathy which promotes a positive relationship between the members and leader (Lieberman, *et al.,* 1973; Johnson, 1982). At times, this relationship may appear strained when the need for control begins to affect the members' behaviors, but the conflicts with a caring leader are not due to a negative relationship but to individual needs at that time.

The leader affects *emotional stimulation* of the members' personal feelings through modeling behaviors, self-disclosure, and confrontation (Lieberman, *et al.,* 1973; Johnson, 1982). Experiential exercises, Gestalt techniques, and psychodramatic techniques are specific modalities which the leader may use to generate feelings within the group. Recall that it is through the awareness of those parts of us that are leaking out repressed feelings that a greater understanding of ourselves as a whole occurs. As the leader picks up nonverbal cues, he may use whatever modality appropriate to help members become aware of feelings.

Executive functions relate to those actions which keep the group on target with its purpose. Facilitating the group's formulation of goals, norms, and general movement through the development of trust, cohesion, conflict, and working phases are all executive functions. The leader must model appropriate communication skills and group behaviors (Lieberman, *et al.*, 1973; Johnson, 1982). Some of these functions were discussed in the previous chapter.

Meaning attribution is a function that gives the members some insight into the reason for their behaviors in the group as it relates to their individual feelings and to the character and movement of the group as a whole (Lieberman, *et al.,* 1973; Johnson 1982). For example, letting the members know that it is natural to feel anxious at the beginning of the group experience is a way of allaying some of that anxiety and making that experience "OK" for the group. The nature of the psychotherapy group necessitates a high proportion of time being spent on meaning attribution, since the goal for members is a change of behavior resulting from increased understanding of one's own dynamics. Time is spent on looking at the process developing between individuals in the group, and the leader focuses more on process than content. All these actions are part of the function of meaning attribution.

The leadership functions which are most needed in the initial stage of the group's development are the executive functions and caring. Phipps (1982) noted that the primary task of the leader is to establish and adhere to the group's purpose. We have talked at length in Chapter Five about how the norms in the group are shaped. Initiating norm development is primarily the leader's responsibility and falls into the category of executive functions. The leader works with the group members to establish a sense of the group's direction or purpose through specific individual contracts and common goals that fit for the group as a whole. The type of group being established determines the amount of energy put into each of the initial leadership functions. A task group will require a high amount of executive function from the leader, whereas a support group would find the initial stage of the group facilitated more by the leader paying attention to caring functions (Loomis, 1979). The high anxiety at the beginning of the group's existence requires the leader to reinforce group behaviors that will reduce anxiety and increase the trust level among the members. Positive interactions between members and with the leader further reduce anxiety. Recall the desire of the group to place the leader in an omniscient role and to become dependent on this person for guidance during the initial stage of group formation. The leader allows some of this dependency initially, realizing that it is part of the group's developmental period, and can be instrumental in bringing anxiety to a healthier, lower level to prepare the group to work in the near future. Thus, the caring functions of the leader at this stage are designed to facilitate the group's growth into a workable force, whether it be for individual growth or task productivity.

Leadership Interventions

The rather limited discussion on functions will be clarified as we talk about actual interventions the leader and group members make to facilitate the group's development. Certainly, the earlier interactions one observes in a group are primarily member-to-leader and back again to member as the leader is seen as the expert on task and group development (Callahan, *et al.,* 1980). Therefore, the designated group leader is making more interventions to fulfill leadership functions than the group members at this point. The leadership functions are never turned over to the members to fulfill but remain with the leader as his or her responsibility. However, as the members become more knowledgeable about how the group functions and begin to model leader behaviors, they are inadvertently helping to fulfill some of the leadership functions. The members will also purposely make certain events happen in the group to influence their peers, some of these also facilitating the work of the group and some being in opposition to the group's designated leader. When a group member tries to redirect the group or challenge the leader, he or she is demonstrating part of the group's necessary development, that of control issues with the leader. If a member picks up a leader role behavior that furthers the group's purpose or goals, this person is making a leadership intervention, helping the designated leader with the group's work. The following are interventions that further the work of the group in its initial stage of development. Some of these would be shared with the group members, although it is less likely at this early stage that the members will be as able to initiate leadership interventions.

1) *Providing for a Comfortable Physical Environment.* It is obvious that a meeting place that is comfortable and consistently used provides some initial stability to the group and relieves some anxiety for members who are worried about finding the room or getting to the group on time. A room change and difficulty in getting to the new one were cited as some of the reasons for the failure of a parenting group for teens (Abbott, 1980). I find a good amount of security in knowing that I will not get lost when I am going to a meeting with strangers for the first time. Just recently, I began an orientation period for a new job in an outpatient clinic. Part of my orientation was to attend several meetings on the inpatient units to understand the transition for the client and to know what the inpatient programs were like. I felt some hesitancy about just walking into a meeting where I knew no one. I took care of myself by scouting out the room ahead of time, deciding how much time it would take me to get there, and trying to find someone I knew who was also going. This helped me feel a little less anxious. One of the meetings I attended was to be an ongoing part of my schedule. The second time I went to the meeting room, some other group was meeting there. It turned out to be the right room, but I was disoriented at first because of the other group meeting there. It seems to me that these experiences point out the importance of orientation for the group members to the physical facilities where the group will be meeting. Perhaps the pregroup interview could be conducted in the meeting room, or the potential group member could be shown where the group will meet. Leaders of support groups may want to schedule a pregroup openhouse for potential members. Support groups often include family and significant others. This would be a good time to meet family members and others who will be attending the group with inpatient or outpatient members. For physical comfort, the temperature, the air circulation, the exit and entrance access, and the chairs the group will use should be checked ahead of time for any problems that would create discomfort for the members. An ideal group room has privacy and accessibility with a limited amount of distractions due to noise, interruptions, and so forth.

2) *Facilitating the Sharing of Expectations, Fears, and Needs.* Most often the members who are experiencing group for the first time do not initially see how their individual needs will be met when they must share the leader's time with many other people. There is great ambivalence to belonging or to investing energy in a process that is not clearly defined (Webster, *et al.,* 1982). Yalom (1975) noted that members could not see how group activities could meet personal needs. One of the ways of

dealing with the members' fears around this issue is to acknowledge their concern as being understandable and then give the group some cognitive data about the ways it can be valuable in a different, yet equally as valid, modality for treatment. Even though members may have had a pregroup interview or screening, the feeling of losing the group leader's full attention is not apparent until the member actually sits in a group for the first time, finally sharing the leader's time with many other people. Yalom (1975) suggested that, in the pregroup interview for the psychotherapy group, the therapist specifically acknowledge that it will probably not be apparent for some time to the member that working on group problems and relationships with other group members will solve one's personal problems.

Group adds a dimension to one's perspective that cannot be gotten from a dyad relationship. If the group is, indeed, a social microcosm, then one may use group as a field work setting for not only trying out new behaviors, but also for being scrutinized by others in an atmosphere where the social norm about not being able to give honest feedback does not exist. I share with my groups the excitement I feel about creating an atmosphere where each person can try out new ways of interacting, gaining support, obtaining feedback, problem-solving, or just spending some time in a setting where it is "OK" to not always be "together" or functioning adaptively. Depending on the group population I am working with, I may not have one group that offers all of the above possibilities. A group of chronic mental health inpatients will be very different from an outpatient support group for new mothers or a staff group formed to complete a quality assurance project. The quality assurance group members, for example, may look forward to learning more about creative problem-solving, something that each member could not experience as richly if trying to do this as an individual.

As the leader attempts to have members talk about their expectations and needs for group, he or she may begin with some nonthreatening introductory exercises that will help the members feel more comfortable with each other. This may be as simple as brief introductions of a demographic nature or a more extensive activity that is experiential in nature. The purposes, precautions, and types of experiential exercises will be discussed in Chapter Nine. I always tell the group about myself and encourage questions from the members if they have concerns about my credentials. Since, in the initial stage of group development, the leader is seen as omniscient, questions to the leader about credentials are probably covert expressions of fear about the "OK-ness" of each other. Chapter Seven presents data on the group themes and the issues most likely to be seen in each stage of development. Sometimes, the leader needs to prompt the group by suggesting that he or she expects that the members will have concerns and that one of these might be how the group will benefit each of them personally. This gives the members permission to have doubts.

If a group has members who have had previous group experiences, these seasoned individuals may be a source of validation about what group is really like. Some experienced members may know how to initiate discussion around these issues. This is a place where the members can begin to share leadership interventions with the designated leader. In the new position I recently accepted, I attend a multidisciplinary staff meeting once a week in which the purpose for the meeting has only vaguely been defined to me. In talking with some other staff after a meeting, I found that the seasoned staff is just as fuzzy about what should happen in our "group" meeting.

As someone who facilitates groups, I know how to focus a group on an issue. If I choose to present my concern about the purpose for our meeting, I will be modeling this behavior for other staff members. I am making a leadership intervention since I am facilitating a discussion of group goals. The group leader should look for opportunities to have members offer interventions to facilitate the group's growth.

3) Reinforcing the Acceptance of Each Member. Being sure that each member is allowed to be heard in the group gives the message of caring and acceptance. In acknowledging each person's right to speak and in letting the member know that he has been heard, the leader is giving the feedback that a message sent by a member has been received by the group leader. Recall that one principle of communications is to not acknowledge with understanding a message that is unclear. It may be difficult for the group leader to also agree with a message that is not part of his or her belief system. However, it is important to let members know that their communications are seen as something they wish to share with the group and that the group has a responsibility to do something with each message. Sometimes, a message is disruptive, off the subject, or an attempt to avoid an important issue. The fact, however, that the person has communicated this is important. The decision about what to do with the message is more complicated. The nurse leader may give the person some feedback about her message, ask individual members to respond to it, or make it a group issue for problem-solving. Throughout the book, we will deal with specific problem issues that occur in a group. It is important for the reader to understand the need for the group leader to "hear" group members from the onset of the group's meetings. Inclusion or acceptance is of primary importance in this initial stage of group development.

4) Maintaining a Directive, Verbal Role. Initially, the leader, as the expert, is placed by the group in the role of being more verbal and directive. In a new situation, having someone take control is generally comforting and anxiety reducing. With certain client populations, a more directive or structured approach may be necessary throughout the life of the group. Children, adolescents, and chronic mental health clients are all groups of people that function best in a group where the leader gives the members a significant amount of direction. Sometimes, the clients will ask the leader for more control if they are feeling at a loss. This can be in the form of a verbal request: "What are we supposed to do in this group?" Nonverbally, the group members may ask for more direction by becoming agitated or restless, becoming physically disruptive (most often seen in children, adolescents, or the client with less ego controls), or seeking attention in various ways, thereby forcing the leader into action. Occasionally, a group member will express anxiety with a latent message hidden in a seemingly innocuous remark, *e.g.,* "I get really upset with my mother's doctor. He won't tell me what to do when she starts having that shaking. How am I supposed to handle that? I've never been in this position before."

This statement, coming from a member in a support group whose mother has cancer, can be looked at from a content level or from the latent level which might mean, "You expect us to know what to do in this group. I've never been in a group before. I'm feeling really helpless." If I were the group leader, I would help her problem-solve about how she could approach her mother's doctor. We might roleplay some assertive responses. Since this is a support group, I would not have permission to explore her personal process that resulted in this maladaptive interaction. She may have difficulty dealing with authority figures or may feel some ambivalence towards her mother. The possibilities are endless, but my contract with her would be to provide assistance in coping. It is in a psychotherapy group that I would focus on her personal process and make the actual handling of the situation secondary. In the support group, after we had dealt with the immediate situation, I would ask her what feelings the situation had engendered for her and if she were having any similar feelings about being in the group.

In the initial stage of group development, the leader should consider sharing the following with the group:

1) what the members can expect from the leader
2) what members can do to let the leader know their concerns
3) what the leader's general style of doing group is like
4) how the individual's needs mesh with the group's needs (This may have been discussed in a pregroup interview.)
5) how the norms for the group are to be established
6) what expectations the leader has for the group's work

The above are just a sampling of specifics the leader might want to convey to the group. The type of group will affect the kind of discussion occurring between the leader and members. The psychotherapy group leader usually allows more anxiety to exist in the beginning stage of group, because this anxiety is helpful to the process of having the members feel a need to explore their relationships with each other and the group leader. A supportive group leader is often working with members who are new to the group process and whose anxiety is high due to the situation which has brought them to the group. In the crisis group format, the time-limited structure and specific problem-solving mode demand the leader be directive throughout the group's life, with the initial directions and guidance to the members being particularly important. A person in crisis has narrowed perception and has exhausted familiar coping mechanisms. Therefore, a member of a crisis group comes with the anxiety of being in crisis as well as the anxiety of joining a group.

5) Limiting Self-Disclosure to Reduce the Anxiety Level. We will be talking about self-disclosure by both the leader and the group members as it develops in each stage of the group's life. Self-disclosure is the process of sharing honestly and spontaneously one's thoughts and feelings. It is dropping one's facade and being an authentic person or being perceived by others as the individual knows himself to be (Jourard, 1971). The goal of psychotherapy is increased self-awareness followed by change resulting from disclosing oneself to the therapist. In group psychotherapy, clients understand that self-disclosure is expected. However, the client still has control of how much he lets others outside of group know him, thus regulating his social image until he is ready for the development of closer relationships in which self-disclosure is necessary (Jourard, 1971). Although the amount of self-disclosure varies according to the purpose of the group, a certain amount occurs in most groups. Of those groups which we discussed in Chapter Five, the task group is probably the only group that demands little self-disclosure.

In the initial stage, the leader sets the tone for the amount of self-disclosure that will become the norm within the group. Yalom (1975), whose focus is the psychotherapy group, saw self-disclosure as a necessary part of the group's work, being a prerequisite for meaningful interpersonal relationships and the process that would most often hook a client into committing herself to working in a group. He cautioned that too much self-disclosure early in a group would often scare other members not yet ready to be so revealing. The member self-disclosing might feel ashamed or regret his disclosure if it were done too early or done to excess.

One of the ways the leader can limit the amount of disclosure early in the group is to be more directive and specific with those norms in which the group members have little input. One of these would be the norm about self-disclosing. As a leader, the nurse might share with the group initially that it may seem hard for members to talk about themselves or share personal concerns with the group. The leader can set the tone for less personal disclosure in the first stage by suggesting that members share a little about themselves that others routinely would know about them but that the group would not, *i.e.,* demographic data. This is helpful in a group where the members are not going to be in therapy but may be needing some emotional support, shoring of defense and coping mechanisms, or will be focusing more on problem-solving or didactic learning. If a member did begin to self-disclose prematurely, it is important for the leader to acknowledge the member's statement and her need to share with the group but also the concern about whether the group would be able to help her at that time. The group leader might suggest some alternative ways for her to deal with the problem and reinforce her desire to disclose as being appropriate later in the group. For the good of the group, self-disclosure needs to be kept at a minimum in the initial stage.

The Middle Stage: Working

Characteristics

Depending on what group dynamics theory one reads, the middle stage of group development has two or more different labels. However, the important processes of this stage are the development of cohesion, the exertion of power and control by various group members, the development of some intimacy between members, the formation of subgroups, and the initiation of the real work of the group (Webster, *et al.,* 1982; Janosik, 1982; Callahan, *et al.,* 1980). This stage shows much activity, much conflict, and a movement toward the group's goals. Each of the characteristics mentioned above will be discussed in detail.

Probably, the most outstanding characteristic of this stage is the existence of conflict within the group. Some of this conflict is directed initially at the leader. Direct anger towards the leader is readily observed. Disguised anger might manifest itself with such behaviors as: bypassing the identified leader by asking certain members to deal with issues the leader would normally handle, talking about "staff" or health professionals in a derogatory manner, and complaining about the way the group is going. The leader is a safer target since she is supposed to be secure in her role, and there is more social distance between the leader and members than among the members. Recall the importance of the affiliation need members have at the onset of group. To be accepted by one's peers is very important. It is, therefore, much better to risk alienating the leader than the members. Generally, anger towards the leader results from unmet expectations about the group. The leader is not allowing the members to be dependent on her, nor is she giving members all the answers to their many questions of how the group works to help them change as individuals or to accomplish the task the group needs to do. Realizing the leader is not a superhuman person the members thought she was adds to the members' disappoint- ment and anger. Yalom (1975) noted that it is important for the leader to differen- tiate between attacks on his person or on his role as the leader. It is important for the leader to allow these attacks on his role to occur and to withstand them, showing the group that hostility can be expressed without destroying those involved. That does not mean that the leader shows no reaction or feelings with such attacks. Letting the group see what their behavior does to others is important learning. It also helps to see the leader as someone with emotions like themselves. If the leader experiences hostility directed towards the individual as a person, there may be some transference or countertransference occurring. The specifics for dealing with this phenomena are discussed in a later chapter. Sometimes, the leader needs to draw out the anger which is probably intended for him but ends up being displaced onto some outside source, such as another system interfacing with the client's care. Some members, instead of getting angry with the leader, will side with him against the more powerful members in the group (Yalom, 1975). If I sense that a group member should be directing some appropriate anger towards me, I will make a comment, such as, "I'd really be angry with me if I were you right now. I've been pushing you pretty hard."

Power or control is a need that the members have, according to Schutz (see first part of chapter) and can also be expressed as anger towards each other. The sources of conflict are too numerous to list, but they may be coming from a member's inter- nal process, *e.g.*, parataxic distortion, a sense of not being "OK" with oneself or others, and so forth, or from one's external environment, such as the deviant behavior of another group member or the frustration of the group time being shortened. There are certain times when conflict is very healthy, as in the exchange of differences of opinion which is giving the group some new perspectives on an issue. The leader must decide when to allow conflict to continue or when to stop conflict if it is being destruc- tive. In the section on leadership interventions, the decision to allow or to stop con- flict will be discussed.

One of the expressions of power within the group is the formation of subgroups. This does not occur until the middle stage when the members are feeling more chal- lenging toward the leader and when there is some intimacy felt between members. The nature of the subgroup has already been discussed. Although subgroups are in- evitable and do signal a new closer alignment among members, which is necessary if the group is to develop, subgroup formation can be devisive to a group.

Intimacy has been identified as one of the needs Schutz said existed for members. Often, a feeling of intimacy first comes to the group after there has been some per- sonal self-disclosure. Another source of intimacy is conflict resolution in which anger has been expressed between members, but the differences have been worked through, and each member has a new understanding or insight into how the other feels. Recall that intimacy needs are met in both the middle and final group stages. The intimacy expressed in the middle stage results more from conflict resolution than from the authenticity that evolves after personal self-disclosure.

Cohesion is closely tied with the phenomena of intimacy and subgrouping. Cart- wright and Zander (1960) defined cohesiveness as the phenomenon of attraction to the group. The group may meet the needs of the individual member, or the group may be a means for helping the individual to meet those needs outside of the group. Attraction increases as members find an atmosphere of cooperation rather than competitiveness. If one has unpleasant experiences in relating to group members, the attraction to the group decreases. In contrast to this, if group tasks are satisfying, and if goals are achieved in the group that cannot be achieved alone by the individual, cohesion remains high in the group. There is a high level of interaction, decision-making, and conflict resolution in a cohesive group (Callahan, *et al.*, 1980). It is interesting that attraction leads not only to intimacy among members but to subgroup formation. Certain members are seen as more capable of meeting their needs, and so a new group is formed (Cartwright and Zander, 1960). Yalom (1975) noted that cohesiveness leads to increased acceptance, intimacy, and understanding for the members as well as to the conditions that further the expression of hostility and conflict. In a cohesive group, the members are able to handle the discomfort of working through the conflict; *i.e.*, conflict resolution is important.

Work for a group may be many different activities and processes, among them the process of conflict resolution, self-disclosure, goal-directed activities, and a high level of interaction. Since cohesion brings members together and imparts a sense of a common goal for which the group is working to meet the members' needs, the middle stage of group is sometimes called the working stage. Depending on the group's purpose for existing, some of the characteristics just noted may not be present in every group which is working. A support group attempts to reduce the amount of anxiety and tension the members feel. For this reason, there would be less focus on conflict, less reason to deal with conflict resolution, and more focus on how the group members could meet each other's needs through supportive feedback and healthy subgrouping as needed. Certainly, negative feedback and conflict could occur in a support group, and the leader would attempt to resolve this in a positve manner through conflict resolution. In a psychotherapy group, the leader chooses to highlight conflict and encourages the expression of negative feelings. In a support group, the focus is on defending against anxiety rather than creating anxiety to further self-awareness. The task group encourages a high level of interaction around goal-seeking behaviors during the working stage. The cohesion that exists due to the interest members have in carrying out a task to meet their needs increases goal-directed behaviors. It is important to differentiate between the expected work activities of different types of groups in order to identify accurately the stage of their development.

Leadership Functions

Emotional stimulation by the group leader allows the group to grow as a unit towards goal achievement and provides the atmosphere necessary for individual growth. The leader's confrontation, self-disclosure, and challenging behaviors all stimulate growth. The leader in a task group might use confrontation to prod the members towards higher task achievement; whereas, confrontation in a psychotherapy group is usually of a more personal nature, such as questioning a member's denial of feelings.

Meaning attribution is a function that helps members evaluate their progress towards individual goals by giving meaning to the experiences members are having in the group and to the movement of the group as a whole. In a support group, this may happen when the leader helps interpret a situation that a member is trying to handle. The feelings the member has around seeing a significant other dying of cancer are related to the coping style the member is using, for example. The leader in a task group might examine why a member is having difficulty with a portion of the task. In a psychotherapy group, the focus is on interpreting the process occurring between members and the behavioral changes members are experiencing.

Leadership Interventions

The leadership interventions that the leader or group members make center around the process of conflict and its resolution, the reinforcement of cohesiveness within the group, the use of self-disclosure to promote intimacy, and the resistances to working. The following interventions are those which are most likely to deal with these issues.

1) Allowing Conflict and Anxiety to Exist in the Context of Adaptive Group Work. It may be hard for the group to tolerate conflict and anxiety for the sake of growth for individuals of the group as a whole. Consequently, some members may try to influence the group to avoid conflict and the anxiety that comes from self-disclosing or taking risks to try out new behaviors in the group. Some of the clues that this might be going on include: 1) the members deny the existence of any negative feelings; 2) members are unusually silent or the group has a low verbal output, especially when this has not been the normal occurrence; 3) the group or its members are unusually compliant and polite; and 4) the group interactions are superficial in content.

Individual members attempting to control the anxiety or conflict might distract the group from a conflict-loaded issue, might steer the group to another subject less anxiety-producing, or might monopolize the group's time with an innocuous problem. One of the interventions the leader might use to focus some of the group's attention to the real issues is to make some process comments. Recall that process has to do with the developing relationship between the members or between the leader and the members. It may be anything not considered content and includes all the nonverbal behaviors one observes. Very often, members who have been in many groups catch on to what process is all about and can make some appropriate comments. The following might be helpful to get the group focused back on the anxiety or conflict going on:

"I'm puzzled by the sudden silence. I wonder what everyone is keeping inside?"

"It seems strange to me that a group of people who know each other as we do have no differences of opinion."

"Sometimes I use laughter to cover up those feelings that are really hard to express. Is that happening here?"

"People look really tight. I guess I don't feel that things are OK today in the group."

The leader needs to decide when it is important to allow conflict to go unchecked; that is, when the development of a conflictual relationship will eventually lead to resolution and growth for the individuals and, perhaps, the whole group. Yalom (1975) cautioned against allowing the unrestrained expression of vengeful anger to occur in the group, but he noted that two people in a conflict with each other are generally expressing the seriousness and importance of their relationship. As long as the parties are exchanging views and attempting to understand the other person's point of view, conflict is healthy. It is often a generator of new ideas or perspectives on a subject and may allow the persons involved to express parts of themselves that others have not seen. Conflict may be resolved with fair-fight techniques, with roleplaying and switching roles, with negotiation, with compromise, or with an understanding that it is acceptable to not agree on certain points and still maintain a relationship. Chapter Eight will deal with conflict resolution. Conflict becomes detrimental when one party is uncaring for the other or the other's point of view, when conflict gets out of control, or when it is obvious that the intent is to destroy the other person. When conflict in a group leads to the group choosing up sides, the issue probably cannot be dealt with in an adaptive way. If members are unwilling to deal with conflict I find it is not helpful to force them.

Anxiety was discussed at length in the section on the initial stage. As the group members become more comfortable with the group and with their roles, they may tolerate more uncertainties within the group. If the leader is late, if she does not give the group an answer to a particular question, or if there are problems in getting the group task done, the anxiety resulting from these occurrences is not overwhelming for the members. The tension created by conflict frequently moves the group towards conflict resolution. In the psychotherapy group, the leader may purposely create some anxiety as a way of moving the group into the process of dealing with it.

2) Monitoring Process and Content. Content and process have been referred to as the "warp and woof of group interaction" (Phipps, 1982, p.160). The association between content and process is an important one. The content is all the conversation that goes on in the group taken in its denotative or literal meaning. Nothing about the content is hidden from the observer's view. The process, however, as described earlier, is everything other than the content that defines the relationship between the members in the group. Much of the process is detected through close observation of the nonverbal behaviors that accompany the content. Often, the content may contain some connotative meanings that would help delineate the process. As the leader "listens" for process by observing the exchange of content messages or the lack of any verbal exchanges, she is asking herself questions to help determine the process occurring. Questions about process relate to why a member is speaking at a certain time, why particular nonverbal behaviors are occurring, what the content has to do with the nonverbal, the timing of particular content presented or issues discussed, what is not being said, and so forth. The following questions are examples of one leader's search for process in a particular group:

- Why did John turn his back on the group after he spoke?
- Why is it that Mary interrupts the male members of the group each time anyone of them talks about relationship problems?
- How does Brett's silence relate to his very verbal behavior of last group?
- How come the group is focusing on issues that cannot be solved during the time we meet together?

Group members may learn to pick up on some process and may make appropriate process comments in the group. The leader, once she has determined what process is occurring, must then decide what to do about those observations. Process relates to the group as a whole or to what is happening with individual members. Therefore, the leader would be looking for group themes or for individual themes, identifying the group's or the member's needs, fears, and so forth. Whether the leader chooses to do anything about the individual or group themes she identifies often depends on the readiness of the individual or group to deal with this information and on the type of group and purpose for its existence. A psychotherapy group would be ripe for such process work, since this is the core of its existence. The support group would probably focus on general group themes at times but not on a lot of individual process to the depth of the psychotherapy group. The task group leader would ignore process unless it was interfering with the task. Identifying resistances to working would be an appropriate theme for the task group to consider. The leader will often verbalize process that culminates in an issue for the group as a whole. The question of leadership, of confidentiality, of trust, and so forth, are all possible group issues. Chapter Seven continues this discussion on group issues and themes as well as individual themes.

3) Reinforcing Commonalities of Individual Concerns and Needs. As the group leader or members are stating issues important to the group or to particular members, they are looking for areas of mutual concern on which the group might focus. The attraction to a group, or the group's cohesiveness, depends on the ability of the group to be an object of need or a way for individuals to satisfy needs related to their life outside of the group (Cartwright and Zander, 1960). It is especially important during times when the cohesiveness in the group is at a lower level that some commonalities of issues be identified. Members who are interested in group maintenance functions, or in helping the group maintain harmonious interpersonal interactions and working relationships, will work on identifying common issues to draw the members together. Optimal group productivity occurs in a highly cohesive group (Callahan, *et al.,* 1980).

4) Modeling and Reinforcing Adaptive Self-Disclosure. It is in the working stage that the leader may allow and encourage more self-disclosure. Jourard (1971) identified those factors most important in determining the degree of self-disclosure: the identity of the person to whom one might disclose oneself, the nature and purpose of the relationship between the people self-disclosing, and the perception of the person to whom one is self-disclosing as to the degree of caring and willingness to reciprocate with the same level of self-disclosure.

Personal self-disclosure is frequently modeled by the group leader. Some examples include the following statements:

"One of the things that really bothers me is not getting feedback from you. I need to know what you are feeling about group, and I'm uncomfortable if I don't hear from you. I suppose it's really important to me to know if I'm making sense to you."

"I've experienced sadness with the death of someone close to me. I felt pretty helpless for awhile. That might be similar to what you're feeling."

"One of my pet peeves is irresponsibility. If I jump on you for that, it's because I think it's important, but I also get angry at irresponsible people so I may not be totally objective."

"I sometimes find it hard to accept compliments. That's something I'm still working on for myself."

Yalom (1975) cautioned the therapist to not self-disclose anything that would be detrimental to the group's work, such as one's favorite members or an impatience with a particular group, and so forth. I have shared with groups my distress at their not being able to work or at the lack of progress the group has made. I have also told particular groups how much I enjoyed them because of the closeness I have found with them. This latter feedback was after the group was over and was to a group of students who had good ego strengths. I feel that the group members are going to sense when I am unhappy with them as a group, and I cannot avoid saying outloud what I feel when this happens. This does not entirely agree with Yalom's advice. I "wear my feelings on my sleeve," as the saying goes, and handle my personal process by sharing it with the group if I feel it is at all obvious. This is my way of doing the best with some of those parts of me that may not be as helpful in my role as therapist/leader but which I like as part of my humanness. In my work with clients who have more fragile egos, I am more careful about how much I self-disclose. I do not necessarily promote self-disclosure by modeling it, but by my modeling I am giving those that are comfortable or willing to take the risk permission to self-disclose. If it is real important to a group's work to have the members self-disclose, I may use an experiential exercise to facilitate this happening. In Chapter Nine, the reader will find examples of this type of exercise.

When I am the leader of a task group, I find it helpful to self-disclose when I see the interaction I am having with a group member is interfering with the accomplishment of the group goals. Generally, such interference is around a misunderstanding. Self-disclosure by the leader in a task group should be limited to that which is needed to facilitate understanding between the leader and members or between members that would help the group perform their task better.

The material being discussed in a support group lends itself to self-disclosure. The goal for self-disclosure in a support group is to release pent-up emotions as a way of coping with stress and to share those feelings to which others may be able to relate, thus facilitating the group's understanding of the particular life situation with which the group is attempting to deal. No intervention is made by the leader to delve into someone's process for intimate material that might promote insight. If a group member comes to some personal "ahas" about his or her process from an experience in a support group, this is a fringe benefit. The leader should, therefore, limit self-disclosure that becomes so personal that it takes the group away from its focus on the life situation experiences common to all. For example, in a group for parents of developmentally disabled children, the nurse leader would not allow a parent to discuss the dynamics of her extramarital affair. If she chose to share with the group that this occurred in a previous marriage after the birth of her disabled child as a way of pointing out the stressors in such a situation, this would be appropriate. The result of this affair on her current relationships and her self-esteem would probably not be helpful to the group. It is up to the group leader to use judgment in deciding when to limit self-disclosure.

The Final Stage: Termination

Characteristics

The final stage of group development continues with the cohesion, increased trust, and the self-disclosure that occurred in the middle stage. It is of prime importance that the leader help the group wind down from the work that has occurred earlier. If the group or an individual member has new issues that were not dealt with before, this is not the time to bring them up. Old issues need time to be finished or as resolved as possible. Recall that the need for affection is uppermost with members during the latter part of the middle stage and in the final stage of the group's life. Those members that have chosen to want closeness rather than distance will need to begin to separate and terminate in this stage. Those that maintained distance will not have as much work to do now. The work of the final stage is termination accomplished by self-disclosure around any left-over feelings, evaluation of what the group experience has meant for the individual, and formulation of how the member has fared as part of a group and what that means in his or her life away from the group which will no longer exist.

Termination in a group is not unlike the termination process between an individual client and the nurse. With both processes, those involved attempt to evaluate the learning that has taken place. The termination phase of the nurse/client relationship is considered one where much may have been learned (McCann, 1979). Such learning includes the affective experience of identifying what the relationship has left each person with regard to memories, level of trust, and feelings of closeness. The increase in the level of anxiety in both the nurse and the client during termination may make them both more receptive to learning. Some of the regression that occurs with individual clients or in a group demonstrates the presence of such anxiety and a need to regress, therefore, to more familiar patterns of behavior. Learning takes place when the client can see that life is filled with the beginning and ending of relationships. As the two exchange shared memories and the feelings they have around these, pain becomes a normal process that the client can begin to accept (McCann, 1979). The termination stage in a psychotherapy group would most likely be very affectively laden because of the focus on affective material throughout the life of the group. A support group might also find the focus to be on feelings and the evaluation of the group according to whether one is feeling better, *i.e.,* more supported, as a result of the group experience.

The leaders of a support group for staff identified a period of differentiation during the end of the middle stage of group and moving into the final stage (Webster, *et al.,* 1982). Here, the group was less dependent on the leaders for support and they were very protective of each other to the point of resisting adding new members even though it was an open group for staff. Since it was a group with persons having good ego strength, the members were able to assume most of the leadership for the group as they began trying to transfer their group experiences to situations that were occurring on the unit. In the last phase, they moved into termination and handled this by regressing some. Once more, they became dependent on the group leaders to be active in the group. To separate, they developed more interests outside the group and devalued the group experience, thus making it less traumatic to leave it.

Not all groups will treat termination the same way. As we discuss the leadership interventions that occur in this stage, we will look at how these interventions might differ from group to group. Some groups will need a longer time for termination than others. In some groups, the process of termination may not be very obvious. The overriding characteristics of this final stage are disengagement in some form and dissolution of the group. Emotions of sadness, some anger towards the leader, and various behaviors to deal with the end of the group, such as denial and evasion, occur (Janosik, 1982).

Leadership Functions

In looking at the characteristics for this stage, it is obvious that members have to have both an intellectual and an emotional understanding of their group experience. Therefore, meaning attribution and emotional stimulation are the two leadership functions that are most important in this stage. Meaning attribution gives a cognitive understanding to the experiences that the members have had in a group (Lieberman, *et al.,* 1973). The emotional stimulation that is needed during the final stage is not the generation of new feelings but the resolution of existing ones by further self-disclosure to uncover those feelings that never got expressed but affect the unfinished business in the group. As noted above, it is the leader's responsibility to see that no new material is introduced during this stage. I have had to be authoritative at times to hold to this rule. I may suggest an alternative place for the member to deal with a new issue, *e.g.,* with an individual therapist; with a doctor, nurse, or other supportive health professional working with this person; or with a follow-up agency contact with the resources to meet this person's need. Although this is often frustrating to a client, it is probably less frustrating than plunging into a new issue and not being able to resolve it.

Leadership Interventions

The first need is to get unfinished business completed. Self-disclosure at this time needs to be an extension of a previous disclosure or, if a new disclosure, something that will help the member and the group understand a process that has already occurred but has been unclear. The following are examples of self-disclosure needed for closure.

Example 1

Colleen and the group leader have had verbal clashes throughout the group's life. It is still unclear to Jean, the group leader, what it is that Colleen and she do that causes them to disagree over very minor points. The group is a task group and has been working on revising the statement of philosophy for the nursing service. Colleen has not liked the wording of some of the statements and challenges Jean's expertise in grammar. Jean tends to become irritated because it has caused what she feels are unnecessary delays in task accomplishment. Various members have seen both points of view, but there seems to be an unusual amount of emotion coming from Jean and Colleen. Since this is a task group, it is not appropriate to explore any parataxic distortion or personality characteristics that might be occurring between them. Jean has decided to model some disclosure that might help finish the difficult interactions between her and Colleen.

"I feel sad, Colleen, that we have been clashing so much in this group. I'm confused about why this has happened, and I feel unable to explore what is causing it, but I wanted to let you know that I don't feel good about it happening. Perhaps we can agree that we disagreed in this group, realizing that maybe we're two people that cannot work together effectively or comfortably."

Example 2

In a support group for clients with terminal cancer, David, the group leader, needs to help Julie feel finished with the coping style she has been using in the group that seems helpful for her right now but has been misunderstood by the other group members. Julie is close to dying and is at peace with this stage of her illness, but her family is not. She has been distancing herself from family as she prepares to die and is being supported in these behaviors by the health professionals that care for her daily. However, many of the group members are not liking Julie's withdrawal, since she has been a very active member in the past and had verbalized extensively in the group. They are feeling her loss, but are not able to connect this emotionally to all the mixed feelings they have about their own situation and about the group. David has decided that the group needs some closure around this issue. Although this is an open-ended group which does not terminate as a whole, Julie is terminating with the group.

"I'm wondering if what some of us have been feeling with your quietness, Julie, is what some families are feeling about several of you as you take more time to reflect on your life and do some of the things you need to do in feeling OK about facing your cancer. Julie, I miss your input in the group because it has been real helpful to me to get to know you better as a person and to see you giving gifts to others here in the group with your insights. I understand your quietness, but I'm sad about it. You've helped me understand something about facing pain, and I really appreciate that. Perhaps some of the rest of you have been thinking about what Julie has done to make this group helpful for you and would be willing to tell her this now. I feel we need to allow you to be quiet if you want to be, Julie. I understand that is what you are doing with your family also, but I wanted to give other group members a chance to talk about this for a few minutes."

The group leader did some modeling in these two examples of the kind of self-disclosing statements that are appropriate at this stage of the group. In both examples, the group leader also modeled "saying good-bye."

The other important set of interventions in this stage helps the group members evaluate their experiences. The leader might model this process by sharing with the group what the experience has meant for him. I have frequently told groups what the experience of leading has done for me. As an elective for the students in my mental health practicum and for other nursing students who wanted to work on their personal process, I offered a group for this purpose. The group was a joy for me to do because I got to know the students better while doing the clinical practice that my heavy teaching load had kept me from doing as much of as I had wanted. I shared all this with the students as we were terminating. I find this type of self-disclosure useful. I think of it as a gift to the group so that they may know what the experience has given me. "Self-disclosure begets self-disclosure" as Jourard said (1971, p.142). In the final stage of the group, this type of self-disclosure is appropriate and can have a snowballing effect on the rest of the members. Anyone who wishes may also continue with other interventions that allow the members to identify specific goals that were reached by the group as a whole or by individual members. A task group will look more at collective group accomplishments, while the psychotherapy group would concentrate almost exclusively on individual member growth within the group experience. For example, a member might acknowledge more ease with handling anger directed at her. Her evaluation of this would be related to how she felt, but it would be in the context of what happened in the group to get her to this point.

As part of the evaluation, members need to see how their learning in group transfers to their outside interactional experiences. The leader might ask members to identify how they will use a certain piece of insight or process that occurred in the group in outside relationships. Although this transference of learning should be going on from the beginning of "aha" experiences in group, it is good to have members make a final summary of this knowledge transfer. Special exercises, such as constructing a time line of one's life at the beginning of a group experience and then at termination will point out to the member how he is seeing his life differently.

Finally, follow-up for future growth is important for individual members. Specific referrals may be made to individual therapists, health service agencies, self-help groups, and so forth. Sometimes members can do all this "discharge planning" for themselves as part of their learning. If the group is open-ended so that members are leaving all the time, one or two at a time, the process the member goes through to prepare for follow-up is a good teaching tool for the rest of the group.

The Overlapping of Stages

Specific processes may signal the movement from one stage of group development to another, but that does not mean that there is a clear break from one stage to the other and never any overlap. One may think of the stages of group development much like Erikson's eight stages of psychosocial development. Even though my daughter is now fourteen and definitely struggling with her ego identity by the importance she places on her image in the eyes of her peers, she surprises me sometimes by really missing her father when he is away and by wanting hugs and kisses from us. Usually, the adolescent is shying away from such open affection from his or her parents. The same is true of the group's development. Although, as soon as some cohesion and trust develops within the group, one sees more self-disclosure, the group may become anxious and less open again: if a new member joins, if the leader is late and disappoints the group, or if some members are not quite as sure of their level of commitment to the group, and so forth. Sometimes growth groups will spend several sessions in small talk and then have some very good self-disclosure occur. However, in the next meeting, the group is back into small talk. Although I know this occurs routinely in groups, I am always newly amazed when it happens. Groups that are terminating may come to an impasse in resolving some old unfinished business, although prior to this difficulty they had been doing excellent conflict resolution. It is the norm to see groups vacillate between stages.

The group leader cannot move a group into another stage before it is ready. I tried to push some of my student groups through the stages of group development during their clinical practicums to acquaint them with this experience. I could determine what stage they were in, and because of the pressure of time, I decided to try and hurry them along. This was not successful, but I did use the outcome, of the students being upset with me, to teach them about how groups operate. We looked at the process and examined what kept the group from moving. All groups will go through the three stages, but depending on the mix of individual members and the process they create with each other, some groups will move more slowly than others. One of my groups of students was very quiet, made up of persons who did not do a lot of verbalizing in the group with each other. Consequently, the group remained in the initial stage for a much longer time. If specific experiential exercises designed to facilitate trust, self-disclosure, or other processes are introduced at the right time, when the group is ready to move into that process, they are quite successful in facilitating the group's movement. However, an exercise that is not synchronized with the readiness for the group's movement often produces uncomfortable results for the group. We will talk more about timing of such exercises in Chapter Nine.

Specific process events can be cited to signify the movement from one stage to another. The end of pleasantries and denial of conflict with one or more members disagreeing or confronting one another or the leader could signify the movement from the initial stage to the middle stage. Likewise, the group's concern for individual members demonstrated by one or more members facilitating another member's resolution of a conflict rather than the leader needing to do this could signal movement into the group's final stage. The group moves at its own pace, but the leader monitors the group's process to identify the stages of development. In the next chapter, we will look at how the group defines itself as it develops into an entity of its own.

REFERENCES

Abbott, M. "Parenting Group for Teen-Agers Fails," *Pediatric Nursing*, 6, no. 5 (Sept./Oct., 1980), 54–56.

Callahan, J., S. Fertig, P.A. O'Dell, and B. Marlowe, "Processing a Task Group: A Continuing Education Committee at Work Planning a Conference," *Journal of Continuing Education*, 11, no. 5 (Sept./Oct., 1980), 8–15.

Cartwright, D. and A. Zander, eds. *Group Dynamics: Research and Theory* (2nd ed.). Evanston, IL: Row Peterson and Co., 1960.

Janosik, E. "Aspects of Group Development: Stages and Levels," in *Life Cycle Group Work in Nursing*, eds. E. Janosik and L. Phipps. Monterey, CA: Wadsworth Health Science Division, 1982.

Johnson, M. "Support Groups for Parents of Chronically Ill Children," *Pediatric Nursing*, 8, no. 3 (May/June, 1982), 160–163.

Jourard, S. *The Transparent Self* (revised ed.). New York: D. Van Nostrand Co., 1971.

Lieberman, M., I. Yalom, and M. Miles. *Encounter Groups: First Facts*. New York: Basic Books, Inc., 1973.

Loomis, M. *Group Process for Nurses*. St. Louis: C.V. Mosby, 1979.

McCann, J. "Termination of the Psychotherapeutic Relationship," *Journal of Psychiatric Nursing and Mental Health Services*, 17, no. 10 (Oct., 1979), 37–39, 45–46.

Phipps, L. "Group Dynamics: Leadership Roles and Functions," in *Life Cycle Group Work in Nursing*, eds. E. Janosik and L. Phipps. Monterey, CA: Wadsworth Health Sciences Division, 1982.

Schutz, W. "Interpersonal Underworld," *Harvard Business Review*, 36 (1958), 123–135.

Webster, S., L. Kelly, B. Johst, R. Weber, and L. Wickes, "The Support Group: A Method of Stress Management," *Nursing Management*, 13, no. 9 (Sept., 1982), 26–30.

Yalom, I. *The Theory and Practice of Group Psychotherapy* (2nd ed.). New York: Basic Books, Inc., 1975.

The Group Emotion: Issues and Themes 7

As an extension of the content presented in the last chapter on the movement of the group, this chapter will focus on the meaning that movement has for the group and its members. The behaviors characteristic of each stage of group development express the needs, wishes, and fears of individual members and of the group as an entity. It is through the leadership functions of emotional stimulation and meaning attribution that the group and its members gain some understanding of what their behaviors mean and how this can be translated into changes and growth for each of them as individuals. Process is the "meat" of any changing that can occur with the individual member. As the leader(s) learn to use process to then facilitate more process or "events" within the group, a therapeutically sound plan develops for the growth of the individual. Group process is a good modality for change, because it multiplies thousands of times over the amount of data one has to work with in human interactions to help the individual understand and begin to change parts of the self. For that reason, group may be as intense or growth-enhancing as individual contact with a counselor/therapist.

In this chapter, we will look at group issues and themes. Issues are more readily observable and identified within the group than group themes. Therefore, we will define these first and then proceed to uncover the more esoteric processes that occur in the group. The issues are those needs or concerns which the individual members as well as the leader want to have the group focus on in order to assure that the group's work gets done. Issues may be task-related or maintenance-related. Task functions have been defined previously (Chapter Five). Maintenance functions are necessary for the maintaining or perpetuation of the group (Wilson and Kneisl, 1979). They have to do with the relationships between the group members which develop during the accomplishment of the group task. Dealing with group conflict, with subgrouping, and with termination feelings are all part of the maintenance functions. In a task group, the maintenance functions exist primarily in order that the task may be accomplished. In a therapy group, the task is to study the developing interactions in the group as to how this relates to the individual member's process. Thus, the maintenance functions would be interwoven within the group task. Just as members may perform some of the task functions, so may members perform maintenance functions (Cartwright and Zander, 1960). Members learn maintenance functions by watching the leader model maintenance behaviors. If a new member joins the group, another member might use an intervention with the new individual that the leader used earlier to help the original members feel more comfortable. He might introduce himself and share some demographic material with the new person. Although overall responsibility for maintenance functions rests with the leader, members comfortable in this role or desiring to grow in their interactional skills will take on such functions. Issues related to the maintenance functions would include the question of trust and confidentiality, safety for risk-taking or self-disclosure, conflict management or resolution, and so forth.

Themes are a little more nebulous to define. Many authors use the two words, "issue" and "theme," interchangeably when talking about the process that occurs in the group. The themes of a group seem to correspond with the various stages of group development and often help define the processes occurring that are indicative of certain developmental issues. For example, a developmental issue that both the members and the leader are concerned about in the middle stage is the handling of conflict within the group. That is a maintenance issue. An individual member theme might be a fear the individual has of losing control of her anger, while a group theme might be the group's desire to overthrow the leader. This covert theme may be expressed in the group by a more overt verbalization of anger at the staff or the system or some other external event that the group may more safely talk about. The individual would express her fear by being very restrained in interactions that are likely to lead to conflict and might attempt to refocus the group on other issues or withdraw or leave the group during moments of expressed hostility.

In the preceding paragraphs, several concepts were introduced rather quickly. We have talked about issues, both those related to the task and those related to the maintenance functions of the group. Generally, task issues are content issues related to the purpose for the group's existence. If the group is a support group for new mothers, issues about mothering might be brought up by both the leader and the members. Thus, the group has both leader issues and member issues. The themes are a more personalized phenomena that express individual secret fears or internal conflicts and processes and collective group fears and processes. Themes may be overt or covert. Overt themes are safer to express and serve to hide covert themes that might be too threatening to verbalize and deal with out loud in the group. Overt themes are also thought to be more acceptable by the group members. The leader must make a decision about making the latent content of covert themes manifest (see Chapter Two). Generally, it is only in psychotherapy groups that much work is done with covert themes, as these require a group contract to deal with such threatening material. The group therapist must make a decision if revealing a covert theme; either that of an individual or of the group would facilitate growth for the members. Latent content containing covert themes is often beyond the awareness of the group leader or only vaguely perceived by him, thereby making it even more unlikely that the material will be made overt. Latent content of covert themes certainly has an influence on the group, since it is a hidden process that is affecting the more obvious processes occurring at the moment. Process, as the reader might be concluding, is multilayered and seemingly endless in its presence. In fact, the amount of data generated by process exceeds the leader's ability to identify and use it all (Phipps, 1982). Although this sounds overwhelming, especially for the novice group leader, I find the idea also very challenging and exciting. It means to me that a group cannot possibly become boring if the leader continually looks for new layers of process. Even if the leader is facilitating a task group in which processing interactional data has very little use to the function and purpose of the group, the leader can still analyze the process within the group for her own learning and growth as a leader. She may need to understand some of the process to make the tasks run more smoothly. She may do something about the process without making it part of the group's awareness. In this chapter, we will look at specific group issues and themes and how they contribute to the process of the group.

Group Issues: Member Issues

Several issues for members relate to their purpose for joining a certain group. If the group happens to be for delinquent adolescents, issues the members might want to consider are: the fact that group membership is mandatory for probation through Juvenile Court, the required behaviors that one must display to get one's probation officer "off his back," control by various adults in one's life, and so forth. Since this is an adolescent group, one of the most significant issues related to the adolescent's development is his identity and how he is expressing this with his delinquent behaviors (Erikson, 1968). Thus, we can assume that underneath these pragmatic issues which the youth might bring to the group are other issues about how to interact with his peers, how to be accepted by others, and what to do about the way he has currently been labeled by society. These issues are more likely to surface later in the group if the adolescent feels safe enough to expose himself.

Each person coming to a group will have needs to be met based on the potential member's idea of what the group's purpose is for being. In a task group to which members are assigned, it might be more difficult for members to relate to the group's goals to the extent that they would have any issues to bring up. If a nurse does not want to participate in writing safety policies for hospital staff, he might address the group with this issue, namely, how does one who is assigned to this group get off the membership list? Other issues could include how resigning from this group would affect one's performance rating by the supervisor; how the group's task relates to his work as a nurse; or how safety policies might benefit his particular unit. Members come to groups with personal issues related to the group's purpose. There are also some universal issues that most members would be interested in with a particular group. If it is a support group, members will be looking for ways to cope with a particular life situation, and will be looking for peers who can share from their experiences in a joint effort to understand the stress they are experiencing. Members joining a self-help group will want to discuss ways of becoming proficient in a particular behavior or set of behaviors.

Safety is a member issue that is especially a concern during the initial stage of group development. Recall that one of the leader's functions in the group is to provide for a safe atmosphere, both in regard to the physical environment as well as in the emotional tone of the interactions between members. This does not mean that the leader guarantees that there will be no conflict in the group or no moments of pain. It is important, however, for the members to know that the leader will help assure that the hurt expressed is dealt with in a caring manner and with confidentiality to the degree that is possible. The members need to know that the group is a place where their emotional needs will be respected and acknowledged as being valid. That does not mean that everything a member says is worthy of spending the group's time or that it will be helpful to the group's work or to the individual's growth. Letting a member try out different communications and behaviors in a psychotherapy group is important. The leader must then decide what limits to set on this as appropriate for the client's and the group's growth. The type of group determines the range of behaviors allowed. For example, if a particular member is having trouble accepting feedback from his peers, that can be disruptive, especially if the group is task-oriented and not designed to deal with interactional conflicts. The leader might work with this person individually or ask him to make a decision about remaining as a member while expressing concern about his need to grow in the area of receiving feedback. The leader needs to protect the group from lost productivity and give the deviant member an opportunity to change behaviors. All these considerations are part of the safety issue of belonging to the group.

Confidentiality, as a part of the safety issue, is not an absolute. Confidentiality should be discussed openly as part of norm formation early in the group. Most often, any group in which members will be self-disclosing has some specifics about the degree of confidentiality to assure a caring, positive experience with the sharing of personal data. I do not agree to blanket confidentiality, because I do not feel I can guarantee that I would not consult with another professional or not share a member's disclosure if it were life-threatening to the person or to someone else. I encourage the group to agree to keep group conversations within the group as a courtesy to each member. If the group does not agree to this, each member knows his or her conversation may be shared by others. As with my unwillingness to assure absolute confidentiality, the members in a group whose peers will not guarantee confidentiality must then decide how much they will share. Certainly, this can have a dampening effect on intimacy.

Closely related to the issue of safety is that of trust and risk-taking. A safe atmosphere promotes trust among one's peers and more willingness to risk self-disclosing, exposing pain, and attempting to change behaviors. Trust is an issue in every group and is part of the developmental work which a group does. The leader can expect to have to deal with this early in the group, and, to a lesser degree, as the group moves into more intimate interactions among the members. Like process, trust is multilayered. It is at many different levels throughout the group's life and also may vary among the individual members in the group. Recall that there may be little trust in one's peers during the initial stage of group with most communications directed towards the leader and with little personal self-disclosure. Trust increases during the working stage where members risk giving negative feedback, getting into conflicts with one another, and becoming more intimate and willing to self-disclose, and so forth. When trust does not exist, it may be an issue. Thus, one would expect the group to talk more about trust during the initial stage of group. Once people are feeling more comfortable with each other in the group, the next layer of trusting is to take risks to self-disclose and make oneself more vulnerable to others. The form this vulnerability takes will depend on the type of group one is in. A task group member will show her vulnerability by risking conflict or disagreement over the group's task. The psychotherapy group considers risk-taking in the area of interpersonal relationships to be the heart of one's work in group. In the support group, members may share some of the negative, scared feelings they are having in trying to deal with a particular life situation. These are examples of the ideal. The group as a whole may show some reluctance to move into this stage of development, or individual members may resist. Generally, the leader deals with the group's resistance by allowing it for awhile as part of the normal developmental cycle and then making the issue part of the group's conscious awareness in order that the group might talk about their reluctance. Sometimes a well-timed experiential technique will help the group take the risk. Sometimes a group will not be very good at allowing risk-taking to occur.

As an issue for individual members, risk-taking/vulnerability may be part of a member's internal set of resistance, or it may just be that a person is slower at moving through the developmental stages. I always allow members to refuse to move or change in group, since I know I cannot change someone who is not ready to change. I will make observations about a member's vulnerability or lack of it and will offer some help in this area, but I let the person decide. Sometimes the cohesion in the group is enough to eliminate the resistance to risk-taking. Very often, individual members may be skilled at helping a peer overcome her resistance. Such leadership interventions by group members facilitates the group's as well as the member's growth.

Leader Issues

Every leader comes to the group with certain ideas about how members should respond in his or her group. Therefore, every leader has an issue around expectations for the group's performance. No matter what type of group it is, leaders want members to participate in reaching the group's goals and in working towards adaptive behaviors in the group. Some leaders will focus more on a finished group product, such as the accomplishment of a particular task. Others will look more for individual achievements by members that mean the group has accomplished its purpose for being. Occasionally, the leader's need to have the group and its members reach certain goals interferes with the group's process of performance. I feel it legitimate and necessary to share my agenda for goal-directed behaviors with the group and to focus on processes within the group which hamper this, but I cannot expect performance from the group which they are incapable of producing. If I find my expectations becoming much different than the group's accomplishments, I have probably incorrectly assessed the potential of that particular group. If we consider again the student group I had (see Chapter Six) which was not moving through the initial stage to working quickly enough, I probably did not have appropriate expectations for that group. Once I had decided that the group was not going to self-disclose as expected but was still just developing trust, I relaxed and formulated a new set of expectations. I decided the group members could learn a lot from analyzing their process and resistances to moving along. This was a very valid goal and was compatible with the stage of development in which the members were. Their analyses could be as superficial or as depthful as they wanted them to be. Being able to discuss what kept them from self-disclosing was a first step to taking that risk. Although the students did not do a lot of risk-taking, their experiences prepared them to more easily move towards risk-taking in another group given the opportunity.

The leader will want to look at trust as an issue to be discussed in the group. From the leader's perspective, trust is a necessary process to prepare the group to do the risk-taking necessary to grow. We have talked about the leader producing an atmosphere conducive to trust. As a group facilitator, I would like the members to trust that I will take care of them and not let them leave group with obvious pain unless they are choosing to do this. The members want to know if they can trust each other, but they need to acknowledge that they trust the leader to facilitate interactions that will be growth-enhancing. Regardless of how close the group comes to self-disclosure with each other and are able to work together, the members need to have a sense of trust in the leader's ability to make group a good experience. Thus, the leader's credentials are an issue with which the leader wants the group to deal. Recall that the members see the leader as omniscient at first, and then gradually decide that the leader is a safe person with whom to express hostility. Manifestations of this hostility include the members' questioning the leader's credentials. Although this may be uncomfortable for the group facilitator, it is an important process for the group to go through. That the members are able to do this signals their acceptance of the leader as a humane and caring person.

The group may test the leader's credentials by asking the leader personal questions, questioning a process that the leader is facilitating in the group, or challenging the leader to handle a certain process in the group. Some of these situations are more covert than others and lend themselves to theme development within the group. It is also difficult sometimes to identify what the group is asking by the process that is occurring. If a group member is questioning the leader about why she is focusing on a particular conflict between two members, the member may be expressing a need to control as well as a need to feel safe with a competent leader. I feel the members' safety is very important to the group's growth, so I tend to deal with any process that seems to be related to my credentials as a leader. Generally, I will make a comment to elicit responses related to this issue, such as:

"I wonder, Teresa, if it is important to you how I handle this situation?"

"What is it that you need to know about me to make it more comfortable for you in this group?"

"I noticed the group became really silent while I was pushing Paul to talk about his mother's death. How did my pushing Paul to work on his feelings affect how you perceive us working in this group?"

Related to the leader's credentials are those fears the leader has that he will expose his incompetence to the group at sometime and may not be perceived as professional by the members. Because the members initially see the leader as omniscient, what will happen if the leader acts as human as the rest of the group? There is a fear of losing control of the group or that too many members will leave and the group will dissolve. Phipps (1982) labeled these fears as a leader issue that occurs quite frequently in groups. This set of fears is such a common one that it has become a leader issue, although I see it handled very differently by different leaders. I usually let the group see that human part of me that makes mistakes, feels unhappy at times, and is not always extremely patient. These are parts of me that I cannot help, and I feel that it is a learning experience for the group if I let my humaneness "hang out." Yalom (1975) talked about therapist transparency and how that exposure of one's realness is often very helpful to the group. In a group with very manipulative clients, I would be more selective about how I showed my vulnerability. Not all people are comfortable exposing weak areas, and it would not be helpful to the group for the leader to do this if he did not want to be so transparent. I find that, when I am more transparent and open, my credentials are not such an issue for me or the group. There are those few members who will use this vulnerability to express hostility towards the leader by hitting the leader's weak spot. Recall the example earlier in the book of my experience in a Gestalt group which I was coleading. The member that screamed at me said something about me that he knew would upset me. I started to cry. The member had just taken advantage of my vulnerability. When my coleader allowed me to talk about my feelings, he was letting me step into a member role for a few minutes. This role change helped me be less concerned about my image as a leader and my credentials with the group. After that, I found it comfortable to step back into my role as a coleader.

Each group facilitator will come with certain content issues that will focus on task accomplishment and will depend on the particular task topic. If the group is formulating a policy for the nurse's role in medication clinics, issues the leader would want the group to address might include: clinical privileges, previous policies, the nurse practice act provisions, and clinic goals. Certainly, the members might have some of these same issues or concerns, but it is the leader's responsibility to see that all issues are covered that might affect the accomplishment of the task, namely, the development of an acceptable written policy. Leader issues related to the task of the adolescent group for juvenile delinquents would cover such topics as self-image, relationships between parents and adolescents, and peer group pressure. The members may not have a sense of the need to look at these particular issues or may not be able to formulate these in an orderly way. Therefore, it is always important for the leader to have specific content issues in mind that the group needs to discuss to achieve its purpose for being.

Group Themes

An Example

The following examples differentiate between overt and covert themes and review some of the data discussed in this chapter and in Chapter Two. I taught my students group process by having them colead a group for chronic mental health clients while I observed from a point outside the circle (Wilson, 1980). In one particular group, a client was talking about his experiences. He was jumping from topic to topic fairly rapidly and becoming very detailed with his story, often going off on tangents with the result that he never quite focused on a unifying series of thoughts that completed his message. The overt theme was sexuality and the difference between men and women. He was talking about several girlfriends he had at various times and then jumped topics to discuss an experience on the beach where he saw many cardboard wrappers from feminine tampons washed up on the sand. Several times he laughed about this and encouraged the other male members of the group to laugh along with him. There was only one female member, along with the two female student nurses coleading the group. The male members outnumbered the females in the room.

Analysis

On the surface, this client was discussing some experiences related to his interactions with women, both with females, themselves, and with inanimate objects that are peculiar to the female sex. His laughter was somewhat nervous in character, thus giving one the impression that this topic was not something with which he was totally comfortable. By looking at both the content level and the metacommunication level of his message, one would conclude his overt individual theme was some discomfort around relating to the opposite sex. If we also look at the group process going on, the overt group theme would be an identification by the group that this was a mixed group and that one set of members, the males, were talking about how they perceived females, particularly as sexual beings.

If I were to call the group's attention to this theme, I would identify it and open up the discussion for a ''here-and-now'' look at what the group members were saying about each other; *e.g.,* that this was a mixed group; that sometimes it was hard for the two sexes to understand each other (How true was this of the members in the group at that moment? What was the comfort level between the male members, the female member, and the two female coleaders?); and that perhaps individual members were wondering how others perceived them in the group. If I wanted to work with the one client who was relating the story to the group, I would deal with the overt message, *i.e.,* that he seemed to want to talk about relationships with women and how that worked out for him. I might ask him to use the group members to test out some of his ideas about relationships since the group was composed of male and female participants.

Origin of Group Themes

The group theme, in this case, sexuality and male-female relationships, is introduced by one member who has a particular need, conflict, or fear in this area. He verbalizes what others may be feeling and have not shared. A process occurs when a group of people is together over a period of time, such as in a client group, which causes individual members to share internal feelings as they respond to the here-and-now situation. It is not even necessary for people to be together any length of time. We all respond to the situations in which we find ourselves according to what in our environment is stimulating us at the time. For example, in working with doctors, a nurse might find herself focusing on avoiding the traditional handmaid role because she has a great deal of emotion tied up with this. She may be attempting to resocialize all physicians, and, therefore, becomes very sensitive to stimuli that have, in the past, resulted in her being caught in this role. If, in reality, the physicians with whom the nurse is working are quite socialized not to expect the handmaiden role, the nurse may be seen as overreacting with her feelings. All members of a group are affected by the group process occurring around them. Thus, an individual member's fear is brought to the surface by some stimuli within the group which triggers this internal awareness. Whitaker and Lieberman (1964) noted this process occurring within groups:

''Whatever is said in the group is seen as being elicited not only by the strictly internal concerns of the individual, but by the interpersonal situation in which he finds himself. Of all the personal issues, worries, impulses, and concerns which a patient might express during a group session, what he actually expresses is elicited by the character of the situation.'' (p. 16)

The members of a group respond to that part of a peer's message which is relevant for them as individuals, and then as a group as the individual concerns shared by many become group concerns. The ''group-relevant'' part of a message ''is defined by the manner in which the other patients react to it.'' (Whitaker and Lieberman, 1964, p. 17). Thus, the individual member's internal processes which are made manifest in the group are the source for the group's themes. Group themes usually extend over more than one session and may reappear at a different level of involvement for the members in subsequent sessions. Usually, the levels move from superficial, safe conversations around a particular theme to more personal, threatening interchanges between members which often elicit painful or negative feelings (Whitaker and Lieberman, 1964; DiMinno and Thompson, 1980). It is most likely, then, that the level of anxiety within a group will increase during that period where themes become the expressions of more painful personal conflicts.

Covert Themes

If we again consider the previous example, a deeper probe into the latent content will reveal covert themes. Generally, I do not focus on covert themes with the group members, but I let such themes tell me more about the possible internal processes of the members. These data help to make me aware of very sensitive areas within the group or with individual members. The client who told his story to the group was, on an overt level, making comments about the sexual nature of relationships, that he had had relationships, and, most likely, had felt a little uneasy and confused at times in these relationships. (Recall the nonverbal nervous laughter.) To go further with the meaning behind his communications, one should consider what the connotative meanings are behind some of his communications as well as the symbolism underlying certain words or phrases or nonverbal behaviors. This requires the therapist/group leader to come with some psychoanalytical background. Such depth of preparation is not necessary for most support groups but would be of benefit in a psychotherapy group. The client in the example might have been saying something about his fears of a sexual encounter, since the tampons could represent the female's menstrual cycle, the unapproachability of the sexual organ, or even the control a female may exert over a male during the menstrual period. To talk about females in the way this client did is somewhat degrading and could indicate the existence of significant anger towards women which he may only have felt safe expressing on a very covert level. Certainly, these are only a few of many possibilities. It is evident that the group leader would not approach a client with these observations/assumptions of his internal process without sufficient data about how the client might react. The leader should assess if this would be helpful material for the client and the group to discuss and should have a good idea about where this intervention would lead and how it would fit in with the goals of the group or the individual client's goals. One way I use what I suspect is a covert theme is to let that analysis help me understand the group's emotion and what underlying anxieties members might be experiencing. The composition of this particular group, being predominantly male, also suggests that the client may have felt a little safer sharing such material where he had more support. It also might be a way of testing out his feelings with other males or a way of seeing how the females in the group would respond to him. His message might have been directed at the two female student nurses and even at me as the controlling person, and also female, in that room. As we discuss all the possibilities, it becomes obvious that more and more levels of process are uncovered as one explores covert themes. We moved from females as sexual beings, to females with whom he may have interacted, to a female member within the group, to the female leaders, and finally to the very important, yet unsaid process, of having a female observer who could hear what was being said in the group but who did not have to share any of herself in a reciprocal manner with the group. Looking at the "here-and-now" process may be a way of dealing with some of the covert material in a less personal and threatening way. One of the female coleaders could ask the group what it was like to have the female instructor sitting outside the circle. This would allow the group to talk about anger, insecurities, and so forth, without having to be very personal. The anger could be directed at a safe person in the room who could handle it easier than any of the females involved in the group process. The group could express themselves without fear of retaliation by anyone else in the group. This analysis of how the covert theme might get expressed in a safer way in the group illustrates two points about covert themes. Generally, covert themes can be expressed more safely by directing the conflict at the group leader who is a less threatening target than one's peers. Since the covert theme is more threatening and less within the members' awareness, overt themes tend to be the group's focus and serve to keep a covert theme hidden.

There is no need for the leader of a task group to look for covert group themes unless some interactional process within the group is interfering with the accomplishment of the task. The leader might be able to understand what process was affecting group members by looking for covert themes. If the group is having difficulty with authority figures as a result of some personal feelings of one or more members that have aroused sentiments within the group, then this group theme would explain some resistance, perhaps, from members in relation to task accomplishment. The leader needs to decide what intervention might make the group's work more productive. Perhaps, giving the group members some control would help deal with some of the antiauthority feelings and move the group towards task accomplishment.

The nurse who is leading a support group needs to make similar analyses of the group process to decide the most helpful intervention. If the covert theme is related to sexual issues not unlike those discussed in the example, the nurse would need to decide how this affected the group's ability to deal with the situation for which the group was formed. If it is a support group for new parents, the sexual concerns most realistic to discuss in this group would be how the couple renews their sexual relationship in between parenting responsibilities, how the couple responds to each other's personal needs during this period, and perhaps, how the parents deal with older siblings' questions related to sex. Although this may not touch on the sexual conflicts of the members, this is not the group where this is an appropriate topic. The nurse leader must make this discrimination. It is not necessary for the leader to understand what covert messages the group is giving out if it is not affecting the group's process around goal attainment. It is very difficult to assess covert themes. If the group leader is aware that they exist and that they express inner conflicts and other personal processes, then he or she can be watching for their development in the group if the manifest content being shared does not seem to account for all the unspoken feelings being expressed nonverbally. Finding covert themes is a leadership skill that comes with supervision and hours of practice with group process.

The preceding paragraphs have presented the process one might use when attempting to discover what underlying themes exist within the group. Whitaker and Lieberman (1964) talked about the approach-avoidance nature of the group's relationship to underlying wishes and fears which make up the covert themes. There is a movement towards and away from the expression and exploration of underlying process. This movement relates to the group's tolerance for the anxiety and conflict which such covert processes cause. Anytime I sense conflict and, particularly, anxiety which I cannot explain by the overt processes going on in the group, I tend to think that a more covert process is occurring. It is helpful to have this sign to prompt me to look further to begin to uncover the various layers of process. The nurse leader who becomes skilled in identifying process will find working with groups to be unlimited in experiences and well worth the investment of the clinical hours to understand the phenomena of process.

REFERENCES

Cartwright, D. and A. Zander, eds. *Group Dynamics: Research and Theory* (2nd ed.). Evanston, IL: Row Peterson and Co., 1960.

DiMinno, M. and E. Thompson. "An Interactional Support Group for Graduate Nursing Students," *Journal of Nursing Education,* 19, no. 3 (March, 1980), 16–22.

Erikson, E. *Identity Youth and Crisis.* New York: W. W. Norton and Co., Inc., 1968.

Phipps, L. "Group Dynamics: Leadership Roles and Functions," in *Life Cycle Group Work in Nursing,* eds. E. Janosik and L. Phipps. Monterey, CA: Wadsworth Health Sciences Division, 1982.

Whitaker, D. and M. Lieberman. *Psychotherapy Through the Group Process.* New York: Atherton Press, 1964.

Wilson, M. "Negotiating Group Process Experiences," *Nursing Outlook,* 28, no. 6 (June, 1980), 360–364.

Wilson, H. and C. Kneisl. *Psychiatric Nursing.* Menlo Park, CA: Addison-Wesley Publishing Co., 1979.

Yalom, I. *The Theory and Practice of Group Psychotherapy* (2nd ed.). New York: Basic Books, Inc., 1975.

Group Decision-Making
and Conflict Resolution   8

    Decisions are often made in a group using the collective expertise of the members. As both a student and an instructor, I have been inundated with assignments both to work in groups for task accomplishment and to study the process of group development. Some of my most painful and most helpful learning experiences have been when I was involved in group decision-making.

    Although group decision-making sounds very task-oriented, it is actually a process that produces, at times, some complex interactions between group members. This process may either impede or promote goal-oriented behavior. A rational problem-solving format is probably most often used in the process that leads to group decision-making. Problem-solving and decision-making are two processes that, together, allow a group to act on a viable solution that leads to goal achievement. Problem-solving allows the group members to define the obstacles preventing goal achievement and to come up with the criteria necessary to generate appropriate alternatives on which the group might act. A course of action is implemented based upon the decision of the group, ranging from group consensus to authority rule. Decision-making, therefore, may not always satisfy the wishes of each group member on how the group should act. It is through the process of arriving at a decision to act that conflict can develop and must be resolved to provide for optimal goal achievement by the group. This chapter will discuss group problem-solving and decision-making and the conditions under which conflict resolution occurs.

    Problem-solving can be done from either a rational or an intuitive cognitive style. The rational mode involves performing a series of discrete steps one at a time which are usually sequential and fit into interrelated categories. The elements of the rational style are able to be separated into neat boundaries explicit in their relationship to each other. Intuitive problem-solving allows for a flow of ideas in which one thought may trigger another, thus increasing the flexibility of problem-solving but also making it harder to have control over the process. Many forms of expression, including images, fantasies, and feelings, allow for visualizing a situation and integrating one's experience into gestalts. Problems are conceptualized in a broader context and are more implicit than explicit (Nugent, 1982). Problem-solving, by being confined to the rational approach, may prevent the group from producing some creative solutions upon which to act. If the group leader recognizes that some persons are more adapted to an intuitive style of thinking, she may be able to harness some of the group's creativity. We will look first at rational problem-solving with its specific steps and then at creative problem-solving using the intuitive style. As an attempt to integrate the material in this chapter, a discussion of the two cognitive styles and how they might be integrated to produce maximum efficiency and creativity will be presented.

    Decision-making frequently leads to conflict as individuals find differences with each other in their value orientation, cognitive style, and goals. Conflict resolution, therefore, becomes an important part of the group process. The latter part of this chapter will present the various approaches to dealing with conflict. In Chapter Six, we talked about the various stages of group where conflict is more likely to occur. It is in the working and termination stage that both decision-making and conflict are likely to be a large part of the group's process. Groups that are unable to deal with conflict in a satisfactory manner or who fail to recognize its existence are less capable of effective decision-making. Unresolved conflict impedes the group's movement towards its goals and generally affects the group members' relationships with one another. This produces a less-than-effective group product. Conflict resolution, in contrast, will often promote a more efficient working group.

The Steps In Problem-Solving

The following are the steps used in the scientific problem-solving method or the rational style of thinking. This process is not exclusive to group decision-making but is an accepted method for either an individual or a group approach for tackling a problem. Although the steps, therefore, are universal in application, examples specific to their application in a group will be given.

Identifying and Defining the Problem

A problem is an obstacle to goal attainment. One sees a discrepancy often between what one wants to occur and what is actually happening. There may also be a discrepancy between the purpose for something and its actual attainment (Erikson and Borgmeyer, 1979). For example, compliance is often identified as a problem in nursing care for a particular client. The nursing staff wants a client to perform postoperative exercises to prevent complications from his surgery, but he is resisting. He may not see that the outcome is related to the actions the nursing staff wants him to take, thereby contributing to a problem where the purpose and the outcome are not congruent for the client. Staffing problems frequently fall into the category of being a "what is" vs. a "what should be." A staff that is short on expertise or manpower prevents the realization of optimal client care. If one's goals are different than another's, the discrepancy between purpose and goal attainment becomes the problem. In a policy-making group, an individual member with a personal agenda different than that of the group's produces a block to decision-making. A member may have a special interest in not having a particular policy adopted. This is quite a common occurrence in the legislature and results in filibustering, outside-group lobbying, and other practices.

Problem-Framing. Problem-framing is a term that describes a way of conceptualizing a problem (deChesnay, 1983). Problem-framing is particularly useful for nurses attempting to define a client's problem list. In individual problem-framing, the ownership of the problem and the expectations for change lie in the person whose behavior has been identified as problematic. System problem-framing changes the problem's ownership from that of the individual to the system of which the individual is a part. The family, the nurse, the hospital, or others interacting with the client must take on the responsibility in conjunction with the client. Individual problem-framing may be attempted first as a way of defining the problem. If this does not lead to a solution, system problem-framing may correct this. The evaluation process has moved away from judging the individual to looking at the effectiveness of the change or solution that was used, *i.e.,* how the system interacts with the individual. Perhaps the family is not supportive of the client's need to be on a special diet. Instead of focusing only on the client's behavior, the staff may decide that the outcome must be that the family verbalize their willingness to buy and prepare the foods the client needs. The problem now becomes the family's interaction with the client.

Evaluating the effectiveness of the change process may lead to reframing the problem so that it becomes a non-problem (deChesnay, 1983). Reframing, another type of problem-framing, deals with images of reality or interpretations one makes as one perceives reality. Reframing changes the meaning of how one is experiencing a given situation in such a way that the new perspective often appears even more appropriate or convincing. It is important that this new perspective fit with the client's view of the world and that it is communicated to the individual in his language (Watzlawick, 1978). For example, a client who experiences his religious beliefs as a powerful force determining his actions in life would not respond to the nurse who tells him to reduce his stress by saying "no" to some of the church's demands on him. However, he might respond to the nurse's suggestion that God wants him to take care of his body and rest it at times. I find reframing particularly helpful with clients who tend to feel very overwhelmed with problems. The sense of having to face problems creates anxiety that prevents the client from taking action. If the problem can be seen as an asset rather than a liability, the client may be more likely to start helping himself.

I recently talked with a man who tended to see even minor inconveniences as major obstacles in his life. The first thing he said to me as he met me was that he hoped it would not rain because he had to take two buses to get home, and he might get wet. His agenda for coming to the clinic that day was to try and get a doctor to write a letter to the welfare department saying that his hiatal hernia prevented him from doing any work to earn his foodstamps. It was the staff's consensus that he would be able to do some of the lighter work the welfare department might assign to him, and the main obstacle to his accomplishing this was the view he had of himself as being "sick" and helpless. His eighty-year-old mother cooked meals for him and financially supported him. I took the approach that he might consider the foodstamp work an opportunity to learn a new skill and test his ability to follow through with some work as preparation for the time when his mother would no longer be able to support him. Initially, all my suggestions were met with "yes, but." I decided to share the observation of this process with him and to suggest that this said to me that he might be part of the difficulties he was attributing to outside environmental sources. I was both putting the problem into a system framework and reframing it to be an opportunity for growth for him. Instead of him being able to blame the environment, much as we health professionals tend to blame the client, I was asking him to consider how his interactions with the "problem" affected its outcome. By my reframing it for him, I became an interactor in the system. I feel I gave him more of a chance to explore the problem and alternative actions. We were acting as a group of two to work on his problem. When we finished talking, he had agreed to think about what I had said.

Groups may be dealing with an internal problem related to their interactions with one another or with one that is related to the particular task/goals they are to accomplish. It is often difficult for the group to conceptualize a problem that deals with its own process. Often the leader or an outside consultant will have to help with this, especially if the group leader is also caught up in the process. In Chapter Fourteen, we will look at how a nurse consultant can help a group to focus on an internal problem.

Once a problem has been identified that is not related to the group's internal process but to its particular task, the group must look at the cause of the problem, the urgency of needed action, and the desirable and necessary outcomes or goals of any actions. It is often helpful to write behavioral objectives. These may be quantitatively observed to evaluate the outcome of any suggested actions (Erikson and Borgmeyer, 1979). A nursing care conference routinely uses this process to formulate nursing care plans for a client. A client-centered problem is an appropriate one for a group of nursing personnel to tackle in a task group format. If the leader of the nursing care conference is an outsider, such as a clinical specialist, the group will respond differently than if the head nurse were leading the conference. With a new or one-time leader, the group members will most likely regress to the point of feeling some of the anxiety about what is going to happen in the group that they felt initially when beginning the group experience. The head nurse will create less anxiety within the group but will also tend to be less objective with the group's internal process. Since the group's focus is on the external task, that of formulating a nursing care plan, the internal process need not be an issue unless it keeps the group from working on its task.

Generating Alternatives

In order to arrive at the best possible action, one needs to have several choices or alternatives available. Going back to the example of a nursing care conference group, one can relate alternatives to a list of possible nursing interventions. The behavioral objectives or outcomes having been operationalized, the group can now consider criterion measures upon which each proposed intervention or alternative will be judged. A set of criteria might include: the number of staff needed for a particular intervention, the length of time the nursing actions will take, the cost to the client or hospital, the level of expertise of staff needed to intervene, and so forth. Criteria suggest potential problems with each alternative. Time, cost, untoward consequences, one's beliefs, or values are all possible constraints (Erikson and Borgmeyer, 1979). One might look at the constraints the client offers to certain interventions that might be chosen. The client may be of a different culture and would reject certain culturally related nursing interventions. Limited resources of equipment would prevent some suggestions from being considered for implementation. The client may not have the resources to purchase the necessary exercise equipment that would help with his postdischarge recovery. Client teaching may have to be modified because of no significant others to monitor the client's continued practice with his colostomy at home. Sometimes the beliefs of the group members will interfere with the selection of alternatives to the problem. If one of a client's problems is isolation and withdrawal behavior related to a recent abortion, a staff member uncomfortable with the value system that allows abortion may not want to consider interpersonal staff supports for this client because of her anger towards this person. The staff group may find itself caught up in an internal values conflict rather than focusing on the needs of the client. The nursing care conference group is a task group and needs to operate like one in dealing with internal conflict. If there is a way to acknowledge the differences in values between group members and then move on to looking for some viable client-centered interactions that one or more staff feel comfortable doing, it seems that this is the most efficient solution. Group members may agree to disagree without derailing the group from its task. However, if an internal conflict prevents the group from staying with the task, it needs to be dealt with in some way. As the group generates alternatives or possible nursing interventions, these might be weighed according to the criteria already established. This provides a more objective view of how viable each alternative might be.

Choosing and Implementing a Course of Action

After analyzing the options by applied criteria and weighing the alternatives against these, one decides on the most desirable alternative or solution. The most effective solution would meet the most criteria and be most accepted by the group. It is interesting that the best solution in terms of the criteria may not be the most popular with the group. For example, a task group of nursing administrators/clinical coordinators and the chief nurse may need to decide on some quality assurance projects for nursing service. The project most likely to meet JCAH criteria may not be the project most enjoyable or most interesting to do. If the unpopular project is chosen, it may not turn out to be as well done because the initiating group is not really behind it. A high-quality solution, therefore, may not necessarily be the solution of choice because of the lack of support behind it. Similarly, a quality nursing intervention, such as one which involves enormous amounts of the nursing staff's energy but gives the most frequent, personal, around-the-clock care to the client, may not be realistic to implement because of the drain on staff and their resistance to working so diligently for one client.

One of the problems with choosing the appropriate solution to a problem is that, oftentimes, one gets caught in thinking that there is only one solution to meet a certain outcome or goal. If this solution seems less than optimal, the individual may become discouraged and decide that the problem is not solvable. Likewise, if a solution is chosen to be implemented and then does not work, the person may decide there is no solution.

The following is an example of the confusion between goals and solutions. A mother trying to work out childcare for her children attempted to get permission from the school districts involved to put her first-grader in the school next door to her daughter's preschool. Both children would then be nearby and close to the parents' work. A few days later, the mother was told that the permission to change districts originally granted was an error. The *one* solution that she had chosen was not working. It was the preschool director that came up with another alternative. She suggested a private school close by, free of city school district requirements. The desired outcome was not that the son be in a particular school but that he be taken care of after school in a setting nearby that was comfortable for him. There is generally more than than one solution to a problem if one defines the desired outcome or goal correctly.

Implementing the solution takes the cooperation of all the parties involved. In nursing care planning, an individual staff person or group of staff takes responsibility for a particular intervention with the client. They are then accountable for implementing the identified intervention. If the staff group is allowed to choose what interventions they would like to implement, they will most likely do a better job.

Evaluating the Results

Criteria for evaluation should come from the behavioral objectives or operationally defined goals. It is very easy to decide if a client outcome has been met if there are measurable actions one can observe. "Demonstrate the technique for insulin self-administration," is much more measurable than "knows how to give himself insulin." "Knows" is not a measurable verb. It is important to look at any untoward consequences of the implemented solution (Erikson and Borgmeyer, 1979). If a client becomes anxious and withdrawn after being taught to take responsibility for his own colostomy care, then perhaps his being taught that right away is not an appropriate intervention. Such evaluation will then lead one back to the beginning of the process, which is defining another problem.

———————————— Creative Problem-Solving ————————————

The intuitive mode of thinking forms the basis for creative problem-solving. In our discussion of reframing, we actually touched on the intuitive mode. By restructuring the client's perception of a situation through reframing, the therapist is required to perceive the problem in a much broader context. Although reframing is included under the rational mode of problem-solving, probably because it fits with the identified step of problem definition and promotes further rational thinking, one may consider the actual reframing as being more intuitive in nature. A therapist using reframing must visualize the client's situation in a way that is less restrictive for the client and which promotes the most adaptive behaviors. Cognitive restructuring is another technique similar to reframing in that one must modify his or her perception of the world. Negative cognitive sets are changed to positive thoughts about oneself and one's capabilities. Goals are seen as a function of internal processes rather than only external events (Granvold and Welch, 1979). The person who is able to see himself as having some control over events in his life that he originally felt helpless about has succeeded in restructuring his view of himself. This technique was used in a support group for post-divorce adjustment where the members needed to regain their self-esteem and sense of control over their lives. The goal was to retrain the members in the way they perceived and defined their divorce experience (Granvold and Welch, 1979). Giving the client a sense of control by changing his self-concept is something nurses do frequently when they help clients experience successes or mastery in a certain area of health prevention, maintenance, or renewal. As with reframing, the basic tool is the rational problem-solving mode done with an intuitive approach by the therapist as to what parts of the client's self might be most vulnerable to some change through problem-solving. Reframing works on perceiving the problem as a non-problem; *i.e.,* the meaning one contributes to one's difficulties changes. Cognitive restructuring gives the person a new set of problem-solving skills by helping that person experience some internal control over things in his or her environment.

The Creative Process

Exercising one's creative processes involves acting in a new and unique way upon familiar material or creating something novel through a unique interaction between the individual and events, situations, or materials in that person's life (Stafford, 1981). Arieti (1976; Stafford, 1981) saw the creative process as an integration of the primary process thinking of the id with the logical mode of secondary process. Recall our discussion in Chapter Two of the creativity of artists and others who needed to be in their id or allow their ego to regress in order to produce works of art. It is obvious that the rational problem-solving approach would not allow regression to primary process thinking where nothing is logical or well-ordered. Those conditions most likely to promote creativity include aloneness, daydreaming, inactivity, and a remembrance of past traumatic events or conflicts in one's life (Arieti, 1976; Stafford, 1981). We might take a lesson from this as nurses when we are concerned with clients who appear to be withdrawing or want to be left alone. Although this is often a sign of depression, it may also be a time-out exercise by the person who is feeling over-programmed by the health team. There are times like this when the client might be doing some legitimate creative problem-solving. It is important for the nurse to check this out with the person and encourage this behavior if it appears to be adaptive. Creativity is probably best done in a permissive atmosphere. It is much easier for me to turn my children loose and let them be creative, because that is the current idea about child-raising. I have more difficulty being permissive with clients. I find my orientation to Gestalt is helpful in giving myself permission to let others be themselves.

The Steps to Creative Problem-Solving

The following may be considered "steps" in the creative process. In talking about a logical set of steps, there is the danger of pushing creativity into the rational mode where thinking follows an ordered set of descriptive actions. It seems that the steps in the creative process have been put into a rational set to attempt to define the process more logically. Although creativity is a process that seems to have some order to it, it is not something that can be followed like a recipe or brought on by planning. In fact, trying to be creative often results in blocking the process (Nugent, 1982).

The following is a description of the internal process that leads to creativity.

1) Experiencing a Felt Need or Orientation to Self-Expression or Stimulation by a Problem Situation. As with the rational approach, the creative problem-solver must first identify an obstacle to goal accomplishment. Generally, there is some awareness of the need for reordering the events or objects in one's environment to produce something unique (Stafford, 1981). The individual moves towards creative problem-solving when he or she feels stale, *i.e.,* wanting something fresh or new to happen with the very familiar events or environment with which the person is interacting.

2) Preparation Through Data Collection and Review to Look for New Relationships in Old Material. This step allows for the reordering of one's perceptions to attempt to see data in a different way. One needs to first gather all information about the problem area, very much as in rational problem-solving. The data are then broken down into what appear to be relevant bits of information with which one might start generating some new thoughts or ideas of how to use these data further (Stafford, 1981). There is a difference here between the generation of alternatives in the rational mode and the generation of ideas in the intuitive mode. Alternatives suggested through intuitive thinking tend to be in greater quantity, with less thought for how they will really fit with the old information, and with a more spontaneous flow. The alternatives to fit the rational problem-solving approach must all be feasible actions that have some credibility from previous use. Those for creative problem-solving need not even be possible as reality is currently defined, but may be some fantastic thought that seems totally illogical. It is through the permission to be illogical that one comes up with new ways to view old objects or events. Idea generation is a much freer process in the intuitive mode of thinking.

An example of how the two modes differ from each other in generating alternatives may be helpful. A multidisciplinary hospital committee has been assigned the task of determining possible uses for an empty wing of the building. If the group were to follow the rational approach to idea generation, only those alternatives that were feasible and possible would be legitimate suggestions. Turning the wing into a video game arcade would violate the rules for logical alternatives. However, this suggestion would be an acceptable alternative if the group were using a creative intuitive mode of thinking. The committee would probably never adopt this suggestion, but the idea might generate some new ways of looking at the old alternatives. Perhaps further thoughts might lead the committee to look at giving the space to the clients, perhaps for some type of project, such as an ongoing craft fair to which clients, their families, or friends could contribute items which could be sold to generate revenue for upgrading patient-care spaces, and so forth. Hospital space is usually not seen as a spot for a business venture but more as a place for equipment or as a patient-care area. Most likely, a daycare center for hospital employees would have been considered an unacceptable alternative in a rational problem-solving approach to space not too many years ago. Its inception may have been the result of some intuitive thinking.

3) Incubation. During this step of the creative process, one is not actively involved in problem-solving at all. In fact, it is detrimental to the creative process for the person to be trying to work further on generating solutions. Incubation is the process of letting up to invite an "aha" or a specific idea that is a feasible answer to the obstacle one is facing (Stafford, 1981). I have often suggested to students that they begin a paper long before it is due in order to add those creative ideas that are required. The new insights one gets from doing research on a subject do not come until the material has been digested for awhile. Often, repetitious thoughts are a sign that it is time for incubation.

4) Illumination and Synthesis. If one has been able to incubate, is patient and relaxed, illumination happens automatically. One may find that "ahas" come at a time least expected, *e.g.,* while lying in bed waiting to go to sleep or at some time when one is feeling very relaxed and not focusing on the problem at all, such as during a long walk or a jog. It is good to have a pencil and paper to record ideas before they are lost. Synthesis is the process of putting the ideas together to make sense of the "ahas" one has gathered (Stafford, 1981). Sometimes modifications need to be made. I find that my initial idea is generally changed before I put a plan into action. For example, I have been doing some creative problem-solving around an inservice I plan to give the staff of an outpatient mental health clinic. The topic is of my choosing, and I want it to be scholarly but also useful and within my area of expertise. The staff in the clinic is extremely varied as to discipline and skills. I had thought about sharing something on Gestalt, but the client population does not seem appropriate for that modality. I could present some theory and practice examples of using an insight-oriented group with a chronic schizophrenic population, but I do not have the statistical data (only my personal experiences) to validate this. I finally told myself to just forget about the inservice since I had exhausted all my ideas. I recognized the need to incubate and trusted that my unacceptable ideas would eventually generate some new solution. I have just recently had an "aha" about this, and it seems so simple and practical! I have been aware of how much this staff group is "not a group," is not cohesive, and spends much time with intellectual activities, attempting to deal with policies that may be beyond their control to change. It seems that they need a positive group experience that would facilitate their sense of well-being and direction as a group. My first "aha" was to share with them my observations of their group process in an attempt to help them start working on some of their problem areas. After some synthesis about this, I decided that the group could not handle my observations and that this would, most likely, make them less adaptive as a group and more reluctant to work. I would be attacking their fragile ego, to describe this process analytically. I could, however, offer the group some nurturing by focusing on improving their trust level and sense of relatedness with one another. I have decided to do some "healing" experiential exercises with them which I see as nonthreatening and most likely producing a positive outcome. My need to refine my first "aha" is the synthesis that is needed along with illumination in creative problem-solving.

5) Evaluation. The creative solution is assessed with the potential for problem areas that could develop (Stafford, 1981). One of the problem areas I am anticipating is possible resistance from the staff when I introduce the group exercises I want them to do. I have decided that I will not consult with the group leader first to ask his permission, but I will assume that, as the person who is the facilitator, I have freedom to structure our time together as I consider appropriate. I also anticipate some individual members not wanting to interact with those with whom they do not feel as comfortable. I have decided I will arbitrarily assign dyads to work together since having to choose partners is sometimes very threatening. If things do not go as I have planned (*e.g.,* some staff are openly resistive), an appropriate intervention would be to ask the staff to look at the process that just occurred as an example of the group's current functioning. I feel fairly comfortable with my evaluation of possible problem areas.

A creative solution or one reached by rational problem-solving has the same chance of succeeding or failing. The quality of each is comparable. It is only the process of arriving at the solution that is different.

Techniques for Creative Problem-Solving

1) Brainstorming. Most readers will probably be quite familiar with this technique, since it has universal application in problem-solving and may even be used as a party game because of its potential for generating some fun. Brainstorming is designed to create a large number of ideas in a short period of time without generating any criticism of individual members' contributions. A problem is introduced to the group. One person is designated as a recorder and must write down every idea suggested without censorship of any kind. The group then ranks the ideas according to some scheme to begin to separate those which are feasible or possible from those which are not.

As with the creative process, the goal is for new solutions to be generated by allowing a large number of ideas to flow and open up new combinations or arrangements of possible solutions. The process of brainstorming may only succeed in an initial generation of solutions. There may need to be another incubation period before illumination occurs. The group may continue to eliminate ideas, combine them, modify them, and so forth. Brainstorming works best when the problem is simple and specific rather than of complex proportions. In a previous example about a hospital committee's work to decide how to use a recently available section of space, brainstorming would have been appropriate. If the problem had been how to determine the future utilization of all space within the hospital, brainstorming would not have worked as well. The latter problem was too complex. If the committee broke the problem down into several steps, such as how would existing space be divided (the process of doing this), what goals does the hospital have for expansion, what might be done with wasted space areas, and so forth, brainstorming could be used on each step. My experience with brainstorming is that it is fun, relaxing, and does often generate some amazingly good solutions.

2) The Nominal Group Process. This technique is similar to brainstorming but has more steps and is a more formal problem-solving process for a group (Cooper, 1982). Each person in the group is working in the presence of the other members but as an individual in generating and deciding on solutions rather than as a group interacting with one another. Each member has an equal opportunity to give input, thus getting maximum participation from each person. Members write their ideas on small cards after being presented with a problem. This is done for the first ten minutes of the group. All ideas are then recorded on a flip chart moving round-robin from one member to another, each person giving only one idea at a time. New ideas may be added as each member gets a turn until all ideas have been exhausted. Each person must clarify his or her suggestion for the group. The suggestions are numbered, and each member then selects the five best solutions and ranks them from one to five. These are recorded on individual cards and listed by rank order for the group to see. Discussion ensues, and after this a final vote is taken to determine the group members' collective decision. The individual quality of this process allows for divergent or controversial ideas to have equal time for discussion. Certainly, this process would not be necessary for all problem-solving but would be most appropriate for those decisions likely to produce strong positive or negative feelings and those creating difficulties in the generation of ideas. A nursing association might use this process to determine program priorities (Cooper, 1982). The discussion by the American Nurses' Association on the appropriate entry level for nurses might be an issue that would lend itself to this type of creative problem-solving.

3) Getting into the Child Ego State. Recall the discussion in Chapter Two on how one's Little Professor operates from the Natural Child and can be quite useful in creating solutions, looking at relationships in new ways, and so forth. Some of the ways I use to get others into their child in order to activate the Little Professor are to have people sit on the floor, to use media that children enjoy (fingerpaints, crayons, etc.), and to provide a nonthreatening atmosphere. The group may share a creative assignment. Among those I have assigned were to write a group poem or to do a group collage. Chapter Nine will present more details on these techniques.

The Rational vs. the Intuitive Mode in Group Decision-Making

Although group problem-solving and decision-making have generally occurred more through a rational approach than from an intuitive one, it is often helpful to use the best ideas from both modes of thinking to reach a group decision. In order for this to happen, the group must tolerate some disorder or ambiguity (Nugent, 1982). Nugent suggested that one of the difficulties of group problem-solving is inattention to the cognitive styles of the members which leads to misunderstandings and inefficiencies within the group. If both styles are used at various stages, each member could make a valid contribution. It is possible that subgroups focusing on different cognitive styles might be formed within each group (Nugent, 1982). Generation of ideas can occur through such intuitive processes as visual imagery, roleplaying, model simulation, and so forth, in order to help members perceive a concept in concrete form. The group can then move to a more rational mode of analyzing the ideas presented. Those group members that are comfortable with both modes of thinking might facilitate intragroup understanding between the two subgroups (Nugent, 1982). It would seem that both modes can contribute to the ultimate solution for a problem.

Advantages and Disadvantages of Group Decision-Making

The group is considered a good source of manpower in which multiple resources can be brought to problem-solving (Nugent, 1982; Cooper, 1982). As we noted above, members will think intuitively, rationally, or with a combination of the two modes, and this can be quite helpful to the ultimate solution of problems. Tasks can be shared by several people. If a problem is solved through a technique such as the nominal group process, all members have an equal chance of influencing the decision (Cooper, 1982). If a group is involved in arriving at a course of action which the group itself will implement, such as a decision to change with step-by-step goals, it is more likely that the change will come about (Lippitt, et al., 1958). Thus, an advantage to group decision-making is involving all those that will actually implement the solution. Wilson and Kneisl (1979) noted the characteristics of good decision-making: decisions put into effect by the group members, the group's time and resources well-used, the decision being of high quality, and the problem-solving ability of the group being enhanced by the decision-making process.

Involving a group in decision-making has its drawbacks when it is necessary to have a unanimous decision, such as in the case of many decisions trial juries must make. If a juror decides to disagree, the jury is hung and a mistrial is often declared. Because this can happen so easily, just one juror hinting at a disageement could reduce the chance of the members wanting to compromise to reach a unanimous decision (Foss, 1981). In a study conducted with jurors using a quorum method for decision-making, one or two jurors unwilling to compromise could not affect a quorum of the jurors ready to reach a decision (Foss, 1981). The power to hang a jury is not unlike that power which rests in minority control by a few members of an in-group who are given the decision-making power for the larger body. The drawbacks of minority control are the possibility of unresolved conflict and resistance to the decision being made by those not included, as well as the disadvantage of not using the expertise or ideas of the entire group. There are times when it becomes unwieldy for a large body to make decisions. Committees empowered to do this can save a group a lot of time and can handle routine matters that the larger group may not need to decide (Wilson and Kneisl, 1979). Certainly, many nursing organizations use the concept of minority control. It is important, however, to understand that there are times when minority control can be detrimental to a group. I have found, from being a head nurse, that it is not always wise to try to expedite a decision by delegating it to part of the larger staff group. If I asked my staff nurses to make some decisions about nursing care on the unit and did not think to include the entire staff in the final decision process, I had difficulty implementing the decision. Although the initial process went more quickly if only a few staff worked on policy, making a decision that the entire nursing staff would have to implement needed to be a decision by the entire staff. Group decision-making frequently slows the process of implementation, but it may be necessary to ensure the successful completion of the process.

Wilson and Kneisl (1979) noted that indecisiveness by a group could be due to several underlying causes, such as fear of the consequences of a decision, the inappropriateness of the method for problem-solving, or a personal problem a member might be having with her loyalty within the group. Certainly, the inability of the group to concur on a course of action, for whatever reason, hampers future actions of the group and those systems it directly affects. For example, in a multidisciplinary setting, it is sometimes difficult to agree on a written policy that describes the functioning of one particular discipline, such as nursing, which interfaces with many aspects of the work done in the clinic. At times, there are conflicting loyalties and agendas within the group, and this delays the decision-making process. It has not been discussed openly what level of decision the group is attempting to reach; *i.e.,* a consensus or simply a majority agreement. A consensus would be more desirable, since this would imply the willingness of each person to give the decision a try. If a consensus is required, that is, support by all the group members for a particular decision, the best solution might not always be chosen. The criteria for acceptance can interfere with the criteria for quality. It is possible, however, that a group can produce a high-quality decision by consensus. This takes much time and energy (Wilson and Kneisl, 1979). Part of the reason a staff group may find that such a tedious process is that many of them look for high-quality consensus and find they must sacrifice swiftness to accomplish this.

Strategies for Dealing with Conflict

Types of Conflict

In those groups where the task is impeded by the inability of the group to function with existing conflict, there are several methods for resolving such conflict. The preceding paragraphs have focused on a group's decision-making process where the attempt is to allow individuality to be part of the group's mode for decision-making. At times, individual differences will overwhelm the group and impede its ability to take action. Conflict within a group can exist on three levels: *intrapersonal, interpersonal,* and *interorganizational.*

Intrapersonal conflict generally relates to a person's role fit. The perception one has of what is expected in a particular role and the actual expectations for the self to perform and reach certain goals must mesh. These two sets of expectations may be in conflict and lead one to exhibit signs of stress and anxiety (Booth, 1982). Strategies for conflict resolution do not deal with intrapersonal conflict. Generally, individual counseling or problem-solving is appropriate for someone experiencing role conflict. Certainly, such individual conflict can spill over into a group to which the person belongs and may manifest itself as resistance to group goals, as parataxic distortion or transference reactions, as withdrawal from the group, and any number of other maladaptive behaviors. Chapter Three dealt with some of this material, and future chapters will also focus on intrapersonal conflict as it manifests itself in the group.

Interpersonal conflict may be caused by an existing intrapersonal conflict that spills over onto relationships with others. If one is feeling hurt, guilty, stressed, or another emotion due to one's difficulty in role performance, the individual may let some of these feelings affect relationships with other group members. Anger or other expressions of conflict directed at another group member may be the result of parataxic distortion where another member's behavior triggers feelings one has left over from a past relationship. Yalom (1975) talked about the mirror reaction, in which a person who is trying to suppress a personal trait he or she does not like sees this same trait in another person and unconsciously reacts negatively to that person. An individual may project some of his or her own but disowned attributes onto others in the group and then feel anger at these individuals. Members in group often come with different life experiences, outlooks, and so forth, thus adding to the likelihood of conflict (Yalom, 1975). Difficulties in communicating, caused by a breakdown somewhere within the message unit, may also cause interpersonal conflict (Booth, 1982). See Chapter One for a review of this process.

Interpersonal conflict can be of value in a psychotherapy group in helping members learn more about their own interpersonal and internal processes. Yalom (1975) described the conflict between two group members as useful if integrated appropriately into the members' experiences. He noted that, when people are angry with one another, that can mean they are important to one another and take each other seriously. It is most likely that unresolved interpersonal conflict will exist in almost any group (Reusch, 1972; Yalom, 1975). This is highly possible if some of the conflict is covert and remains so due to the group's avoidance of such latent material. If the conflict is preventing the group from getting its work done, or it has become unproductive for the individual's learning, it must be resolved. Chapter Eleven will discuss conflict resolution in interpersonal situations.

Interorganizational conflict, or the conflict between groups or subgroups, occurs most frequently in settings where the bureaucracy is greatest and where groups exist with each other in interdependent positions. The activities of one or more groups or subgroups directly affect another group's ability to attain goals (Booth, 1982). In this situation, conflict resolution, or the elimination of the obstacles between these groups that are preventing the realization of the group's goals, is necessary. The rest of this chapter will focus on the various modes of conflict resolution used for this purpose.

Conflict Resolution

The four major modes of conflict resolution are confrontation, bargaining, force, or accommodation. Two other possibilities, avoidance or unilateral action, are ways of dealing with conflict but not in the sense of involving both groups in some type of action with which either has any control.

A unilateral action has one making a decision without input from anyone else in either group (Booth, 1982). If the President, involved in a conflict with Congress over possible action on a piece of legislation, ignores his Cabinet in making a decision, he has made a unilateral move. Obviously, the advantages of group decision-making have been lost.

Not addressing the conflict, or avoiding it, may just delay the inevitable and generally turns out to be very frustrating for one or both groups (Marriner, 1982; Booth, 1982). Frequently, one group outstrips the other in power and may then choose not to deal with the issue, leaving the other group at a loss. The most familiar example may be that conflict that occurs between a group of nurses and nursing service. If the nursing administration decides not to deal with the issue, the group of nurses is left without recourse (Booth, 1982). These nurses must wait until their power base increases before they can again present the issue. It is possible that, through this setback, the group becomes stronger, assuring that the nursing administration will not be able to avoid a conflict and its eventual resolution in some form in the future. The following four processes allow for some resolution of conflict:

1) Confrontation or Collaboration. This process is known as a win-win situation because both sides will most likely experience a satisfying solution (Marriner, 1982). Each group generally has equal motivation to reach some resolution, with an equal power base from which to work and the time to reach a long-term solution. The issue is understood by both groups, and a solution preferred by each side is discussed (Booth, 1982). Collaboration occurs in the form of problem-solving with each side attempting an assertive, cooperative approach (Marriner, 1982). The reader might recall the discussion in Chapter One on fair-fighting with couples. The process, although exaggerated in its steps because of the assumption that couples frequently do not listen to each other, is a form of confrontation for resolution of problem areas.

2) Compromise or Bargaining. This process is only partially satisfying to both sides and is considered a lose-lose situation, where the groups tend to have equal power bases, and expediency of resolution is important (Marriner, 1982). Booth (1982) suggested that bargaining was a skill underused by nurses in dealing with physicians. The power struggles that sometimes characterize physician-nurse interactions certainly might be postponed in favor of bargaining with each group getting some of what they want. Expanding the stereotyped picture of physician-nurse conflict to male-female conflict, one tends to think of the male group as having had more experience with bargaining as a way of settling conflict in male-dominated work groups of management and unions. I prefer to approach conflict with a physician group as being a unique process each time, since no group is exactly the same as another. I need to guard against becoming very subjective in my viewpoint of what I fantasize the physician group might want from the "nurses." Unfortunately, since I feel the need to address this in the chapter, I must have some emotions tied up with the issue of physician-nurse interactions.

Although bargaining is considered a lose-lose resolution, it is an important process when there are divergent goals or values existing between groups attempting to work together. The problem-solving approach with open communications as seen in collaboration is most effective when the conflict is around perceived rather than real incompatibilities of values or goals (How, 1980; Booth, 1982). How noted that groups might have difficulty identifying goal incompatibility or value differences because of the fear of censure by others. When arguments are restated several times, or the communications become derogatory or contain moral overtones, this is probably an indication of incompatibility and the likelihood that an optimal solution will not be found (How, 1980). Once incompatibility is acknowledged, the groups or subgroups can begin looking for a compromise that would be minimally acceptable by both sides. Sometimes priorities need to be identified in terms of what a group will not accept and what would be the consequences of not reaching a compromise, *i.e.,* not taking any action. Finally, there is the option of third-party intervention (How, 1980). How's discussion of the communication myth, that open communication leads to increased understanding and resolution, has application for any interaction. I tend to self-disclose and attempt the most open communication possible with most people. I have found that I am sometimes disappointed by the response of the other person who refuses to self-disclose or further the relationship between us. I have had to modify my approach and still feel uncomfortable knowing that some others do not value open communications as much as I do. It has been an important lesson to learn.

3) Force or Competition. The group with the most power uses that to gain the optimal goal at the other group's expense. This is a win-lose situation and obviously may lead to other conflict or problems in the future (Marriner, 1982; Booth, 1982). Recall the discussion on types of power in Chapter Four. Competitive power was described as having both positive and negative effects. If competition incites the other group to increase its power base for future encounters, the growth of this group might change the outcome of later conflicts. Certainly, the use of force to win a conflict in an interorganizational situation must be carefully considered.

4) Accommodation or Smoothing over a Conflict. This is another situation of unbalanced power in which the group with less power neglects its own needs to meet the needs of the other, or neither group acknowledges differences great enough to cause conflict. Conflict may be perceived as bad and its opposite, harmony, perceived as being most important (Marriner, 1982; Booth, 1982). Notice that accommodation is a process that does not lead to complete withdrawal from conflict resolution but greatly minimizes the differences between conflicting groups. Again, this appears to be a short-term solution for conflict resolution.

Conflict resolution is a process that most often uses a rational problem-solving mode to reach a conclusion. However, the intuitive mode may be very useful in helping groups come up with some creative approaches to resolution. With this idea, we have come full circle from looking at problem-solving as a way of generating alternatives to allow group decision-making actions and then considering these same processes in dealing with conflicting actions that groups wish to take in reaching their goals. Both rational and intuitive approaches may serve all the processes in group decision-making and conflict resolution.

REFERENCES

Arieti, S. *Creativity the Magic Synthesis.* New York: Basic Books, Inc., 1976.

Booth, R. "Conflict Resolution," *Nursing Outlook,* 30, no. 8 (Sept./Oct., 1982), 447-453.

Cooper, S. "Methods of Teaching Revisited: The Nominal Group Process," in *Journal of Continuing Education in Nursing,* 13, no. 2 (March/April, 1982), 38-39.

deChesnay, M. "Problem Solving in Nursing," in *Image: The Journal of Nursing Scholarship,* 15, no. 1 (Winter, 1983), 8-11.

Erikson, E. and S.V. Borgmeyer. "Simulated Decision-Making Experience via Case Analysis," *Journal of Nursing Administration,* 9, no. 5 (May, 1979), 10-15.

Foss, R. "Structural Effects in Simulated Jury Decision Making," *Journal of Personality and Social Psychology,* 40, no. 6 (June, 1981), 1055-1062.

Granvold, D. and G. Welch. "Structured Short-Term Group Treatment of Post Divorce Adjustment," *Educational Journal of Group Psychotherapy,* 29, no. 3 (July, 1979), 347-358.

How, M. "Conflict Resolution and the Communication Myth," *Nursing Outlook,* 28, no. 9 (Sept., 1980), 566-570.

Lippitt, R., J. Watson, and B. Westley. *The Dynamics of Planned Change.* New York: Harcourt, Brace and World, Inc., 1958.

Marriner, A. "Managing Conflict: Comparing Strategies and Their Uses," *Nursing Management,* 13, no. 6 (June, 1982), 29-31.

Nugent, P. "Management and Modes of Thought," *Journal of Nursing Administration,* 12, no. 2 (Feb., 1982), 19-25.

Reusch, J. *Disturbed Communications.* New York: W.W. Norton and Co., Inc., 1972.

Stafford, L. "On Promoting Creativity," *Journal of Nursing Education,* 20, no. 7 (Sept., 1981), 27-30.

Watzlawick, P. *The Language of Change.* New York: Basic Books, Inc., 1978.

Weeks, G. and L. L'Abate. *Paradoxical Psychotherapy: Theory and Practice with Individuals, Couples, and Families.* New York: Brunner/Mazel Publishers, 1982.

Wilson, H. and C. Kneisl *Psychiatric Nursing.* Menlo Park, CA: Addison-Wesley Publishing Co., 1979.

Yalom, I. *The Theory and Practice of Group Psychotherapy* (2nd ed.). New York: Basic Books, Inc., 1975.

FIGURE 8.1 THE RELATIONSHIP BETWEEN GROUP PROBLEM-SOLVING, GROUP DECISION-MAKING, AND CONFLICT RESOLUTION

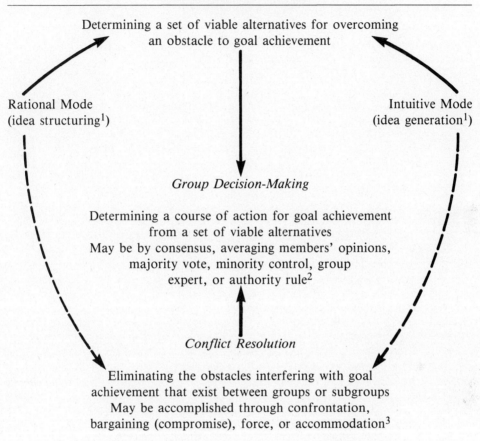

Group Problem-Solving

Determining a set of viable alternatives for overcoming an obstacle to goal achievement

Rational Mode
(idea structuring[1])

Intuitive Mode
(idea generation[1])

Group Decision-Making

Determining a course of action for goal achievement from a set of viable alternatives
May be by consensus, averaging members' opinions, majority vote, minority control, group expert, or authority rule[2]

Conflict Resolution

Eliminating the obstacles interfering with goal achievement that exist between groups or subgroups
May be accomplished through confrontation, bargaining (compromise), force, or accommodation[3]

– – – – – – Either mode may be useful in conflict resolution.

SOURCES

1. Patrick Nugent, "Management and Modes of Thought," *The Journal of Nursing Administration,* 12 (Feb., 1982), 19-25.
2. Holly Wilson and Carol Kneisl, *Psychiatric Nursing* (Menlo Park, CA: Addison-Wesley Publishing Co., 1979), pp. 443-444.
3. Rachel Booth, "Conflict Resolution," *Nursing Outlook,* 30 (Sept.-Oct., 1982), 447-453.

Supplemental Learning Activities

5-8

1. Identify the possible norms operating in a group in which you are currently a member (*e.g.,* a professional organization, a staff group, a social club, etc.).

2. The following is a descriptive account of a group meeting. It is a growth group made up of staff working in a mental health unit who have joined the group to learn more about their own process. Identify the following:

a) The characteristics or needs expressed by members that indicate the group's developmental stage
b) Current issues before the group
c) Overt themes and possible covert themes

Group Summary

Evan was new to group today but plunged right in to ask the group for feedback about himself. He had some difficulty getting out what he wanted to say, and he shared with us that he had rehearsed his presentation/questions to the group. The group was very slow to respond to Evan's request for feedback. When I asked him if he had gotten what he had expected, Evan said he had expected to hear how he should change, but he had not.

The group quickly moved to a discussion about being in the service. Kevin shared that he had initially thought of his time in the service as really not part of the business of his life as he perceived it for the future. He saw himself getting on with life after his time was over. "But this is life too," was his next comment. Many of the group members participated in this discussion. The question of whether to go for promotion or not and the problem of having to tell people what to do were topics discussed. The conclusion was that these problems were not peculiar to the service.

I suggested that perhaps the group's avoidance of their "here-and-now" process with each other had to do with a fear of finding out that we all did not always agree. Brad shared that he would feel hurt if someone said something to him that was negative or changed his image of that person. I asked the group to consider what it would be like to discover that not everyone in the room always felt the same way, got along, or agreed with what others said. Brad suggested that Evan, being new, might be a factor in the group's not discussing more issues.

Kevin began to disagree with Brad about the issue of positive strokes. Brad's position was that there was a lack of them among the staff.

Brad then talked about how he always had to take charge of getting people to group. Jim asked the group why we let Brad do this and how come it even needed to be done. I asked Brad how he let that happen since it sounded like he was saying he did not want this role. Kevin told Brad he appeared to take on too much worry, anxiety, and responsibility for getting things done. Brad shared that in the past he had gotten messed up because others did not follow through with their responsibilities.

Jim and Kevin both seemed to feel that Brad did too much or took on too much responsibility.

Group went over at least five minutes. I had a hard time getting Kevin and Brad to stop discussing the above issue.

3. Since the steps to rational problem-solving are so familiar and automatic to many people, it is only through analysis of a problem situation that one is able to clearly identify the process of rational problem-solving. The following paragraph describes a problem situation. Attempt to work with this situation using the analysis key presented below. The key is suggested as a reference for those readers who may want to teach problem-solving in a group. Adolescents might find such a didactic presentation helpful and less threatening than the confrontation they frequently receive from adults.

The Situation

The raise you expected in your job did not come through. You were counting on that extra income to pay for the portable TV set and stereo which you just bought on sale and charged. Now you have a bill for the merchandise but no income to pay for it. The sale was final, and the merchandise is not returnable. What can you do?

Analysis Key

Step I: Problem Identification and Definition

Identification: Anxiety, uneasiness, inability to act, awareness of an obstacle to doing something one had planned

Ask: What part do my actions play in not being able to do what I had planned? What part does the environment (other people or things) have to do with things not working out? It is important to identify the role of the "self" in the problem that is occurring.

Definition: Ask how often? when? where? with regard to the problem situation. Identify specific actions the "self" does to perpetuate the problem. Identify other actions (the environment) that occur which further clarify the problem situation.

Step II: Generating Alternatives or Solutions

Identify a measurable goal or outcome that should occur if the problem is solved.

Suggest several possible solutions, making sure that one does not confuse a solution with the goal.

Step III: Choosing the Solution

Develop a way to measure or rate each solution by objective criteria. Criteria could include: cost of implementation, time involved in implementation, unwanted consequences of the solution, degree of congruence with values or beliefs, difficulty of implementation, comfort level of implementation, and so forth.

Rate each possible solution using the criteria agreed upon. The best solution may not always be the one that is rated the highest on the objective criteria that have been chosen. Sometimes a person will choose the solution that fits the criteria most important to that individual, although other solutions may be meeting more of the objective criteria. Sometimes a person will choose a solution that is difficult to implement, but that will help that individual grow in some way. Solutions should always meet the goals the individual has for problem-solving.

Step IV: Implementing the Solution

List the actions necessary to carry out the chosen solution. It is best to be as specific as possible with each action to be taken. Consider other individuals whose actions are necessary for the implementation of the solution. If others are involved, the solution will depend on actions with which you may have no control. It is probably best to have as much control as possible over implementing a solution to your problem, because you can take responsibility for your own behavior.

Step V: Evaluating the Outcome

Has the problem situation changed so that you can accomplish your goals or at least identify that this problem is no longer an obstacle to goal attainment? Objective measure of problem-solving includes the following.

a) Look at the desired outcome/goal you wanted to reach by problem-solving.

b) What specific action can you observe about yourself or your environment (other people's behavior, events, etc.) that tell you your goal or expected outcome has or has not been reached?

c) Are there any unwanted consequences from the solution you used? How does this affect the outcome/goals you had for solving this problem?

If the solution implemented has not solved the problem or has caused too many unwanted consequences, systematically go through the first four steps in problem-solving to see if you need to revise or work any step over again.

4. Try solving the problem situation listed in Exercise 3 using the creative mode for problem-solving by engaging in a brainstorming activity. Compare the results and the process of each mode. Which mode feels most comfortable to you? Analyze the mode of thinking you use for daily problem-solving.

Part Two

The Practice of Group Process as a Therapeutic Agent for Change

Part Two focuses on the practice of group by the nurse leader in both client- and staff-centered groups. Having developed a theoretical and structural basis for this practice in Part One, Part Two looks at the process of engaging a variety of group populations and presents some techniques for advanced practice with group process elements. It is suggested that the reader use those parts of Section One or Two which fit particular practice needs. Section One will address the needs of those nurses who will be structuring supportive groups for clients and looks at how the nurse can facilitate group interaction between different staff/peer subgroups. Section Two offers material for the nurse who has had some group experience and wants to develop more specialized practice skills.

In an attempt to meet the needs of the advanced practitioner wishing to engage in the consultation or teaching of group process, a chapter focusing on these topics has been included. The novice group leader who is seeking some consultation may find this section useful for understanding the process from the point of view of the consultant.

Section One

Special Techniques
and Group Populations

Specific Experiential Techniques and Their Application 9

Although this chapter may be used as a recipe book of various experiential exercises designed to enhance the movement of a group or individual members towards goal attainment, the basic purpose of this material is to describe the process of using other than a verbal mode to facilitate cognitive, affective, and behavioral insights for the client. As a clinician, I find I have gone from grasping onto such techniques to ensure that "something" would "happen" in the group I was leading to allow experiential activities to "flow" into the group process as it seemed appropriate. Those times I have found it most appropriate to use experiential activities are: 1) to overcome a process that is blocking group movement; 2) to sharpen or clarify a specific process element; and 3) to create a process that will allow new growth within a group.

The novice group leader will frequently think of experiential techniques as existing alone or apart from the group's developing movement. Perhaps this is analogous to the nursing student who focuses on a particular technique, such as suctioning a tracheostomy or monitoring chest sounds. It is less likely that these measures will be conceptualized by the student as part of a particular client's total nursing needs, since the performance of the techniques are specific actions the student must learn to do. The experienced nurse will perform such actions when her assessment of the client's condition tells her this would add to the well-being of the individual and not just when a nursing procedural manual suggests they be done. The novice group leader might be tempted to read this chapter as a procedural manual. Certainly, it is only through some "hands-on" experience that one becomes comfortable with specific group techniques. It is helpful to observe an experienced group leader or to work as a coleader with someone who has used such techniques before. If the reader will focus on the process of assessing the readiness for using experiential techniques and the purpose for their use, the tendency to learn the "how to" or the procedure, only, may be avoided. This chapter will discuss the process of incorporating experiential exercises into the group's movement. Specific exercises with which I have worked or observed being used by other group leaders will be presented. Since there are endless ways to engage a group experientially, it would be impossible to discuss all the techniques available. A more helpful plan seems to be to share those that have worked for me. The exercises have been classified according to their purpose within the group.

━━━━━━ The Process of Experiential-Based Learning ━━━━━━

An experiential exercise is any process done alone or with other individuals that promotes the awareness and expression of "here-and-now" feelings, "ahas" (cognitive insight in a "here-and-now" context), and actions that signal behavioral changes.

Very often, another medium of expression other than the verbal mode is used, although verbalizing is a part of most experiential exercises during the time when the participants share their "ahas" verbally with each other. This might be called processing, feedback, sharing, or another term peculiar to the particular exercise.

Experiential learning that results from a particular exercise involves a universal set of steps that one can identify when any such learning takes place. The following is a brief description of these steps (Shropshire, 1981). Leader preparation as well as cautions are discussed later in the chapter.

1) The experience phase consists of the actual exercise in which the group or individual members participate. The novice group leader will be most concerned about this part of the activity because this requires the leader to know how to facilitate the actions necessary for the experience to occur. However, this is the most unpredictable part of the exercise, because each group or individual participating does so a little differently. The leader must be prepared to handle resistances, anxieties of the participants, steps that do not work as well *in vivo* as they sound on paper, and so forth.

2) Publishing feelings, the next step, may actually occur simultaneously with the performance of the activity, or it may occur only at the end. Participants share their reactions to what they have just experienced. This is often a spontaneous communication and is not complete for the person, since the reaction to the experience has not been put into perspective with the individual's "self." Recall the discussion of the Gestalt experience. The awareness and heightening of the "figure" does not make a completed gestalt. It is not until the individual has fit the figure back into the "ground" or the whole self and has done something with this new awareness that there is closure. The initial reactions participants have to an experiential activity do not provide closure for them.

3) Processing is the "key" to experiential learning (Shropshire, 1981, p.6). It is here that the "ahas" occur for the individual or for the group as a whole. New insights about oneself or one's interactions with others is part of a cognitive process of learning. Yalom (1975) called this motivational insight, because an emotional experience has led to the individual's understanding why he or she behaves in a certain way. It is interesting to note that experiential learning incorporates the affective, behavioral, and cognitive modes of experience to facilitate growth for the individual or the group. The activity demands an affective response. This leads to new behaviors or to a sharpening of certain behaviors that heighten the affective experience. One's cognitive mode then processes it all. Processing involves a group discussion of the activity and one's reactions and behaviors to it.

4) Generalizing allows the individual to translate the experience to his or her world outside of the group. If someone has just discovered that pressure to compete with others leads to feelings of inadequacy and interpersonal withdrawal, other competitive situations in one's life will now have more meaning, and one's behaviors around these situations can be more easily understood. If the processing in Step Three has produced a collective awareness and understanding about a particular piece of group process, generalization can still occur for the individual. If the group has discovered it is not cohesive because of a lack of trust between members, each individual can begin to think about his or her trust level with others and how that occurs outside of the group. Since most therapeutic groups provide for a social environment with

member interactions being similar to one's interpersonal experiences outside the group, it should be quite easy to generalize about one's learning.

5) Once a connection has been made by the individual to one's world outside the group, the person can start applying what he or she has learned to extragroup experiences. The person who feels a lack of cohesion among her peers at work can take a look at how trusting the individuals in this group might be. Perhaps she would like to take the risk to demonstrate more trust with one or more of her peers. The application phase is one of planning to initiate new actions in one's world outside the group.

Purposes for Experiential Learning Activities

I use experiential activities when one or more of the following conditions exist in the group.

1) There appears to be a block for one or more members or for the group as a whole in their movement towards the group's or the individual's goals. Blocks may result from an individual or the group using one or more defenses to prevent awareness for themselves or others. Intellectualization is frequently a defense which members use to avoid feelings that might eventually lead to motivational insight. Intellectualization allows one to separate a painful emotion from the event to which it belongs. Rational explanations make it easy for the person to avoid the feeling state of the situation in which they have been involved (Wilson and Kneisl, 1983). Recall the discussion in Chapter Three of intellectualization as a form of resistance to "here-and-now" feelings. The example given there illustrates the process of intellectualization. A group is very good at using this defense as a collective body. One person may focus her anger on the system she is in, making rational comments about the bureaucracy for which she works. Others may become more global and talk about the political system, a particular government agency, or even the garage mechanic's attempts to undermine the state inspection system. The group has now stopped working on its goals and is intellectualizing. The member originally bringing up the negative emotion of anger has no opportunity to deal with her feeling in a satisfactory manner. The group has colluded with her (probably not within conscious awareness) to keep the negative feeling at a safe distance.

I find that a similar process can occur when I allow people to verbalize too much. This leads to rumination instead of active problem-solving. A member may start talking about his difficulty with the chemotherapy he is taking and might begin to problem-solve about this. However, if he becomes aware of his hopelessness around his illness, he may slip into a verbal rumination of his problems. To let him continue would not be helpful for him or the rest of the group. Frequently, such ruminations are catching, and other members of the group will become verbally repetitious without direction.

A colleague and I recently started a group for clients who are at the stage of their life to start working on their life review. The life review is an intrapsychic process in which there is a gradual return to consciousness of past life experiences, especially those which still are causing some conflicts for the individual. It is an attempt at resolution of these conflicts in preparation for one's death. Reminiscing helps one perform the life review (Blackman, 1980). We had planned to structure many of the groups around some experiential exercises that would promote this internal process through some reminiscing and some more action-oriented exercises. The group did a pencil-and-paper exercise to draw the most important event in their lives, the most disappointing, and so forth. The presentation to the group of each person's individual drawings led to a discussion of the military, since these group members were all veterans of World War II. The reminiscing was very appropriate initially, each group member sharing experiences of combat, his familiarity of the aircraft used on the various fronts, and so forth. One member became preoccupied with his combat experiences, and he began repeating these experiences over and over without coming to any conclusion about their meaning for him. Other members started engaging in the same process. At this point in the group's interaction, the reminiscing had ceased to be therapeutic, since the ruminations were preventing members from resolving any feelings they had about their combat experiences. One member had gotten emotionally ill during his initial enlistment and could not relate to the others' experiences. The group's ruminations prevented him from talking about how it felt not to be in combat or sharing feelings with the other members. The group leader might attempt to stop the ruminations and resolve some feelings around the process the group had just experienced—a sense of isolation by one member and the others not being aware of how their behavior was affecting him or their own resolution of feelings. This would require the group to move from one style of verbalizing to another that could allow awareness and problem-solving to take place. Sometimes that is hard for group members to do. I have found that to move into an experiential activity is more effective at breaking the ruminating behaviors and making the process that has just occurred more real for the group.

One exercise that might be helpful is to have the member who felt isolated from the group actually isolate himself physically. He would have to experience physical distance from the group, helping him to better understand and express the psychological distance he was feeling. We will talk more about this exercise and others that use kinetic techniques to promote motivational awareness.

Another instance where experiential learning might be used is to compensate for a block in the group's cognitive abilities. For a group of clients that are cognitively impaired, such as those made up of aging clients that need structure in the areas of memory, judgment, and so forth, reality orientation exercises provide such a structure (Tappen and Touhy, 1983). A group of developmentally disabled clients would also experience some cognitive impairment and would do best with kinetic therapies that focus on simple physical activities that promote awareness of feelings. The cognitively ordered verbal procedures of most groups are also too frustrating for adolescents who are more action-oriented (Winn, 1982). The adolescent is still developing his cognition and needs more concrete structure, thus making kinetic techniques helpful.

2) A current group state exists which needs to be emphasized, sharpened, or clarified. Frequently, this will involve making a phase of the group's development more a part of the group members' awareness. If the group is in the first stage of development, the issue of trust is an important dynamic operating in the group. Although the members are not verbal about their lack of trust with each other, the fact that there is a hesitancy to self-disclose and take other risks of one's person in the group testifies to the need for developing trust with each other. There are many experiential exercises that meet this need.

The development of cohesion is a normal part of the group's movement. Although it is unwise to try to move the group through its stages faster than its readiness to do so, there is a place for exercises that are timed to coincide with the group's readiness for a certain phase of its development. The experiential learning that takes place is merely highlighting the current process occurring in the group. It is the leader's responsibility to know when the group is beginning to experience a certain stage of development. We will talk extensively about cautions for the group leader later in the chapter. Experiential learning activities may be developed for any stage of the group's development.

Experiential learning also helps to heighten a moment of motivational insight or a process element occurring at that moment in the group. The family group provides a wealth of process in which experiential activities are particularly appropriate. The positions of closeness or estrangement, dependency or interdependence, and so forth, as well as the hierarchical position of family members within the family system and in relationship to outside systems, may be highlighted in a family sculpture. Each individual forms early kinesic or muscular images of himself and his identity as a part of a family. Kinetic techniques allow the individual, in physically placing himself and his family members in positions that represent their roles in the family, to be free to change old images and experiment with how new roles in the family would feel (Winn, 1982). Thus, a family who verbally talks about feelings of estrangement between its members will be able to check out the truth to this feeling with a physical sculpture. Frequently, I have seen families who discover that the overt feelings are not always the ones that show up in the sculpture. One family I worked with did a sculpture in which Dad placed his wife and their son close to each other, although the conversation in family meetings had centered around the son "getting his act together" so he could be independent of Mom and Dad and out of the family system. Each family member has a chance to make the family constellation any way this person sees it or would like it to be. Most often, a family will do several sculptures, showing the current state of their relationships with each other and then what they would like the family relationship to actually be. This experiential exercise definitely highlights what can sometimes be a hidden dynamic within a group. Exercises that point out covert themes are helpful if the theme is something the group is able to accept and attempt to work through. The reader will recall that many covert group themes are never actually brought to the awareness of the group. The group leader must decide what processes are therapeutically safe to highlight for the group before attempting the experiential exercise that might lead to such awareness.

   3) There is a need to create a new process within the group, either to facilitate the group's goal attainment or to handle an unexpected event within the group. Occasionally, a very devastating or scary event will take place within the group, and an experiential activity facilitates the resolution of the feelings that have been created by the earlier process. Just verbal exchanges may not completely work through the process, since defenses such as intellectualizing are available to group members to take the edge off of the uncomfortable feelings. In the senior life review group, one meeting was spent talking about suicide, since one member was currently suicidal and another member had not resolved his depression over the suicide of his son. The group had begun with an exercise about hands and what emotions they depicted as expressed through a series of pictures. The rest of the group members tried to give

words of comfort to the other two, but most of the group began to withdraw verbally after seeing this as not working. A sense of aloneness pervaded the group. It seemed appropriate to do something collectively as a group with our hands to facilitate a sense of closeness and caring. We decided to hold hands and silently pass along a "good thought" by squeezing the hand of the person next to each of us. Not only did it help deal with an unexpected group process, but it moved the group further towards one of its goals which was to facilitate a supportive relationship with one another. The experiential activity did this more succinctly, yet appropriately, than would a discussion.

Cautions for the Group Leader

As mentioned earlier in the chapter, experiential learning techniques require an experienced group leader who is prepared to handle the developing process of such activities. It is not enough to know what steps one needs to take to perform a certain activity. The group leader is introducing new process and must be able to handle the outcomes of this process with the group. I learned to use experiential techniques by trying them out only after experiencing many of them as a member of a training group. It is suggested that the nurse leader learn to intervene experientially by going through the five steps of the experiential learning model as a group member first. One may do this also while coleading a group with a more experienced leader.

The American Nurses' Association's Congress for Nursing Practice refers to the practice of psychiatric nursing as not only a scientific approach embracing the theories of human behavior, but as an artistic endeavor involving the personal use of the self (Wilson and Kneisl, 1983). This personal element, I like to think, characterizes the approach all nurse group leaders take, using the personal part of the self to empathize with the group members enough to sense when another process must be introduced into the group to facilitate the group's learning. Just as the nurse makes an individual intervention with a client who has just been told about his terminal illness, so this same nurse needs to sense the appropriateness of making a group intervention to support the members' needs to grow, either by resolving an issue, making a feeling state more prominent, or providing an atmosphere that feels safe for growth to occur. The process in the group helps the nurse leader decide what intervention is appropriate. Very often, an experiential activity will serve the purpose nicely. Certainly, there should be a balance between verbal communications in the group and more action-oriented activities. I have not experienced a group that could operate without a little of both. Even a psychotherapeutic insight-oriented group that generally relies on the clients to be verbal to facilitate motivational insight uses some experiential activities when members touch each other or allow silence to exist to facilitate new process in the group. Experiential activities need not be fancy to be helpful to the group's process. The following are a list of cautions the group leader needs to understand to successfully use experiential learning activities.

1) Assessing the Group or Individual Need Accurately. If the group leader follows the conditions under which experiential activities may be helpful, as discussed earlier, he or she will know if an activity should be tried. Activities are done as early as the first group meeting to facilitate a stage of the group's development. Members who know each other's names the first group meeting and something about each person might feel more secure in attending group the next time. I often ask a group what they would like to do when it appears there is an impasse or the verbalizations are feeling repetitious and boring. If I am not sure an activity would be appropriate or wanted by the group members, I will share with them my perceptions of the group's process, offer some suggestions, and let the group decide. How much decision-making the members are able to do depends on their ego strength. Even a group of very regressed clients should have a chance to verbalize how they feel about an exercise. I usually decide for a group when I know the group definitely needs an experiential activity to help the process along. It is only when I am unsure that I ask for input from the group. I use their perceptions to validate my own.

Some activities should come from the group members themselves. An art therapist worked with a group of very depressed clients who were required to attend her group in order to be exposed to some different stimuli. However, they did not have to participate if they did not want to do so. In fact, it is not possible to force a depressed person to participate. The therapist initiated several different activities including movement to music and poetry reading hoping to get the clients involved. Eventually, several clients wanted to select the records to be played and to structure their own movements to the music (Wadeson, 1982). A group of authors suggested that, very often, the activities selected for seniors are condescending and controlling, sometimes furthering the infantization of the older adult. Therefore, child-like activities should always come as suggestions from the group members, thereby ensuring that the members were ready to do such things (Tappen and Touhy, 1983). The group members are the leader's most accurate source to assess the need for experiential activities.

2) Matching the Exercise with the Presenting Need. A lengthy discussion of specific exercises that work for specific needs the group might have is discussed in the next section of the chapter. It is important to remember that the leader should only choose those exercises which he or she feels skilled enough to facilitate (Shropshire, 1981). The group cannot profit from a poorly led experiential activity. I would feel more comfortable not dealing with a group process experientially if I could not determine how I would facilitate a particular exercise. Verbally intervening in the process might take longer but would be the best choice if the leader did not feel skilled in doing an experiential exercise.

3) Understanding the Purpose and Goals for the Exercise. Most exercises have identified outcomes that should occur if performed properly with a group that needs the outcome that the exercise is designed to produce. For example, some exercises promote trust among the group members. The blind walk is an example of this. Pairs work together with one person being blindfolded and the other person guiding the first around. The partners then switch roles to give each member a chance to experience the blind walk. Obviously, trust is required between the pair for the two to get through the exercise without trauma. Through the process of two people spending time together, some self-disclosure might occur between them. This is not a specific outcome for this exercise but a byproduct that can occur. Another result could be a decrease in the level of trust between partners if either member is not ready to trust the other. Experiential activities are chosen for the process or outcome they facilitate. An exercise in frustration may be just for that purpose, to have the group experience a frustrating process. Frequently, training in small group dynamics for managers or others in areas of industry consists of many experiential exercises designed to point out certain dynamics that may occur in a group. These exercises are process- rather than outcome-oriented. The outcome is to have an experience with a particular group process, such as a *laissez-faire* style of leadership. How the group deals with the process they are experiencing is their learning. In the experiential learning activities that follow in another section of the chapter, expected processes and outcomes will be discussed.

4) Expecting the Unexpected and Using These Outcomes Adaptively. There are times when even a correctly assessed need for a particular exercise leads to an unexpected outcome. One member may react with more feeling or with different feelings than is the norm. In the exercise we used with the senior group, where they were to talk about any feelings or associations they had to pictures of hands doing different things, I never expected the conversation to focus on the suicidal ideation of one member. I was aware that another member had lost his son to suicide by a self-inflicted gunshot wound, but I also knew he was well-defended against talking about this. I do not think that he would have if the other member had not unexpectedly focused on the hand with the gun and shared with the group how he often thought about this. The desired outcome of the exercise had been for the group to share some "here-and-now" feelings by reacting to the pictures and perhaps to reminisce, about some period in their lives, what some of these feelings brought to their awareness. The member who talked about suicide certainly shared "here-and-now" feelings, although they were more intense than I expected from a group who had only met three other times. One unexpected outcome was that the member whose son had shot himself shared indirectly how suicide affects those family members surviving. He did this by telling the other member that it would be very hard on his family if he shot himself. An unexpected outcome for the group was the successful management of some very frightening feelings and a resultant increase in cohesiveness among the members. As we closed the meeting, one client reminded the group about confidentiality. This was the first time a member had initiated a discussion of the group's norms. This said to me that he had some identification with the group and was concerned that all the members share his investment in the norms.

The group leader needs to stay flexible about the outcome. If something happens that was not supposed to occur, the leader needs to go with the new process. The group has a need to deal with whatever comes up, so the outcome that never materializes does not mean the exercise was not helpful for the group. I consider unexpected outcomes as more information for me, the group leader, as to what the group needs. If an exercise produces no outcome except resistance, that is an important piece of information about the group and is "food" for some work with the members. One may not finish the exercise or may have to do something different with the exercise than was planned, but this makes the activity just as valid. In our group, we ended up focusing on one member's pain and did not have an opportunity to pick up on some of the statements by members that could have led to some reminiscing. That does not matter. The leader should come to a group expecting the unexpected and having a variety of ideas about the possible unexpected outcomes for the exercise. Taking her cues from the members, the leader should be ready to change the focus as necessary (Wadeson, 1982).

5) Preparing the Individual or Group Sufficiently but Not so Much That the Outcome is Defined. One should give explicit, clear instructions to the group about what they are expected to do. The steps the members are going to have to perform must be clearly defined before the exercise starts (Shropshire, 1981). However, an outcome that is defined for the group ahead of time takes away the spontaneity of the activity and precludes the occurrence of any other process that might be just as important or more so for the group's learning. If we had told the senior group that they should try to reminisce as feelings became apparent to them when they looked at the pictures of hands, we would not have heard about one member's current pain, nor would we have had the opportunity as a group to support this member in his pain and come closer together in the process. It takes practice to describe an activity to a group without programming them for a specific outcome. New exercises might be tried on one's colleagues initially to see if the instructions are clear but do not reveal the expected outcome.

6) Timing the Exercises for the Most Adaptive Outcomes. If a group is not ready to self-disclose, planning an exercise with self-disclosure as the goal will not facilitate this process. In fact, the group might become frightened about such an expectation and express this by getting angry at the leader or joining together in resistance maneuvers. Either process is still very workable, but it will not accomplish the specific outcome for which the exercise was designed. One can always have the group examine their response to an exercise that did not work. If the timing was wrong, both the group and the leader can learn something from this.

I used a self-disclosure exercise for a laboratory class session on group dynamics. The nursing students were divided into several smaller work groups which had been together since the beginning of the quarter. The groups had been formed to give the students an experience in being part of a small group and studying their dynamics. I had decided that most of the groups would be ready to experience some self-disclosure. One group had not moved far enough into the working stage to feel comfortable with the exercise I had given them, although each group could do as little or as much self-disclosure as it wished. This group was apparently even threatened by that choice, and expressed some really negative feedback to me about how I should not expect this of them. I had them analyze their process with me and with each other. Although their group process did not go in the way I had planned, I perceived them as learning something from this exercise. I also learned that I cannot just go by a timetable of when I think a group's development indicates a readiness for a new experience. I need to have more information directly from the group's process to determine the stage of its development.

Spontaneity is also important for timing. The more spontaneous an activity, the more successful the process usually is for the group (Shropshire, 1981). Just as one can introduce an activity before the group is ready, one can also be late for a process or do too much preparation for it. I find I can be most spontaneous with an activity when I have tried the activity before, know how to use it, and know what the outcomes most likely will be. I do not start doing activities on the spur of the moment until after I have a good understanding of how to predict a group's readiness level for a certain activity. As a cotherapist working with another group leader, I feel that it is helpful to observe the more experienced person introducing some spontaneous activities. The novice leader might try thinking of times when activities would be helpful and test out these perceptions with one's coleader to see if they were accurate.

7) Allowing Sufficient Time for Processing the Outcome. Processing is the most important step in experiential-based learning. Once feelings have been shared in reaction to the exercise, the leader has the responsibility of helping members make sense of what they experienced. I do not feel comfortable ending this phase until I sense there is no unfinished business (see Chapter Three) that the group or an individual member needs to handle. Sometimes an activity will create anxiety for members, and this may not be alleviated until those members have pondered their feelings or even discussed them in subsequent groups. I depend on the individual to let me know if he or she does or does not need any more processing at the moment. The senior group which my colleague and I have been coleading closed a meeting with many members feeling unsettled about the "heavy" discussion we had experienced together. As part of our processing that group, we had members talk about how it was for each of them, and we acknowledged their feelings of helplessness, validating those feelings as being reasonable and understandable. Quite a while before the group was due to be over, I began asking people to talk about how they were feeling and had them try to make sense of that. I feel strongly that group should stop at the time it is scheduled to be over, since not keeping to this rule encourages members to introduce heavy material at the end of the group and control the group's time in that way. One way of handling the need for more processing time is to acknowledge this with the group and problem-solve about what to do. Getting the group involved in this may help the members' sense of relatedness with one another. Empathizing with the anxiety members feel at not finishing their processing is also important. Working with experiential activities, the leader begins to accurately assess the amount of time needed for processing. I usually try to err on the side of having too much time rather than too little.

Rogers (1970, p.57) suggested that the leader make process comments "sparingly," since such comments make the group members self-conscious and give them a feeling of being watched. Feelings that come from the members about their experiences and that are then processed by them are more natural and also more important (Rogers, 1970). The leader also needs to be aware of the importance of providing a climate of acceptance for the discussion of feelings and processing, even if some members have minority opinions (Shropshire, 1981). The reader is reminded that modeling by the group leader, with regard to expression of feelings, "ahas," and so forth, in a personal way with material that is appropriate to share with the group, is a good way to help the members begin processing.

8) Retaining One's Objectivity as the Facilitator. Carl Rogers (1970) noted that the group leader should not avoid sharing personal feelings if these feelings are affecting the facilitation of the group. He felt that this might actually help the group become more expressive, but cautioned that personal problems should not be shared if they are severe or in any way detrimental to the group. If the group leader does share personal material, it is helpful to have a coleader who may remain objective to oversee the effect of the self-disclosure on the group members. I participate in the experiential exercise with a group when I feel it would be helpful to model and share my humanness with them. I am usually familiar enough with the exercise that I know what my responses have been, what my feelings are, and what all this means for me. Therefore, I have already processed and can remain objective while the group processes. There are certainly times when I choose not to be part of the process of the activity, such as when I anticipate the group will have a particularly strong emotional reaction to the exercise. I want to be able to remain objective to help the group process. The more I know about the outcome of an activity, the better I can anticipate the reactions to it. It helps to have been a participant in the activity at least once before facilitating it, but it is probably not wise to participate the first time one does facilitate. The leader needs to observe the group and be ready for unexpected outcomes, and this requires objectivity.

A Potpourri of Experiential Techniques

The following are a sampling from among the almost endless possibilities for experiential-based learning activities. They are organized according to the major outcome one might expect in using them with a group. Many yield more than one outcome affecting the group's process. It is possible, for example, that heightening awareness of one's own process and that of the group's might also lead to conflict resolution as two people in the group use this knowledge in their interpersonal exchanges. Increasing the group's trust level may also make it easier for the group to begin to self-disclose. Psychodrama, a specific technique, has a very personal effect on the protagonist but will also stir up feelings in the audience that may lead to those members wanting to work through some individual dynamics.

I have chosen to discuss those activities with which I am personally familiar. There are numerous bibliographical sources of experientially based learning activities. Another source is one's personal creativity and observing others at work in groups. Many of the activities presented here may originally have been in a different form and have been tailored to fit my personal needs as a group leader. Whenever possible, I will give the original source. Most experiential activities have a touch of the group leader's personality. I would have difficulty doing an activity with which I would be uncomfortable as a participant. Therefore, I choose techniques that I have actually experienced or could see myself experiencing.

Warm-Up Exercises

Generally, these are used as ice-breakers, much as some people use ice-breakers at a party. Support groups are frequently made up of people that have never been in a group before and who may be feeling some anxiety on attending their first meeting. The psychotherapy group usually works best with its members having to deal with some anxiety. However, a support group has as one of its goals the alleviation of the members' anxiety. Being able to dialogue with the other group members in a nonthreatening way is important. Therefore, I often use get-acquainted warm-up exercises to help the members of a support group feel more comfortable with each other. The adolescent group is another appropriate place for action warm-up activities. Physical activity is a coping mechanism for adolescents, since it gives them a sense of control over their environment (Langford, 1981). Warm-up exercises are often action-oriented. Since the peer group is so important for the adolescent, a technique for making that peer group get acquainted is important.

A very simple warm-up that prepares a group to be more in their Child (see Chapter Two) and, therefore, more ready to experience and share feelings, is batting at balloons to keep them up in the air. This is done as a group with the members usually bumping into each other as they try to keep the balloons aloft. A group of nursing students and I tried this with staff at the hospital where the students were having their mental health clinical experience. The staff was made up of adults of all ages who were initially very resistant to the activity. At our gentle insistence, they tried it and ended up laughing with us. The students then presented an experiential inservice.

Rogers (1970) suggested an activity in which group members mill around introducing themselves with a handshake, eye contact, and first names. They must then stop using words but continue with the other two actions. Finally, they must stop shaking hands and find another way to say "hello." I would not use this activity with a group whose members might not feel safe enough with the demands for so much nonverbal behavior. A growth group might respond to this activity without the anxiety that a support group would have, since the expectation for joining a growth group is that one will be willing to try new experiences.

I have done a variation of this activity incorporating some nonverbal behaviors but also giving the members a physical prop for support. This activity originally came from Jones and Pfeiffer's *A Handbook of Structured Activities for Human Relations Training* (La Jolla, CA: University Associates, 1979). These handbooks are published each year and contain some excellent suggestions for experiential learning. I generally modify them slightly to fit my personal group needs. In the activity, the group members are given paper and crayons and asked to put on the paper something that is personal about themselves which they are willing to share with others. I have them either pin the paper to themselves or tie it around their neck with string and mingle with each other showing their picture but not talking. They are then to select three other people (or however many the leader would choose for a small group) with whom to have a verbal dialogue to exchange information about themselves. The small group may then join another group of equal size and repeat the process until all group members have met each other.

Verbal introduction between pairs is another method for warming up. After the partners meet, each can then introduce the other to the larger group. Verbal introductions in which each person shares with the group his or her nickname and its origin is both fun and informative. I did this for the first time at a church planning workshop. Even though we all knew each other slightly, sharing nicknames was a unique way to present a different side of each of us to the others.

As a warm-up for an adolescent group, the members pair off, take five minutes to share personal interests, and then join into groups of four with each person introducing his or her partner to the group. The person doing the introducing stands behind his partner and assumes this person's identity in a roleplay (Langford, 1981). Adolescents like to roleplay, but being able to "hide" behind the person one is roleplaying is less scary or risky. The adolescent may roleplay himself as a variation to this. The members may also be asked to put themselves in a particular body position that tells the rest of the group something about each of them.

Exercises to Heighten Awareness of One's Own Process in a Group

Kinetic Exercises

Experiential awareness leads to insights which are more powerful than those that one could gather from an interpretive comment (Schachter, 1982). Experiencing says more than talking. Kinetic psychotherapy uses social interactive games that appear to be nonthreatening but that actually stir up those emotions most often present in a threatening real-life situation (Schachter, 1982). Games, although a natural as therapy for adolescents and children, allow adults to experience regression of the ego and the emergence of a more creative self for problem-solving. Games offer a permissible atmosphere to try out new discoveries of the self and new behaviors. As activities for therapeutic group experiences they need to be easy to learn and have outcomes appropriate to the goals for the group (Nickerson and O'Laughlin, 1982).

An example of a kinetic therapy game is called "freeze tag." One person in the group must try to "freeze" the others by touching them with a plastic ball. If the person is to get free again, he must ask another unfrozen member to tag him. The participants experience needing to ask for help from each other. The group leader observes the action and stops it when she senses the need for members to publicize their feelings. Individuals are encouraged to share any feelings directed at another person immediately with that person (Schachter, 1982). There are endless possibilities for games which stimulate one's emotions in a safe therapeutic atmosphere.

Movement Therapy

The process of placing members in a physical space that fits their psychological relationship to the group uses the principles of kinetic psychotherapy. Placing a member who is feeling isolated outside the group and having him "break in" to the group's circle of members who have joined hands is helpful to focus on the feelings of isolation and rejection. Very often, the group will let someone break the circle and come in without much difficulty, because rejecting someone is uncomfortable for the group. Family sculpture is another form of kinetic exercises. I have used several movement techniques I learned in a series of inservices given by a movement therapist at the hospital in which I worked. Movement therapy is always done to music. Very often, the rhythm of the music adds to the emotions experienced by the group. The movements are not organized as games but are more free activities that individuals could experience singly or, at times, with a partner or a group of people. The solitary or dyad activities are done in a group. One might compare the solitary activities to those which occur when toddlers experience parallel play with each other. Each toddler is doing a solitary activity but seems to take comfort in the presence of the other children also engaged in solitary play.

Movements might include a series of fantasies in which the individual must climb in or out of something, assume a body position to fit with one's fantasy or one's feeling, and so forth. Other solitary activities include exploring space with one's body and keeping one's eyes closed while reacting physically to such words as *pound, scream, wiggle,* and *scratch.* Dyads may mold each other into a sculpture. The one being molded must submit to his partner's placement of his body.

Passing on a movement is a popular exercise for a group. Each person takes a turn being "it" and must decide on a movement that he or she wants to do to the music. The rest of the group copies the action. As a new person is tagged, that member now has the leadership of the group and must think of a movement. Other group activities include lifting one member and rocking this person back and forth, holding hands together and melting to the floor, and sitting in a circle and throwing pillows back and forth to one another.

Another type of movement therapy is improvisation. This is a process of free association in which the person allows his or her body to physically move in an unrestricted, spontaneous way. The movement promotes awareness of emotions that may have been repressed. Publishing one's reaction verbally then leads to some processing of the activity and some new insights (Balazs, 1982).

Behavioral Rehearsal-Roleplaying

In Chapter Four, behavioral rehearsal was discussed as a way of trying out new behaviors for one's interactions with others. Behavioral rehearsal allows an individual to try out more than one role or way of interacting and to, therefore, increase the repertoire of possible responses to a situation (Reakes, 1979). For the individual, taking on the role of another person or taking on a new role for himself may evoke new feeling states or old ones that had been repressed if the roleplay is directed towards that end. In a group, behavioral rehearsal allows members to vicariously experience every other member's role response to a problem (Reakes, 1979). Roleplay used as an experiential activity may be structured as a sociodrama or a psychodrama.

A sociodrama describes an interpersonal situation that depicts the portrayal of a set of roles common to a group of people. For the adolescent, this might be conflict with one's parents or an authority figure. For a nurse, it might be an interaction with a noncompliant client or with an aggressive physician. Through sociodrama, individuals may play roles that normally would be in conflict with their own. They also may try out more expansive role behaviors to add to their normal role performance. Sociodrama explores one's role behaviors rather than the individual's intrapsychic phenomena. A group of critical care nurses experiencing work-related stress participated in a sociodramatic roleplay. One of the exercises required a nurse to roleplay a terminally ill client interacting with staff (Stillman and Strasser, 1980). In a group experience for fathers who were having conflicts with their adolescent sons, the members roleplayed father/son interactions that depicted conflicts with their own fathers when they were adolescents. This helped each member have more empathy for the problems of their sons (Ravbolt and Rachman, 1980). A unique sociodrama for a group of women trying to understand their female role in society was to roleplay such scenes as two infants conversing about their gender and how it was acquired, housewives totally absorbed in their daily household chores, and a scene with a sexually aggressive male interacting with a very passive female in stereotyped male/female role behaviors (Mindek, 1979).

Psychodrama uses roleplaying as a basis for helping the individual explore personal issues. The technique requires that a trained psychodramatist lead the group in a series of connected roleplays that recreate one or more scenes of the protagonist's life in a "here-and-now" presentation. The protagonist is that person from the group whose personal issues the group sees unfold on the "stage" (Fine, 1979). Process events are explicitly presented, allowing the protagonist to "experiment with, develop, and expand role repertoires" (Fine, 1979, p.441). One sees the subjective reality or intrapsychic world of the protagonist as it develops through a series of roleplays designed to allow past, present, and possible future events blend together in a "here-and-now" drama (Fine, 1979). The reader might be reminded of Gestalt, the technique for presenting intrapsychic material in a "here-and-now" framework while dealing with past events in the present in order to complete some unfinished business. The individual experiences personally meaningful "ahas" or insights from the gestalt. Both Gestalt and psychodrama are spontaneous therapies. Fine (1979) noted that enacting possible future events in a psychodrama is not for behavioral rehearsal but is for expanding one's repertoire of possible roles.

The process introduced by Moreno (1946, 1959, 1969) as psychodrama is a therapeutic group method based on the language of the theater (Fine, 1979). The rest of the group acts as the audience for the protagonist and takes on various auxiliary roles in the drama. A warming-up process in which the group discusses its goals and may be asked to experience a guided fantasy or other directed activities focuses the members on personal feelings and, perhaps, some unfinished issues. The protagonist frequently emerges as the one most in need of some "working through." As part of my introduction to psychodrama, I was the protagonist at an inservice given to the nursing staff by two experienced psychodramatists. I was aware of some ambivalent feelings, having just returned to work after the birth of my third child. Life was very hectic for me, and I suppose I was "ready" to do something about trying to understand my overlapping roles as career person, mother of three, and wife. Our group warm-up consisted of several of us chatting about our daily lives. I recall being very surprised when the director asked me if I wanted to be the protagonist. I suspect he had sensed my readiness to work. He had me pick a scene from which to start the drama. The director observes both the audience and the protagonist for their ongoing reactions to the drama and helps the protagonist select an opening scene and members of the audience to play auxiliary roles (Fine, 1979).

Role reversal is an important technique in psychodrama. The protagonist switches roles with the auxiliaries to help them learn how to play their roles according to the protagonist's perception. The director may have the protagonist switch roles to experience new emotions as a different player in his life drama, to see the situation in a different way, to allow some reduction in the dissonance he may feel in having sensed ambivalent or opposing aspects of himself, and to help the protagonist gain control of scary emotions by switching roles to drain the intensity from his feelings (Fine, 1979).

Remembering that the goal is to enhance the "here-and-now" process of the event the protagonist is playing out, the director uses other techniques to promote self-awareness (Fine, 1979). Some of these the reader will recognize as dramatic terms: the soliloquy, in which the person can express out loud one's inner feelings; the aside, to voice feelings that would normally be inappropriate to say out loud; and various interventions by the auxiliary players. To be an auxiliary, one must be able to empathize and pick up nonverbal cues from the protagonist. Often, the director teaches group members to do this by modeling the role of the auxiliary. Group members learn to be sensitive to each others' feelings and reactions to the drama when the director, protagonist, auxiliaries, and audience process the drama with a feedback session at the end. In doubling, the auxiliary duplicates the protagonist's movements by standing behind or alongside of him and subjectively identifying with him. The double may mirror or amplify what the protagonist does in order to help the protagonist be more aware of his feelings and their expression (Fine, 1979).

Psychodrama is a sophisticated technique requiring the experience of a trained director and the intense participation of all the members of the group. Although I had several months of weekly psychodrama experience as a director and member of a group, I learned not how to be a trained psychodramatist, but how difficult the technique was to direct and how unskilled I felt at doing it. However, I did learn a lot about my own process. Psychodrama is an excellent technique for adolescent groups to experience. It provides both structure and action for the adolescent client (Stein and Davis, 1982). I attended a workshop on group techniques for adolescent clients. An intriguing way for the adolescent to deal with body image problems is to put on trial that part of her body about which she is most sensitive. The adolescent enacts a psychodrama by choosing a judge, jury, attorney, and so forth, to bring the body part to trial. The reader is directed to further readings about psychodrama to have a more complete picture of this technique.

Exercises for Conflict Resolution or Release of Tension

Protective techniques that allow one to express anger or other negative feelings include the following which I have used with both groups and individuals.

1) *Bataca Swords.* These are pieces of styrofoam which may be used by a couple embroiled in aggressive feelings towards one another (see Chapter One) or by any group that needs to get rid of hostilities. They may engage in a mock fight without hurting themselves or others.

2) *The Body Bag or Punching Bag.* One does not need an authentic body bag for this exercise. Frequently, big pillows are used with good results. An individual or a group may use the bag or pillows to pound on, thereby letting out any pent-up anger, irritation, and so forth. It helps to fantasize about the object of one's hostile feelings. A group of adolescents throwing soft sponge balls at one another may express anger safely. If the game is stopped when the adolescents are letting out their strongest feelings, there is the opportunity to have a verbal session exploring alternatives for getting rid of the anger the group is currently feeling (Stein and Davis, 1982).

3) *Physical Motion.* When one is rocked, lifted, or moved in another soothing way, this creates a sense of peace which can promote reduction in tension. I have used the rocking exercise with group members who seemed to be feeling needy, yet would not ask for help from the group. As a movement therapy, the person is picked up gently and rocked from side to side like a baby. The individual must be well-supported in order to completely relax. A parachute is a good medium for a group to use in tossing someone gently about. It is big, yet light, soothing, and fun.

Exercises to Promote Trust and Self-Disclosure

Many dyads have experienced the blind walk where it is necessary to completely trust one's partner. This exercise would not be appropriate until group members have spent enough time with one another to have shared demographic data and have some basis for trusting each other. The blind walk solidifies the individual's ability to trust. The group would probably be ready to move into more personal self-disclosure after this exercise. Rogers (1970) perceived this exercise as being useful to test one's attitude towards dependence on another.

Passing a member around the group while he or she has eyes closed is another exercise that requires the person to have a beginning level of trust before doing this. The group forms a tight circle around the individual and then passes that person around, allowing the member to fall backwards to be caught before falling to the ground. A variation of this is to have the group members lie down and lift their hands over their heads. One member may be passed down the line over the others with the motion of each person's hands. Since there is a great deal of touching involved, members who are not comfortable with this much invasion of their personal space would probably not feel positive about participating in the exercise.

Exercises to Promote Cohesion among Group Members

Group-building exercises help strangers get to know one another faster than if their interactions were not as focused. For example, in one exercise, each member chooses as a partner someone he or she does not know. The leader outlines particular information the partners should share with one another. These may be pieces of demographic or personal self-disclosure related to one's likes and dislikes, one's concerns, one's feelings, and so forth (Browne and Jacobson, 1981). The dyads then form groups of four with each person introducing his partner to the other dyad. The groups may then increase to eight and repeat the process as many times as is necessary for the group's size. Closure should be done by the facilitator with some processing of the exercise (Browne and Jacobson, 1981). Recall the group-building exercise for an adolescent group discussed earlier in the chapter. Rogers (1970) identified group-building exercises as important in industry for effective working relationships.

New games allow for cooperation rather than the competition most people associate with a "game." Passing a member over the heads of a group lying down was presented as a trust exercise. It is also a new game. The parachute is frequently used for new games as is a huge foam rubber "earth" ball which people can roll on or to one another. A new game for adolescents is called the "car wash." Two lines of adolescents facing each other two feet apart are the washers. One member is the car. He or she crawls between the two lines and is rubbed and patted on the back, arms, legs, and head. The whole group takes turns getting to be washed (Langford, 1981). As with this new game and several of the others, the group must be comfortable with touch.

Other group techniques to increase cohesiveness include throwing a ball of yarn to one another while disclosing some demographic or personal data about oneself. The member holds onto one end of the yarn and throws the ball to another person in the group. Eventually the group makes a "spider web" of the yarn, a symbol of their unity as a group. I first saw this done by one of my students with a group of very psychotic individuals that had not been together more than one other time. It worked marvelously! I have since used it many times myself.

Groups may do creative projects together, such as a group mural, collage, or poem. The possibilities for such projects are endless.

As a group leader, one may create or find experiential techniques for almost any group process problem. I find using such activities greatly expands my possibilities of facilitating a helpful group experience for others.

REFERENCES

Balazs, E. "Movement Therapy in the Classroom," in *Helping Through Action: Action-Oriented Therapies,* eds. E. Nickerson and K. O'Laughlin. Amherst, MA: Human Resource Development Press, 1982.

Blackman, J. "Group Work in the Community: Experiences with Reminiscence," in *Psychosocial Nursing Care of the Aged* (2nd ed.), ed. I. Burnside. New York: McGraw-Hill Book Co., Inc., 1980.

Browne, S. and M. Jacobson. "Teaching Mental Health Principles Through Continuing Education," *Journal of Continuing Education in Nursing,* 12, no. 2 (Mar.-Apr., 1981), 7–14.

Fine, L. "Psychodrama," in *Current Psychotherapies* (2nd ed.), ed. R. Corsini. Itasca, IL: F.E. Peacock Publishers, Inc., 1979.

Langford, R. "Teenagers and Obesity," in *American Journal of Nursing,* 81, no. 3 (Mar., 1981), 556–559.

Mindek, L. "Inpatient Psychiatric Women's Groups: The Concept of Sexuality," *Journal of Psychiatric Nursing and Mental Health Services,* 7, no. 4 (Apr., 1979), 36–39.

Moreno, J. *Psychodrama: Volume I.* New York: Beacon House, 1946.

Moreno, J. *Psychodrama: Volume II.* New York: Beacon House, 1959.

Moreno, J. *Psychodrama: Volume III.* New York: Beacon House, 1969.

Nickerson, E. and K. O'Laughlin, eds. *Helping Through Action: Action-Oriented Therapies.* Amherst, MA: Human Resource Development Press, 1982.

Ravbolt, R. and A. Rachman. "A Therapeutic Group Experience for Fathers," *International Journal of Group Psychotherapy,* 30, no. 2 (Apr., 1980), 229–239.

Reakes, J. "Behavioral Rehearsal Revisited: A Multi-Faceted Tool for the Instructor," *Journal of Nursing Education,* 18, no. 2 (Feb., 1979), 48–51.

Rogers, C. *Carl Rogers on Encounter Groups.* New York: Harper and Row, Publishers, 1970.

Schachter, R. "Kinetic Psychotherapy in the Treatment of Families," in *Helping Through Action: Action-Oriented Therapies,* eds. E. Nickerson and K. O'Laughlin. Amherst, MA: Human Resources Development Press, 1982.

Shropshire, C. "Group Experiential Learning in Adult Education," *Journal of Continuing Education in Nursing,* 12, no. 6 (Nov.-Dec., 1981), 5–9.

Stein, M. and J. Davis. *Therapies for Adolescents.* San Francisco: Jossey-Bass, 1982.

Stillman, S. and B. Strasser. "Helping Critical Care Nurses with Work-Related Stress," *Journal of Nursing Administration,* 10, no. 1 (Jan., 1980), 28–31.

Tappen, R. and T. Touhy. "Group Leader-Are You a Controller?" *Journal of Gerontological Nursing,* 9, no. 1 (Jan., 1983), 34–38, 44, 59.

Wadeson, H. "Combining Expressive Therapies in an Effort to Survive on a Depressive Ward," in *Helping Through Action: Action-Oriented Therapies,* eds. E. Nickerson and K. O'Laughlin. Amherst, MA: Human Resources Development Press, 1982.

Wilson, H. and C. Kneisl. *Psychiatric Nursing* (2nd ed.). Menlo Park, CA: Addison-Wesley Publishing Co., 1983.

Winn, W. "Physical Challenge Approaches to Psychotherapy," in *Helping Through Action: Action-Oriented Therapies,* eds. E. Nickerson and K. O'Laughlin. Amherst, MA: Human Resources Development Press, 1982.

Yalom, I. *The Theory and Practice of Group Psychotherapy* (2nd ed.). New York: Basic Books, Inc., 1975.

TABLE 9.1 A SAMPLING OF EXPERIENTIAL EXERCISES

Type of Exercise	Expected Outcome
Warm-ups	
Batting balloons	Become acquainted; move into Child Ego State
Saying "Hello" nonverbally	Prepare for self-disclosure
Saying "Hello" with crayons and paper	Become acquainted
Verbal introductions in dyads	Become acquainted
Sharing nicknames	Become acquainted
Verbal introductions in dyads with roleplay	Become acquainted
Kinetic techniques	
Freeze tag	Awareness of the process of asking for help
Family sculpture	Awareness of one's position in the family system
Breaking into the circle	Awareness of being isolated
Movement Techniques	
Fantasies	Awareness of one's immediate feelings
Exploring space	Letting "go" to explore unknown space
Dyad sculpturing	Experiencing the feeling of controlling others or being controlled
Passing on a movement	Experiencing directing or controlling others
Lifting and rocking a member	Experiencing giving up control to others
Improvisation	Awareness of one's immediate feelings
Protective techniques	
Bataca swords	Safe expression of anger
Body bag/punching bag; pillows	Safe expression of anger
Lifting and rocking a member	Reduction of tension
Parachute toss	Reduction of tension
Behavioral rehearsal	
Roleplaying	Increase repertoire of possible responses to situations
Sociodrama	Expand repertoire of role performance
Psychodrama	Explore individual intrapsychic phenomena within one's role
Group building	
Verbal exchanges in dyads	Increase group cohesion
New games	Increase group cohesion
"Spider web" and yarn	Increase group cohesion
Group mural, collage, poem	Increase group cohesion
Blind walk	Promote trust and self-disclosure
Passing a member around	Promote trust

The Staff Task Group 10

───────────────── **Introduction** ─────────────────

The task group has been described briefly in Chapter Five. Since most nurses end up being both a member and a leader of a variety of task groups, it seems appropriate to describe more fully the structure, both formal and informal, of the task group. To be an effective member or leader, one needs to understand the informal communication channels and leadership power structure that frequently affects the quality and quantity of the work accomplished by such a group. Nurses serve on both nursing and multidisciplinary task groups. The multidisciplinary group adds the dimension of other disciplines' slant on a shared task or problem, thereby creating more information the nurse must process and understand. If the task group is controlled by upper-level management, such as a medical, nursing, or hospital administrator, the formal structure becomes more important and must also be understood by the nurse member. This chapter will present theory from group dynamics to explain the formal and informal group structure, and will provide several examples of task groups whose structures vividly illustrate the process identified in theory. As both a member and a leader of several staff task groups, I am still learning how to be most effective in accomplishing goals in a group task format. It has helped me to synthesize the information I have gotten by both experiencing membership and observing the group process in other task groups. The nurse who can successfully operate in a task group has an important tool for effecting change in nursing practice.

A task group is formed for the purpose of accomplishing a specific goal, that goal being the reason for the group's existence. Although all groups have goal-directed activities, the goals may be more process-oriented in nature, such as those which a support group or a therapy group might have. Some staff task groups are formed because of the existence of a particular staff that makes up a unit or has a particular working relationship. It is understood, then, that periodically this group will have specific tasks to perform in the carrying out of their duties as staff of a unit or section of a hospital, clinic, or other health facility. Some staff task groups exist on an on-call basis to perform a particular duty when that duty is needed. For example, a group of one's peers who meets at specific times to select colleagues for meritorious performance might not then meet again until circumstances occur to warrant such action. Some staff task groups are formed for one particular job and then are disbanded after that is accomplished. The task groups in which nurses will always be participants are those groups formed as a result of a particular working assignment with others in a unit or with a certain population of clients. These groups will be discussed in detail. Some of the other staff task groups that perform specific one-time or ongoing tasks will also be discussed.

───────── **Areas of Practice Using a Task Group Format** ─────────

Any large health care agency, such as a hospital or health department of a county or city, will most likely have some agency-wide committees on which nurses might be asked to serve. Many of these will be multidisciplinary in nature whose nursing representative may only include a nursing administrator as a member or as the chairperson. Directors of various services may meet to plan the budget, discuss personnel ceilings, determine professional practice standards for physicians, nurses, and so forth. Some multidisciplinary committees, such as safety or quality assurance, will ask nonsupervisory as well as administrative personnel to be members. The staff nurse could ask to be a member of such a committee. Nursing service may have its own quality assurance committee made up of staff as well as supervisory nursing personnel. Other committees are peculiar to nursing service and include groups dealing with developing educational programs, revising nursing policies or procedures, or passing on professional qualifications for promotions and the hiring of nurses.

Those staff task groups peculiar to the unit, working area, or client population with which the nurse interacts may include nursing staff, a multidisciplinary staff, or, at times, some client members. All inpatient units have an implied existing task group with all the nursing staff as members and the head nurse as chairperson. There may be other nurses on the staff, who, at various times, take on leadership roles in this group. Nursing issues for the unit are brought to the attention of the nursing staff group, and nursing care conferences and care planning would be some of the major tasks that this group would tackle. Many client-care areas will also form a multidisciplinary task group from the total staff that are working with clients. Multidisciplinary planning meetings with regard to client care, policies, and so forth would be worked out in this group. In an outpatient client area, there is more likelihood that the staff group will be multidisciplinary. Very often, clients are included in their own care conferences or planning meetings, at least at some point in their care, and then the client would become a temporary member of the staff task group. It is frequently the practice on mental health units to form client governments and to have staff and client representatives do joint planning for parties, outings, and the day-to-day functioning of the unit. This is an important part of a therapeutic community or similar therapeutic milieu where clients take major responsibility for the management of the activities of daily living. A preventive health clinic or community walk-in medical clinic may invite client representatives to sit on staff task groups to participate in planning for clinic expansion, to help with problem-solving, and so forth.

With the variety of staff task group committees on which nurses may function as members or leaders, the nurse becomes an important participant in policy formation and all aspects of health practice planning and problem-solving in health care delivery.

The Structure of the Staff Task Group

As described in Chapters Five and Six, every group has a uniform structural framework that includes a normative system and an executive system held together through the communication patterns developed in the group as the group members relate to each other as parts of a common system. The structure of the task group is particularly important in the way it affects the group's ability to complete its work. The group's movement toward its goals, or its locomotion, is determined to a great extent by what happens to the group's internal structure as it is formed (Phipps, 1982). Groups may have a variety of power structures that carry out the executive functions and control norm development, but the way the leadership is structured is particularly crucial in the task group since the group's leaders have the potential to affect goal accomplishment. In order to have power in a group, one must be seen as occupying a high-status position. In this position, one can control the flow of communication to the rest of the group and the accessibility of members to one another. Sociometric data about how central or isolated members are in relation to each other give the observer clues to the communication patterns in the group (Phipps, 1982). These are the dynamics of the structure which we will discuss in more detail as we look at how a task group operates to get its work done.

The Power Structure

Since the persons in high-status positions end up with the most power in the group, it is important to understand how status is assigned. Status is a vertical ranking of the position of members (Phipps, 1982). If status in a group is determined externally to the group, it is normally assigned to a value the external community puts on status. This is *ascribed* status. *Achieved* status is given through group consensus and is conferred by the group's internal value structure (Phipps, 1982). In a multidisciplinary group of physicians, social workers, nurses, occupational therapists, and so forth, the physicians would most likely be the members to be granted high-status positions based on their standing in society at large (ascribed status). Physicians are generally more highly valued than other members of the health team in relationship to the ascribed status accorded them in the community, based on their education and responsibility for the health care of the client. A multidisciplinary clinic may not start until the physician arrives, and the physician's available practice time affects the hour parameters set up for the client's care. Members of other disciplines may earn status in the multidisciplinary group through special contributions to the group or other actions that the group recognizes as noteworthy. This is achieved status.

Although status and its associated power are frequently factors in the determination of the leadership of a task group, small groups who are initially leaderless may eventually make the leader the person who initiates most of the work on the task as the group is being organized (Phipps, 1982). The leadership may also relate to the expertise being offered in the group, the leader being the person most capable of contributing to the realization of a completed task. The leadership would then rotate among those capable of goal production for the group. However, high-status members, regardless of their expertise, frequently dominate a group, influencing the other members to conform (Schmitt, 1982). Most readers undoubtedly have seen a health team being led by an incompetent member who, because of his or her status, has kept the leadership role regardless of an inability to accomplish group goals, which in this case might mean that other group members cover up for this person's mistakes, especially if these affect the quality of health care provided. Schmitt (1982) noted that nurses, because of the split they encounter in providing both physiological assessment under a medical model and independent nursing practice with a nursing model framework, often have difficulty dealing with a physician in authority who is also not an expert. Task group leadership through status only is often detrimental to the goal performance or the group.

——— Leadership in Nursing Staff Task Groups ———

In a nursing management staff group, the leadership frequently arises from the status of the nurse members. The nurse administrator has both increased status through nursing's hierarchy and the power of a position that dictates a leadership role in multiple staff committees. An educational committee might have either the inservice coordinator or another administrative person that handles this responsibility, or a clinical nurse specialist as chairperson. The clinical nurse specialist most often does not hold an administrative position but has status due to his or her expertise in a specific area of nursing. When the assigned leader comes also with expertise, there is less reason for the group to award achieved status to someone else within the group.

Two examples from my own practice illustrate both a nursing task group functioning very well with the defined leadership structure and one which accorded the defined nurse leader with neither much ascribed nor achieved status. Unfortunately, the second group did not have a person to deal with maintenance issues, of which there were many in this group, and the group was not able to be task-oriented due to the lack of an effective power structure. The group members never dealt overtly with their discomfort at the lack of leadership.

Example 1: A Facilitative Leadership Structure

The "leadership group," of which I am a member, is made up of all the mental health clinical specialists, the head nurses from the mental health units, and the mental health nursing supervisor. The latter member is both the designated leader by her administrative status and position title, and the group's chosen leader because of her achieved status of expertise in mental health nursing practice. Since the group membership is comfortable with the formally defined leader, there are no attempts to set up a new leader. However, all but the new, orienting members are capable of assuming the leadership when the chairperson is gone, which is quite frequently. All the members enjoy a degree of achieved status in other groups in which they are leaders or members and seem to use the "leadership" group more as a support group to provide them with ideas and ways of coping with the problems they encounter in other groups they must lead. The leadership group's defined task is to perform those duties that allow the mental health nursing part of the hospital to achieve a high standard of nursing care. Supervision of other nurses, training for nursing staff, and the definition and problem-solving of administrative issues and policies are dealt with in this group. It appears to be one of those task groups whose members take responsibility for the maintenance issues in the group. Therefore, a separate leader to handle socioemotional issues is not necessary (Phipps, 1982).

Example 2: An Inadequate Leadership Structure

A unit nursing group making up the staff on a female mental health inpatient unit where I placed students for clinical experience had a series of ascribed leaders who were all head nurses placed in the leadership position because of their staff assignment. The two that I knew were very different leaders. One kept herself in her office doing paperwork while several of the staff nurses assumed any leadership tasks necessary for the care of clients. The head nurse did accomplish the "paperwork," something that was highly valued in this clinical agency. After the head nurse retired, one of the staff nurses who had been a leader in clinical nursing assumed the head nurse position. She continued to be interested in clinical issues but gradually spent more time away from the clients and other nursing staff attempting to do the many administrative "paperwork" duties she was assigned.

Since the head nurse had worked with me and my students, she was supportive of a project I negotiated with her and the head nurse of a second unit in the agency where I had also placed students. The process of negotiation was actually with the entire nursing staff of both units; however, I mistakenly thought that the support of both head nurses meant that the project would go smoothly for us. My students and I negotiated permission to do a student-led group which changed the treatment focus on the units since the nurses were not actively engaged in leading therapy groups (Wilson, 1980).

What I had not assessed was the source of the power under which the head nurse on the woman's unit operated with her staff. I expected she would have received some status from the staff nurse group which she led initially because of her position as head nurse. However, because of the inability of the head nurse to change the low ascribed status generally accorded all nurses on the unit by the other staff disciplines, the nursing staff group seemed to give her little ascribed status in their own group. Her mental health nursing skills were, in several areas, greater than those of the other nurses, but this was not a value widely held by the nursing group who were mostly non-mental health nurses. Since she did not have ascribed status from the nursing group, her efforts to send me female clients for our group were not supported by the other nurses.

I encountered a series of passive-aggressive behaviors by the nursing staff. I found I could not get a set of female clients to come to our group, even though none of the staff members was objecting openly to our doing the group. One staff nurse would tell me we could take a client, but she could not be found when it was time for group. Another staff nurse refused to give me permission herself, saying that she was not the regular staff nurse responsible for the clients we wanted in the group. The head nurse wanted us to have female clients, and she sent several to us, only to be reprimanded by the social worker group leader for doing so (Wilson, 1980). The fact that the head nurse had little ascribed and no achieved status with the unit multidisciplinary team certainly was a factor in this process.

There was not another identified leader in the staff nurse group, but several nurses operated at times in a controlling manner with the group. The group had no member dealing with relationship issues in the group, and these were avoided most of the time, therefore, adding to the inefficiency of this group as a successful task group. The group members operated as individuals in their approach to nursing care and did not identify any specific goals towards which the nursing staff group could work. This was a group in which task commitment was low, and there was no socioemotional leader to facilitate more viable relationships in the group and free up energy for more task commitment. Such a group needs a leader who could spend time in member relationships and identification of a central task (Phipps, 1982). It was obvious that when the head nurse could not free any female clients for our group, she was not supported by the other nursing staff in a task she had identified as being important.

— Leadership in Multidisciplinary Staff Task Groups —

As noted earlier, ascribed status is often a factor in the leadership of multidisciplinary staff groups. However, other members may earn status through that accorded by the group members. For nurses, the lack of ascribed status they have experienced in multidisciplinary groups is gradually changing for the better. Several factors are responsible for this. The nurse has developed a set of behaviors that have not always been associated with the practice of nursing but which are now being taught in undergraduate nursing programs (Mauksch, 1981). The practice of health care has also changed to provide a more comprehensive multidisciplinary approach to the client's care, as practitioners attempt to treat the client as a whole person. This has made a difference in the way the client's care is recorded (the POR system) and in the practice of nursing (Devereux, 1981). We will discuss these factors as they relate to the changing status of the nurse.

Mauksch (1981) identified four behaviors, now formally being taught to nursing students, that have made a difference in how the nurse is perceived by the physician and the health care consumer. These behaviors are: risk-taking, assertiveness, accountability, and autonomous intervention.

Risk-taking requires that the nurse assert his or her position that may not be recognized by others in order to establish a more collegial or peer relationship with other health professionals (Mauksch, 1981). Mauksch noted that one sign of this was the first-name basis on which physicians and nurses now interact, which has not always been true. In establishing a working relationship, the nurse needs to take a risk to interact with the physician in the same way she would in any other collegial relationship. Nurses must take risks to share observations about clients, using a knowledge base to provide observations that will be pertinent and correct in relation to theory. In sharing such observations that present one's point of view of the client's needs, it is important that these observations are backed by theory. Such nursing assessments are part of the client's data base.

Assertiveness speaks to the nurse's sense of self-worth and trust in his or her nursing judgments enough to share them even in a situation where they might be challenged by other disciplines. Part of this assertiveness is also choosing to not make up for the deficiencies of other health care workers yet insisting on priorities of the client's care which the nurse sees as essential (Mauksch, 1981). Not covering for another discipline does not mean the client suffers, but the nurse speaks out about the deficiencies of service in order to insist that they be corrected while not taking over responsibility for their correction himself. One's assertive energy is well-spent if the nurse can get social service to see a client for a social service need rather than trying to meet this need, however inadequately, with the client herself. If the nurse can establish this as an ongoing happening, that social service takes on this responsibility, then she will have accomplished something for all clients that come along later with this same need.

Although accountability has always been part of the nurse's actions, particularly in the area of administration of medications and the practicing of invasive treatments, Mauksch (1981) noted that accountability to the client had been less than adequate in nursing's tendency to yield to institutional guidelines, such as not telling the client what medications he was taking, or not suggesting that he had a right to question a physician about a treatment he did not understand. Nurses are recognizing that they must fight what have been traditional rules in order to provide for the client's best interests. The nurse has become a client advocate. This may mean that a nurse would question a client's participation in a research study if it were not going to provide any benefit for the client. The nurse, in being accountable to the client, makes sure the client has all the information necessary to make a wise decision about his health care.

Autonomous intervention by the nurse is seen in the independent practice elements which the nurse may use with clients. Committees within the health agencies that meet to discuss nursing practice and the interventions that nurses may do independently reflect the autonomy which nurses are gaining (Mauksch, 1981). As a clinical specialist in mental health nursing, I am granted a list of clinical privileges based on my nursing knowledge, such as the practice of individual and group therapy, in the setting where I work. It is important for nurses to make other disciplines aware of those areas that involve nursing judgments and which may be considered autonomous interventions by the nurse.

The events that have taken place within health care settings that have led to a more collegial relationship between the nurse and other disciplines include the development of clinical privileges and protocols for nurses, the switch to a primary nursing focus in many inpatient settings, the use of the problem-oriented record system, and the joint practice of physicians and nurses in client rounds and in quality assurance projects (Devereux, 1981). With one nurse taking responsibility for the client's total care, the physician can go to one person, the primary nurse, to discuss a client's status. The POR system demands collaboration between the many health care disciplines, since all entries about the client are written on one problem sheet and one set of progress notes. Although it is difficult to find time to dialogue with everyone involved in the clients' care, it forces this process to occur.

Nurses, therefore, probably do have more ascribed status in many health care agencies than has been true in the past. The identified leader in a multidisciplinary staff of an outpatient mental health center has traditionally been a psychiatrist, psychologist, or social worker. It is my bias that a masters- or doctoral-prepared mental health clinical nurse specialist would be as capable of directing a mental health center. It may be that in other areas of nursing the nurse will more readily find a place of leadership with a multidisciplinary team. This would probably be in some aspect of preventive health practice not so filled with tradition as the leadership in community mental health centers.

It is possible for the nurse to achieve some status by using those behaviors cited that contribute to an increased ascribed status for nurses. This will lead to a more visible position within a group of which he or she is a member. The multidisciplinary staff group of which I am a member has a psychiatrist as the identified leader. I have a strong desire that nursing be a voice in this group and am aware that I must do certain things to achieve status in the group in order to establish a power base for this to happen. The head nurse on the unit where I attempted to gain female clients for my group did not establish a collegial relationship with the psychiatrist. She infrequently offered an opinion on a client's status based on her nursing assessment, although she did make accurate assessments for nursing interventions when assisting the nursing staff with a problem client. She acted autonomously in deciding female clients could attend our group, but she had not established a credibility for these autonomous actions with the psychiatrist or social worker.

The Informal Power Structure

Informal ways that staff can influence the power structure in a staff task group may be described as what Shostrom (1968) called actualizing behavior. An actualizer is one who sends and receives messages honestly while risking the self to do this. Shostrom described a manipulator as, "a person who exploits, uses, or controls himself and others as things in self-defeating ways" (p.11). "Actualizing behavior is simply manipulative behavior expressed more creatively." (Shostrom, 1968, p.9). He seemed to be talking about how the actualizer learns what manipulation is but remains honest in his dealings with others as he interacts in a way that might cause another person to respond favorably to what the actualizer would like to see happen in that interaction or particular relationship. Peterson (1979) listed the tools of power as: 1) credibility, a broad term having to do with honesty, openness, directness, and competency in one's area of expertise; 2) persuasion, one's ability to present arguments in a logical, orderly manner; 3) interpersonal relations with others up and down the hierarchy of a system; and 4) access to the informal communications network and to membership on committees whose recommendations are being accepted. Peterson talked about knowing the informal system and identified those areas where one could be most influential. However, she also described credibility as being most important. It seems that Shostrom and Peterson both identified creative actualization as a type of positive manipulation, or, as Shostrom said, creative manipulation. Each of us learns to time our interactions with others in a way that will create a favorable outcome. For example, one does not confront another person if it seems that, at the moment, the individual is too upset or angry to be able to hear feedback without becoming defensive. It is best to wait for a more appropriate time when the person would most likely be receptive. Working informally in a formal structure involves understanding where the power lies in a group, when people will most likely hear ideas with an open mind, and so forth. For example, the director of the setting in which I work is more responsive to someone who approaches him individually rather than confronts or questions him in an open meeting. I have observed that the psychiatrist I work with has a great deal of access to the director and is able to be heard and get things done each time he interacts individually with him. It appears that the director sees him as a peer. I have shared with the psychiatrist I work with some of my concerns about policies in our work setting, and these have gotten passed onto the director. It is important for nurses who are members of multidisciplinary staff groups to assess the degree of status they have in the group and how they might increase that status in order to have more power to determine what happens in the group that affects the client's care. As a member of a task group, the nurse needs to speak up in meetings using a credible knowledge base and looking for areas where he or she can add to the success of the group's task accomplishment.

The Power Structure in a Multidisciplinary Management/Staff Task Group

When the group members are not only staff but also management from other areas of the health agency, another layer of complexity is added to the power structure. In a committee made up of members from nursing, medicine, and management, the director of the hospital, if a team member, has obvious ascribed status, especially if this person happens to be a physician also. A hospital administrator who is not a physician may not present with as much ascribed status as the physician administrator. Most often, the nurse members of such committees are those in administrative positions that also come with some ascribed status because of this. The staff nurse will usually be a member of a multidisciplinary management staff group concerned with safety issues, quality assurance, or other health concerns within the agency which staff working directly with clients would see as important areas of management.

The dynamics involved in assessing the power structure revolve around a multilayered membership. Not only are there the dynamics of several disciplines vying for power, but there is also the factor of the formal agency leadership structure with which to deal. The nurse should consider both these factors when determining how influential he or she might be in such a group. It would be important to look for informal relationships existing between group members as a way of assessing the informal power structure which can often be an effective position from which to attempt some influence in the group. For those staff nurses who find themselves working on a multidisciplinary management/staff task group, it will be a challenge to determine the informal power structure of the group and to work on achieving some status within this group.

——— The Communication Structure of a Staff ——— Task Group: Types of Communication Channels

The power structure of the task group influences the type of communication that occurs between the members. The existence of a status hierarchy interrupts the flow of communications between different status levels and requires sociometric choices to be made between members within the same status level (Cartwright and Zander, 1960). Recall that sociometry measures the amount of attraction between members or the degree to which members are liked in the group. The amount of communication or interaction between members is a measure of the sociometry for the particular group. If members are restricted to interacting only on one status level, this can hamper the work performance of the group. A member who does not feel free to exchange an idea with the group leader because of status restrictions most likely loses interest in the group's task. I found our nursing staff task group generated excellent ideas about nursing interventions for clients during nursing care conferences. I encouraged nursing assistants as well as staff nurses to take an active part in the problem-solving in these meetings and specifically looked for ways to stroke contributions made by staff who would be seen as members of a different status level in a group where the head nurse has both ascribed and achieved status. Although I was dealing with different levels of status, I attempted to overcome this with an all-channel communication network.

All-channel communications operate without restriction. The nursing leadership group made up of clinical nurse specialists and the head nurses on the mental health unit described earlier in this chapter operated on an all-channel communication network even though the nursing supervisor, as leader of the group, had ascribed as well as achieved status. There was both a willingness on the nursing supervisor's part to provide for open communications in the group, and a blend of ascribed and achieved power among the members of the group. The sociometric diagram of this group would probably show a fairly even distribution of interactions between and among the members of the group.

Two other communication networks illustrate a more restricted set of communications (Guetzkow, 1960). In a circle configuration, one may only communicate directly with that member to the right or the left. Any other communications not in the member's direct channel must be relayed through someone else (Bavelas, 1960). The wheel has the "spokes" able to communicate only with the "hub" of the wheel (Guetzkow, 1960). This depicts severe communication restrictions in what would be a very authoritarian power structure. Either network would be extremely difficult communications under which a task group might operate. Obviously, there would not be the means for having a discussion by the whole group together on task-related problems. Nursing staff task groups need to be careful to avoid the "hub" communication channel, since there is a built-in hierarchy that makes it possible for the head nurse to isolate him or herself from the rest of the staff and encourages the staff nurses to do the same with the auxiliary nursing staff. A multidisciplinary management/staff task group might find a similar occurrence if the management head is very conscious of using the ascribed status that he or she has to limit communication flow between group members and control access to the top. Not being available except during committee meetings is one way to control the communication flow. Equally frustrating is when the management head sends an assistant to act in his or her behalf as chairperson of a meeting. No members are able to confront the committee group leader directly about a task or directive but must deal with the intermediary.

A multidisciplinary staff task group has a defined quality to its communication structure because of its unique task. Normally, a multidisciplinary team operates most efficiently in a clinic setting where each member is there to offer a specialized service to the client. Because a multidisciplinary team consists frequently of specialists of different disciplines that are working in a parallel or sequential manner for the client's care, communications need to focus on coordination and collaboration of tasks (Schmitt, 1982). A psychiatrist and I do a medication clinic together one day a week for some chronic mental health outpatients. Although we have worked out a system of assessing clients in separate offices at the same time to allow for a faster flow of numbers of clients, we have different but coordinated tasks to accomplish. He needs to make the final determination of dosage for a long-acting antipsychotic medication administered to clients, and I frequently will do diet counseling, problem-solving, or stress management with the clients while administering the medication. I make a nursing diagnosis, and he makes a medical diagnosis, yet we work together very well. Part of the ease of our working relationship is the amount of achieved status he gives to me while downplaying his own ascribed status as a physician. I also accord him achieved status as I observe his very caring and thorough work with clients. We are collaborating on looking for ways to reduce the dosage levels of the antipsychotics we give to clients to allow clients to function as free of medication side-effects as possible. In order for collaboration and coordination to take place in a multidisciplinary staff task group, the communication channel needs to be as open as possible to allow for the discipline representatives to have free access to each others' ideas on task accomplishment.

Forming A Task Group

Definition of the Tasks to be Performed

In order to enhance the group's commitment to task accomplishment, the group leader needs to spend time defining specific elements of the tasks to be performed and goals to be reached. In assignment of task duties, the leader generally needs to be directive, thereby assuring that all tasks are assigned and understood by the group members (Phipps, 1982).

The leader needs to be competent in the tasks which the group is to perform (Calkin, 1980). As a clinical specialist, I found my credibility and base of power with those nursing staff groups with whom I worked to be based on their having seen me perform nursing interventions with clients. If I were meeting with a staff to plan particular interventions for a client, I could relate to the staff nurse's frustrations since "I had been there" also. If a task group is to tackle a particularly big job, such as writing a set of standard care plans for a set of identified problems, it helps if the leader has a concept of what the finished product should be like. The leader must be able to define both the outcome and the process of how the task will be done. The first step might be a literature search to gather as much information as possible for the specific problem to be addressed. The group leader does not necessarily have to be an expert on the problem, for example, of dysfunctional grieving for the group to be able to respect that person's leadership. However, the leader should know where to get the necessary information and should know the process for identifying behavioral goals, nursing actions, and so forth which are part of the standard care plan.

Membership of the Group

Membership refers to both the size of the group and the characteristics of the members. The preferred number of members on a task group is five. This allows for the most productive work being done (Lancaster, 1981). If the group gets larger than about seven members, communication begins to be centered on one person who holds the power in the group. If the group is smaller than five, there are more opportunities for power conflicts between the members (Lancaster, 1981). Less time and energy are left for task accomplishment.

It is important to consider the effects of a membership that allows for persons of different status to be part of the group. In our discussion about ascribed and achieved status, we identified the different membership structures and the leadership that was specific to these groups. For example, a multidisciplinary group most often is led by a member of the discipline with the most ascribed status. This person might also earn achieved status from the group members. However, even if this is not the case, some groups are willing to base leadership on ascribed status alone. In what is known as a leveling effect, those persons that occupy the highest status are the ones that dominate decision-making and to whom the other members will often yield. A group made up of nursing administration and staff nurses might have the staff nurses being hesitant to disagree with nursing management (Lancaster, 1981). Obviously, it would take members who could earn some achieved status in the group to balance a membership where the leader holds ascribed status to allow for more thoughtful decision-making. If one is calling a group together to perform a particular task, it seems logical that input from many different individuals is desired. If the membership is too weighted with those having ascribed status, the group's decisions are probably not going to reflect ideas from the whole group due to the leveling effect.

The Structure of a Meeting

A task group leader is usually called a chairperson. It is that individual's role to assist the group towards the best conclusion or decision in the most efficient way. The chairperson clarifies, moves the meeting with the planned agenda, and summarizes the decisions or conclusions the group has made. This also means imposing the group's will on any member that attempts to divert or delay the group's accomplishment of the task (Jay, 1981). In some groups, there is a person that fulfills the maintenance functions in the group, thereby freeing the task leader to concentrate fully on accomplishing the group's goals. It would be the maintenance leader's function to work with those members that seem to want to divert the group from its task. A skilled chairperson will elicit from those members that seem adept in interpersonal relationships help in the area of the maintenance functions of the group.

Jay (1981) suggested several nonverbal behaviors by the chairperson that would serve to limit the discussion and discourage digression from the task at hand. Impatience is shown by leaning forward, fixing one's eyes on the speaker, tensing the muscles, raising the eyebrows, or nodding briefly. I find myself leaning forward most often to show impatience. I believe I use this gesture also when I am about to interrupt someone who is droning on without getting to the point. I also will reach out and touch someone if I am about to speak and I feel it is very important that they understand what I am trying to say. If the leader wants to encourage a member who is offering an idea to the group, it is good to allow that person plenty of time to speak (Jay, 1981). I encourage someone with an idea by asking that person to clarify certain points, or I will frequently repeat parts of what the individual has said.

Most task groups function best with an agenda of what the group meeting is going to include. This should be distributed prior to the meeting in order for members to be prepared to discuss agenda items. It is important, then, to stick to the agenda for the meeting and to allow discussion only on agenda items (Lancaster, 1981). Exceptions to task groups using an agenda would be a client-centered conference or an informal staff meeting. The purpose of an agenda is to help the members run smoothly through the tasks the group must accomplish. Time is an important element for the chairperson to control, since most task groups allow only a specific amount of time to meet and accomplish their tasks. The meeting should start on time and end on time. This gives the members a message to not be late or risk missing some important business. It also gives members the sense that the chairperson is aware that their time is, indeed, valuable. Allotting a specific amount of time for each agenda item is helpful, and a timekeeper might be appointed to remind the group when a discussion is going beyond the time allotted. Just how rigid the chairperson wants to be about time depends, most likely, on the character and progress of the group. If a discussion is productive but runs over the time allotted for this, one would want to continue the discussion as long as it is helping the group accomplish its task. If members tend to digress from the task or have side conversations, more active intervention by the chairperson is required.

Some digressions may be maintenance issues, such as an interpersonal conflict or individual need one member has to monopolize or divert the group. These socioemotional issues are often best worked with outside the group, although immediate intervention may be necessary to get the group back on its task. A comment to the members in conflict, such as, "Perhaps you and Donna could discuss your differences outside the group and at this time just acknowledge that you need to disagree," would be sufficient to redirect the members. A difference in philosophy often leads to conflict. Since this is not something that is quickly resolved, if ever, the members who disagree might need to just acknowledge this as a difference between them. Misunderstandings as a result of a breakdown within the message unit/feedback cycle require immediate assessment and intervention to correct the problem, *e.g.:*

"We're really getting caught up in the details of how to change the careplan. I noticed that none of you were answering my question. I was asking you what process we needed to suggest to each staff unit to get them started on revising their particular set of standard careplans."

The group task will move along more smoothly if non-agenda items are not allowed to be discussed. Finally, giving the group a summary of what has been decided and who has agreed to do what task is helpful. Most task groups also keep minutes (Lancaster, 1981).

A task group that seems to slow down because of a lack of ideas or answers to particular problems needs some stimulation. Brainstorming is an excellent technique to facilitate creative problem-solving. Recall the discussion of brainstorming and problem-solving in Chapter Eight. Many of the suggestions in that chapter work well in a task group. Brainstorming energizes a group and provides new ideas for task accomplishment.

The interpersonal process of the members of a task group is not of particular concern to the chairperson unless that process becomes disruptive. We identified conflict as one disruptive interpersonal process. Another process would be self-disclosure to the extent that this caused members to abandon their task in favor of interpersonal rewards. Certainly, group members should feel comfortable enough with one another to work together productively. The major reward for membership in a task group is task accomplishment and not interpersonal growth. If the members are allowed to spend time self-disclosing rather than working towards the group's goal, this is detrimental to the group. Somewhere between conflict and interpersonal closeness is a friendly yet superficial manner of relating that probably works best for members in a task group.

Process Elements

Recall the discussion of conflict resolution in Chapter Eight. While those ideas help the group deal with overt conflict, the prevention of unnecessary conflict is also important. Communications that prevent defensiveness facilitate the group members working in an open, goal-directed manner with one another. Using descriptive words prevents defensiveness (Chiavetta, 1982). Notice the difference between these two messages:

"I can't tolerate your lateness. That just shows how interested you are in the work of this group." (judgment of late member's motives)

"I get upset when you keep coming to group late. We don't seem to get started unless you're here. I'm worried that we won't get our work done without your input." (description of effect lateness has on the group)

There are two other important phenomena that frequently occur as part of the process in a task group as it works on goal accomplishment. The existence of hidden agendas and the possibility of *group think* are important elements that can affect the group's task accomplishment.

A hidden agenda is a member's private goals or motives for the outcome of a meeting and is always kept from the awareness of the group (Lancaster, 1981). Recall the discussion in Chapter Two on latent content. Many times a hidden agenda is operating on this level. A hidden agenda might be that a member has a fantasy about dating the group leader. When conflict erupts between this member and another female in the group who is working well with the male chairperson, the manifest content might be that the two have different ideas about how to accomplish a particular task. However, latent content may include an imagined idea by the group member that the other female wants to have a relationship with the group leader as well. Most of the other members and the leader will not have any idea what the latent content is and will not guess that one member has a hidden agenda. Hidden agendas are more evident at times of conflict within the group. If the group's task is proceeding well, the hidden agendas are not as readily apparent (Lancaster, 1981). When group conflict seems on the rise, it may be that a hidden agenda is part of the impetus for the conflict. Lancaster (1981) said one cannot force a hidden agenda to surface, and this process may only be dealt with as it becomes evident in the group. As cues are leaked from the person with a hidden agenda, the group has more of a need to deal with this process. In our example, the female member wanting to date the chairperson of the group might start giving this person extra attention while ignoring other male members. The hidden agenda is now manifest content. Once the leader has a sense of what the agenda might be, it is appropriate to share this with the member since it interferes with the group's goal accomplishment. With this particular agenda, the group leader might choose to talk with the member outside of the group.

Group think is a term that describes an inappropriate conformity to the group's norms. Group think occurs more often in groups where there is a push for group consensus rather than for another form of decision-making. If there is too much cohesiveness within a group, members may not want to risk disagreeing (Rosenblum, 1982). Unfortunately, uniformity within a group is also important for the accomplishment of certain tasks since too much deviation leads to difficulty in goal achievement. Cartwright and Zander (1960) talked about the group pressures that occur to support one another's opinions in order to reach a consensus. Such pressures have "no bases in logic, objective reality, or evidence of the senses, which enable a person to arrive at a judgment or opinion he feels is appropriate" (Cartwright and Zander, 1960, p.170). Cues to the existence of group think include a decrease in spontaneous questioning by members, an increase in silence, and a hesitancy for members to play devil's advocate (Rosenblum, 1982). Some suggestions for combatting or preventing group think include the following (Rosenblum, 1982).

1) The resources within the group should be used to their fullest with everyone given a chance to speak and to be heard. It is helpful to seek as many expert opinions as possible.
2) The leader should allow for as many alternatives as seem reasonable to be considered. There should always be more than two.
3) The members need to reassess the decisions made in the group based on any new input that is received. If new subgroups are frequently formed to review all information, more people are considering the facts.
4) Members must consider challenging the information being presented. It is very important to consider the ethical implications of one's decisions, even if all the group members consider themselves to be moral individuals.

I find it helpful to ask for feedback from group members on how they feel the group has been going. This may be done anonymously by written notes handed to the chairperson. If the leader is indeed interested in the best possible goal achievement, he or she will be willing to enlist feedback from members. It is easier to give truthful responses if this is done anonymously.

Terminating the existence of a task group is usually done automatically when the reason for the task group's formation no longer exists. The goal has been reached or tabled indefinitely. Since interpersonal relationships have not been the focus within a task group, there is less need to disengage from one's fellow members. However, I feel that at anytime I sense a closeness among the members of a group, regardless of the group's purpose for existence, I want to provide some time and opportunity for termination. Chapter Nine included some ideas for focusing experientially on relationships. Some task groups continue in existence without meeting until a new task requires regular meetings again. Sometimes the membership may change during a time when the group is not meeting as individuals change positions and are then not eligible for membership in the group. Obviously, there can be very little termination for such members.

The task group will be one that most nurses will have experienced as both a member and as a chairperson at one or more times during their career. Being an effective member or leader provides satisfaction for the individual and task accomplishment for the group.

REFERENCES

Bavelas, A. "Communication Patterns in Task-Oriented Groups," in *Group Dynamics: Research and Theory* (2nd. ed.), eds. D. Cartwright and A. Zander. Evanston IL: Row, Peterson and Co., 1960.

Calkin, J. "Using Management Literature to Enhance New Leadership Roles," *Journal of Nursing Administration,* 10, no. 4 (Apr., 1980), 24–30.

Cartwright, D. and A. Zander. *Group Dynamics: Research and Theory* (2nd ed.). Evanston, IL: Row, Peterson and Co., 1960.

Chiavetta, L. "Group Communication: When I Speak No One Listens," *Nursing Management,* 13, no. 5 (May, 1982), 36–37.

Devereux, P. "Essential Elements of Nurse-Physician Collaboration," *Journal of Nursing Administration,* 11, no. 5 (May, 1981), 19–23.

Guetzkow, H. "Differentiation of Roles in Task-Oriented Groups," in *Group Dynamics: Research and Theory* (2nd ed.), eds. D. Cartwright and A. Zander. Evanston, IL: Row, Peterson and Co., 1960.

Jay, A. "The Meeting Chairperson: Master or Servant?" *Journal of Nursing Administration,* 11, no. 5 (May, 1981), 30–32.

Lancaster, J. "Making the Most of Meetings," *Journal of Nursing Administration,* 11, no. 10 (Oct., 1981), 15–19.

Mauksch, I. "Nurse-Physician Collaboration: A Changing Relationship," *Journal of Nursing Administration,* 11, no. 6 (Jun., 1981), 35–38.

Peterson, G. "Power: A Perspective for the Nurse Administrator," *Journal of Nursing Administration,* 9, no. 7 (Jul., 1979), 7–10.

Phipps, L. "Group Dynamics: Leadership Roles and Functions," in *Life Cycle Group Work in Nursing,* eds. E. Janosik and L. Phipps, Monterey, CA: Wadsworth Health Sciences Division, 1982.

Rosenblum, E. "Group Think: One Peril of Group Cohesiveness," *Journal of Nursing Administration,* 12, no. 4 (Apr., 1982), 27–31.

Schmitt, M. "Working Together in Health-Care Teams," in *Life Cycle Group Work in Nursing,* eds. E. Janosik and L. Phipps. Monterey, CA: Wadsworth Health Sciences Division, 1982.

Shostrom, E. *Man, the Manipulator.* New York: Bantum Books, Inc., 1968.

Wilson, M. "Negotiating Group Process Experiences," *Nursing Outlook,* 28, no. 6 (Jun., 1980), 360–364.

Structuring a Group Experience for the Client Population

11

--- Introduction ---

In this chapter and the next, we will look at the process of forming a client group in either an inpatient or outpatient setting. Agency constraints and supports, the milieu, the role of the nurse leader or observer and other staff, the physical setting for the group, client selection and preparation, and curative group factors will all be topics addressed in Chapter Eleven. Chapter Twelve will examine the structure of the teaching-supportive group for various client populations, including the chronic client. The nurse in practice, depending on his or her theoretical preparation, available supervision, and agency support, may have the opportunity to attempt one or more client group leadership experiences. Beginning nurse group leaders need regular supervision time, preferably from a clinical nurse specialist with a graduate degree in mental health nursing and experience as a group leader. The roles of the supervisee as well as the supervisor are discussed in Chapter Fourteen.

--- Structuring an Inpatient Group: ---
Assessment of Factors Affecting the Group's Structure

The Treatment Philosophy of the Agency

The attitude of the health care agency towards time spent on treating clients using a group modality is significant for determining the success of such interventions. A system not supportive of a group experience can result in less-than-effective group treatment outcomes and a negative experience for the staff involved (Loomis, 1979; Marvin, 1982). Both economical and political restraints may interfere with the feasibility of providing group treatment to clients (Loomis, 1979). The experience and educational level of staff, the number of staff, and the influence of a medical school and its training needs are all examples of how the economic and political climate may affect group practice in an agency.

Marvin (1982) suggested a need for the following information that would help the potential group leader assess the position of the health care agency on group treatment as a viable modality: 1) the treatment modality most favored by the agency; 2) the attitude toward group intervention by those people in administrative or power positions in the agency; 3) the type of group interventions favored by both the prospective client population and the health care agency (If the clients are thinking of group as an intensive psychotherapeutic experience and the agency is set up for only short-term stays, there would be an obvious discrepancy in the two groups regarding their expectations.); 4) any disparity that might exist between the group leader's approach to group interventions and the expectations of the client population and/or the agency (The group leader might want to combine both teaching and supportive elements in a couples group for new parents. The parents may feel threatened with a group experience that focuses on personal data as well as didactic material. The agency might want to combine pre- and postnatal couples in the same group and use a didactic mode only for a limited number of sessions.); and 5) the group outcomes or goals expected by the agency or community (Is the community expecting less alcohol-related accidents if an ongoing group is established for those found guilty of driving under the influence of alcohol? Does the agency expect the community to fund part of this program?).

Beliefs about Group as a Treatment Modality

There are many outcomes one can expect from group treatment depending on how the group is structured. Loomis (1979) identified the following as possible group outcomes: insight into one's personal process with others; didactic learning, particularly about health issues; behavioral change; and maintenance of one's current level of functioning in order to prevent rehospitalization. Maintenance implies little growth or expected change in the client and usually describes that client population which is considered chronic (Loomis, 1979). One frequently thinks of the chronic mental health client as someone with a psychosis that remains status quo as long as the client is compliant with taking antipsychotic medications. Other clients, such as those with chronic pulmonary disease, diabetes, hypertension, arteriosclerotic heart diesease, or an organic mental syndrome, may also be considered for a group that would help these individuals with compliance in their medical regime.

Maintenance may sometimes be used synonymously with compliance, but other goals associated with maintenance groups may actually make possible some growth or new learning for the client. Teaching clients to make the most of life within their limitations is a part of maintenance and may be considered growth-enhancing if the individual member finds life easier, more fulfilling, and so forth, as a result of the group experience. Learning to change one's physical environment to accommodate limited mobility or a disabling outcome of an illness is an appropriate teaching topic for a group of chronic clients. Experiencing a new hobby or other leisure-time activity may be very helpful for the chronic mental health client who needs more structure in the day to maintain contact with reality. Socialization is an important goal of many different types of groups, but it is particularly important for the chronic client who has withdrawn from social contacts because of his or her illness. Some groups for the chronic mental health client are focused on resocialization skills as the primary outcome for the group members.

An outcome which is very important for clients experiencing a crisis is learning that leads to new effective coping mechanisms. As discussed in Chapter Five, the support group as well as the psychotherapy group provide for this goal for their members. Emotional support expressed within a climate that allows for members to talk about their stresses and receive validation of the crisis symptoms they are feeling is certainly an important goal for the support group. When a member finds others in the group who have had similar feelings or experiences, this also provides validation as well as new learning on how to deal with particular crises.

Most groups provide for more than one outcome for their members. However, one goal may have more importance within the group than some others. The reason groups are identified according to type as described in Chapter Five is to specify that outcome which is central to the group's existence. Different health care agencies may favor one group outcome as being more important or cost-effective than another. The psychotherapy group which focuses on personal growth through insight into one's process with others requires a significant amount of time and therapist energy for this to happen. Many agencies do not keep clients as inpatients long enough for a psychotherapy group to be feasible. Therefore, this group modality is most often found in outpatient settings. If recidivism is a problem within a health care setting, an outpatient group to maintain client compliance with medications and treatments may be highly desirable. Frequently, such outpatient groups will be set up specifically by inpatient staff to keep clients in the community. Alcohol treatment programs, drug treatment programs, and mental health units often provide an outpatient experience as a routine part of the client's discharge plans. Supportive groups may be considered a luxury by some agencies, and staff time is not available for this type of group. Since client teaching is part of the nursing process, many agencies will decide on a group structure for many of their teaching activities. Sometimes this is for economical use of the staff's time. However, it is often believed to be a richer learning environment for clients. Certainly, if eight clients can be treated in one hour by two staff members, this is more economical than one staff person spending an hour with each of these clients individually. Time must also be allotted for the coleaders to get together to plan group and discuss the group's development as well as the group members' progress.

It is important that the group modality not be considered less effective than individual treatment. I see the two modalities as providing for different outcomes for the client, and I often work with clients that are experiencing both modalities concurrently.

"Group work should not be regarded as a second-rate treatment but as a complex, demanding process capable of maintaining functional behaviors and of producing therapeutic change when the group is well-grounded in theory and organized with care." (Marvin, 1982, p.118). As Loomis (1979) noted, it is the group process as well as the leader's interactions with members that provides for the positive benefits of group treatment. Some health care agencies see the economics of groups for treatment purposes as the reason for their use. My bias is that group benefits may outweigh the benefits of individual therapy for a client, and I see the economics as an extra that certainly may help sell the idea of group to an agency.

Some outcomes could not be achieved through individual therapy. For example, the emotional support and validation for one's feelings during a crisis are only available to any extent through a group medium. An individual staff person may provide support for a client, but one individual's input is not as valuable usually as that of several others who have also been experiencing similar feelings. The learning accomplished in a group may also often be superior to that of an individual encounter. Other members asking questions and offering information they have learned from their illness help a new member facing that same illness problem-solve for those difficulties which others have encountered and handled effectively. An individual teaching session allows the client more personal time with a staff member, but does not offer the wide range of learning experiences and first-hand information that a didactic group for clients all dealing with the same illness might offer. It is not only economics, therefore, that should be an agency's criteria for considering group treatment for clients.

Training and Educational Level of Staff Participants

As mentioned in the Introduction, the nurse who leads a psychotherapy group needs to have preparation at the graduate level with a masters in mental health nursing as a clinical specialty. This meets the American Nurses' Association standards of practice (Wilson and Kneisl, 1983; Marvin, 1982). Since most psychotherapy groups exist in outpatient settings, the inpatient agency may not find it necessary to have masters-prepared nurses to function as group leaders. However, a beginning group leader needs supervision, and this should come from a staff person qualified at the graduate level, whether this be a clinical nurse specialist, psychologist, social worker, or other prepared person. Agencies may also employ an outside consultant part-time for their staff learning to lead groups. Many general hospitals have access to liaison staff or other consultants who may work with staff learning to lead a group. Very often, the social work staff takes on the role as group leaders in the medical-surgical areas of a hospital. The number of trained people available is certainly a factor in considering group as a treatment modality. I feel it is important that nurses request appropriate consultants for supervision before taking on a group and that they negotiate with the administration to receive the support they need. The role of the clinical nurse specialist as a consultant may also include supporting staff in their negotiations with the administration for appropriate group supervision. This role is discussed in detail in Chapter Fourteen.

The Roles of Staff Participants in a Group

Besides the role of group leader, there may be roles for staff who are observers only or who are participant-observers. Another leadership role may be that of co-leader. The nurse may assume any one of these roles within the group. Very often, these roles are shared by staff of different disciplines, and the observer role is frequently related to situations where groups are for treatment as well as the training of staff. Although several authors (Marvin, 1982; Phipps, 1982) identified the co-leadership role as having three possible structures, that of observer-recorder, junior-senior coleader, or an egalitarian coleader, I do not see the observer-recorder role as being one of coleadership.

Observers may sit outside the group within view of the group members, or they may be in another room observing behind a one-way mirror. For ethical reasons, the group members must know they are being observed and must agree to this. I always share with group members the reason for the observation, *i.e.*, that the observers are paying attention to what the leader or leaders are doing in the group and are looking at how the group is developing as a means of learning more about groups and of helping the leaders who are facilitating the group. If clients have any hesitancy about this process, I do not allow observers. It has been my experience that most of the time, once the group members understand that they, personally, are not the focus of the observation, they are willing to have observers. In doing an inpatient group with students, I had both students and interested staff sitting in the same room as the group but outside the group circle (Wilson, 1980). The clients were at different stages of acute psychosis, and their ability to reality-test varied. Even those clients who were suspicious of others tolerated me as well as students and staff observing. Since the model at this agency was that students from many different programs and of different disciplines consistently observed in groups led by various staff, it may have been that the clients had adapted to this invasion of their privacy. I noticed that in the groups led by staff, the staff person never asked the clients' permission to have students attend the group. Students sat right in with the clients in the body of the group, and some staff expected the students to participate. This participant-observer role will be discussed shortly. It is important to note that observers affect the process within the group, especially if they are in the view of the group members. One-way mirror observation is less disruptive to the group process and seems to be a more ideal model for group observation. As a trainee on a family study unit designed specifically to train family therapists, I found the one-way mirror observation to be extremely helpful for my learning. Frequently, several trainees and a supervisor would view a family session together and discuss group process as it was unfolding before them. Families that came for therapy understood that training was an important part of the unit's reason for existence and had to agree to being observed. However, the outcome for the families was the input of several skilled family therapists in the work the trainees were doing with them.

In an article by LeSor and Phanidis (1982), several models for observers were discussed. In attempting to follow the principle that feedback is most effective when presented as close as possible to the situation with which it is related, the observers made contact with the group leader right after group. The observers were to help both the group leader and the members look at the group's development, but the time elapsing for the members before they received feedback varied with the model used. In one model, the observers met with the leader for a post group discussion, and the leader would share some comments with members in the following group meeting. Another model allowed the group members to listen while the observers talked with the group leader about the session. Members were then allowed to make comments about this process at the next session. The most direct feedback model provided for the observers to join the group during the last five minutes of the session to make comments on process and problem-solve with the group members about the group's development.

The participant-observer role requires the individual to focus primarily on group process as an observer but to offer comments to the group and interact with the group members also. As noted above, this role was the one used by the inpatient agency where I had students. I have seen this role used for trainees or visitors to a group when the group members requested that the observer also participate or when the group supervisor felt it important to give the leader process input while the group was meeting. Unfortunately, participant-observers sometimes forget or hesitate to participate. This may be awkward for both the group leader and the clients who are wondering what the observers sitting in the group are thinking. Recently, I had a psychology intern request to observe the group I was doing that was process-focused and goal-directed towards reminiscing. When I consulted with the group members, they requested that the new person sit in and participate. He agreed but did not say anything during the entire session. As I was attempting some closure with the session, I requested some input from him. He gave the group members some very caring and pertinent feedback. I found myself wishing I had called on him sooner. My style is to wait for someone to speak, especially if I have told him this was my expectation. I frequently found that my students did not interact with the groups to which they were assigned as participant-observers, and this was my impetus for starting my own training group (Wilson, 1980).

The junior-senior cotherapy model provides for one leader as the senior therapist and is usually used for training purposes. "This approach is commonly used in agency settings, because it provides in-service training of new personnel and nonprofessionals under the guidance and watchful eye of an experienced group leader." (Wilson and Kneisl, 1983, p.512). Leadership in this model may be with people of different disciplines, and it is not unusual to find a clinical nurse specialist coleading with a psychology intern or social work student who is learning the leadership process. Berne (1966) noted that coleaders do not have to have the same level of expertise, but their duties should be well-defined. Problems can occur when the junior leader experiences growth in leadership abilities but the group is not able to give this person the status that should go with this growth.

The egalitarian model of coleadership provides for two persons of a similar level of expertise (Wilson and Kneisl, 1983; Phipps, 1982). Both may be training to become group therapists, or both may be experienced in facilitating a group. Egalitarian cotherapists are frequently of different disciplines. This is often helpful in providing the group with two different slants on the way behaviors, feelings, and one's health status are perceived. In a support group for clients with cancer, a nurse might focus on health habits and provide knowledge about medications and treatments while a social worker would have more expertise on community agencies that could be of help to the client and his or her family. Both coleaders would share the responsibility for facilitating the group's development and perceiving and assessing the group's process. However, their specialized areas of expertise add another dimension for the members to use. Some agencies prefer to allow only one leader per group because of the economy of using one staff person instead of two (Wilson and Kneisl, 1983). The time spent by coleaders developing their relationship with each other and discussing the group is considerable and certainly another economic factor. The quality of the group experience for clients is certainly enhanced with a coleader situation. Chapter Thirteen will present in detail the coleadership process and the many complementary roles coleaders may take to facilitate the group process.

Daily Schedule of the Unit Activities in Relation to Group Time

On mental health units, group time is a planned part of the schedule from the point the staff decides that groups will be part of the treatment program for clients. Groups may be changed, discontinued, or added; but as long as the staff agrees that time should be allotted for group, a slot in the schedule should be found for a new group without too much difficulty. When a group is started in a medical or surgical inpatient area, it is more difficult to work in a time for this (Loomis, 1979). Clients may be off the unit at radiology, nuclear medicine, or having a variety of treatments that frequently take precedent over a group experience. Depending on the degree of involvement the staff feels with the group and the agency's philosophy about this as a worthwhile modality, group leaders may meet with a variety of active and passive resistances. Even when staff are committed to holding the group, scheduling may be a problem. If family will be coming for the group, it may be necessary to meet in the evening. Some creative problem-solving might have to occur with scheduling.

The Physical Setting for the Group

Berne (1966) described the ideal physical environment for a group. The room should be free of physical distractions and sound-proofed from external disturbances as much as possible. Size and privacy are important as well as a configuration that allows for members to sit in a circle. Berne suggested a therapeutic distance of a little less than an arm's length which leaves each member free for normal leg and arm movements without needing to be concerned about encroaching on another's space. Sitting around a table allows members to create a physical barrier between one another, gives clients a crutch for leaning, and hides part of the person's body. All this allows protection for members that prevents therapeutic use of nonverbal behaviors and may siphon off some of the anxiety necessary for members or the group to work. Certainly, this is particularly true of a psychotherapy group. I find a table to be very distracting, and it prevents members from reaching out to one another to share an intimate moment or provide some physical support.

Confidentiality and the integrity of the group is an important issue for members (See Chapter Seven). If there is not a private place for the group to meet, confidentiality is in jeopardy. Staff on the unit must be supportive of the group leader's efforts to ensure the preservation of confidentiality in respect to the group's work. Just making sure that the door is closed to the group room when the group is meeting seems very simple and routine, but I am shocked by some practitioners who leave a group exposed by not shutting a door. It would seem that the group might get the message that what any member might have to say is not important enough to ensure privacy. I am very direct with staff about how important I see that courtesy of making the group room private.

When students are participating in a group or attending a group as observers, the members need assurance that those visiting the group will maintain confidentiality about what goes on. Sometimes members do not directly tell visitors this is important to them, but they may express this through the theme that develops in the meeting. Perhaps the group talks about the confidential relationship with their doctors, or a member relates a story about a breach of trust between himself and his father when he was a child. Both these topics reflect the group's concern about the present possible breach of trust. Instead of saying this openly, the members develop it through an overt theme that the leader should pick up and articulate for the members to help them talk openly about their concern for confidentiality. When a psychology intern was visiting our senior process-oriented reminiscence group, the members did not directly ask the intern to maintain the integrity of the group. However, one member talked about how wonderful he thought the group was because everyone could say what they felt and know it was going to be confidential. As I was closing the group, I turned to him and said I thought that when he talked about confidentiality within the group, he was intending to tell our visitor that he would like this new person in the group to maintain this important norm. He agreed emphatically.

—— Negotiating A Group Experience for Clients —— When the Existing Program or Staff is Not Supportive

There are times when the health care agency or unit staff are not in favor of a group treatment program. In other instances, the staff may want to start a group but find their current program does not easily accommodate a time or a place for group. The latter problem is probably the easier of the two to work out, since staff and agency support are the major factors in assuring a successful treatment program. If the staff feels that group is important, they will find a way to adjust the current program to accommodate a group.

Change theory from a systems point of view, described by Lippitt, *et al.* (1958), offers some help for the practitioner attempting to introduce group treatment into an existing agency/staff system. To illustrate the translation of change theory into practice, two examples from my own clinical experience with the change process will be discussed. Most likely, many practitioners have initiated change without being aware of the steps they were using. Although I had studied change theory in graduate school and had applied it to clinical situations with individual client systems, I did not attempt to translate this theory for work within a larger system until much later, after some trial and error. Attempting change in as large a system as an agency can be intimidating but is very worthwhile.

Problem Awareness

The first step in the change process is the development of an awareness for the need for change in the client system. The system may seek help after feeling a need, although this probably occurs more with individual clients than with an organizational system or a group. With clients who are noncompliant, the need is not usually initiated by them but by the change agent or a third party. A parent, police officer, or social worker may see that a client gets to a clinic or is hospitalized if this person is in danger of harming himself or others. Adult protective services may get an elderly person hospitalized who has not been taking care of herself and who may be very ill physically. The change agent may be the first one to be aware of a difficulty and may bring this to the client's attention directly or may try stimulating awareness of the problem within the client system. Stimulating a voluntary desire for help without forcing this requires some creative problem-solving by the change agent. In the two examples which I am going to discuss, one situation for change was the result of a third party intervening to put me and the client system together. In the other, I attempted to stimulate awareness of the problem within the client system.

Example 1

One of the mental health inpatient units in the hospital where I worked had a reputation for being an undesirable place to send clients or staff. As a locked unit, it accepted those clients most psychotic, requiring seclusion at times, and needing a great deal of one-to-one attention by staff. The unit also accepted transfers from the rest of the hospital when a client needed a locked area for any extended period of time. The psychiatrist spent little time on the ward and avoided any working relationship with the nursing staff. In analyzing the power structure on the unit, it appeared that the social worker possessed the most power. He used two offices to see clients and receive phonecalls, his own outside the ward door and the head nurse's office on the unit. The social worker also ran the one meeting on the ward and held the only group, not allowing nursing staff to participate in any organized treatment plan for the clients. There was no therapeutic method for deciding when clients would be put in seclusion or removed. The high level of energy from the clients and lack of a structured treatment program gave one the feeling of the unit always being in chaos. As a substitute weekend supervisor for the nursing office, I made rounds on the ward. Although I had a key, no one but the ward staff members were allowed on the unit without an escort to the nurse's station by a male staff member. Most of the time, the nursing staff stayed in the office, and the clients remained in the dayroom with minimal supervision.

At the time when I was asked to transfer to this unit as the head nurse, the psychiatrist had resigned, and the nursing supervisor was in the process of revitalizing the nursing staff with persons interested in creating a treatment program for the unit. Another psychiatrist had been temporarily put in charge of the unit. He was very interested in making the ward a therapeutic place for clients to be. The social worker continued to operate as he had, probably because there was no permanent head nurse to attempt to regain some of the physical space belonging to the nursing staff as well as the right to determine a nursing treatment plan for the clients.

In analyzing the situation according to change theory, the client system or the problem that needed changing was the ailing nursing staff. I am focusing on this aspect of the change because it was the nursing supervisor, as a third party, who asked me to be a head nurse on the unit to institute a viable nursing treatment program. The psychiatrist was also already acting as a change agent, but his position was temporary. He, the nursing supervisor, and myself were to interview new psychiatrists for the ward chief position. It was unclear what resolution there might be with the social worker. Lippitt, *et al.* (1958) talked about vested interests in the client system that were motivated to prevent awareness by the system of problems. The social worker on the unit had, for a long time, joined forces with the psychiatrist who later resigned in an effort to continue the status quo on the ward without any outside interference. Although the nursing supervisor was aware of the problems, she was powerless to do anything as long as the psychiatrist and social worker controlled the unit. Her major area of power was with nursing staff. She had to negotiate with the medical staff and social work department with any problems coming from these areas.

Example 2

In Chapter Ten, a description of the units on which I placed students and the power structure of the nursing staff group was described in length. It is this system to which I would like to now refer again as an example of a change initiated by my stimulating an awareness of a difficulty (the learning experiences for students) in a client system, which in this case was the nursing staff. I do not believe the nursing service was aware of the inadequacies, both in the type of learning experiences and in the amount of experiences available for the number of students they were trying to service. One of my goals with students was to teach them to recognize and facilitate process interventions with clients. I felt that a group experience would be a rich area for the students' learning. Initially, there was one process group available which could take only two students at a time. This I shared for part of the time with an instructor from another school. When that group was closed to us at the clients' request, I made a decision to bring the inadequacies to the staff's attention (Wilson, 1980). I had already decided to request that the students and I do our own group where I would have complete control of the learning experience. By deciding the direction of the change, I was already moving into Phase 3 of the change process (Lippitt, *et al.*, 1958).

It was my perception that the underlying power within the multidisciplinary team that practiced there was with the psychiatrists, who had strong ascribed status (see Chapter Ten) in this agency that functioned from the medical model. The social workers, who were the group leaders, had ascribed status because of their education and position. Therefore, the social workers claimed that power not used by the psychiatrists. I wanted to instill within the nursing staff an awareness of the power they did have in defining the scope of nursing interventions, including the nursing students' learning experiences, to the rest of the staff (Wilson, 1980).

Lippitt, *et al.* (1958) talked about using a leverage point to gain accessibility to the client system to allow the change process to begin. Eventually, the leverage point should lead to the final change goal. My leverage was the fact that, through no fault of the nursing staff, the one process group experience for students had been closed to us. I knew the head nurses felt badly that this had happened (Wilson, 1980). I was counting on their readiness to problem-solve with me around this dilemma.

Establishment of the Change Relationship

A group is one system that is particularly susceptible to pressures for change exerted from the outside (Lippitt, *et al.*, 1958). I felt that the pressure for what I represented, the preparation of future nurses, was an excellent force to motivate the nursing staff to engage in the change process with me. My role as a change agent was to create a special environment or situation which would lead to new learning by the students. This, I hoped, in turn would create new behaviors within the nursing staff leading to their taking more responsibility for their own learning and for their modeling these new skills for students. By inviting the staff to attend a student-led group, I hoped to facilitate their own learning about process and their assertiveness with the other disciplines on staff (Wilson, 1980). I went through a lengthy presentation of my problem to the staff. I felt that my having been in the agency for over a year would facilitate their acceptance of me and what I had to say.

In the first example, I became a change agent on the locked acute unit by being put in the role of the head nurse and becoming what change theory calls an "autonomous subpart to help provide internal strength" (Lippitt, *et al.*, 1958). Prior to my appointment, I had dialogued with some of the staff about the problems they saw on the unit, some of their dissatisfactions, and so forth. This helped me to assess several of the areas that Lippitt, *et al.* (1958) described as important for the change agent to consider. These included the capacity and motivation of the client system to accept and use help. Resistance is often centered in the fact that the person as the change agent and his or her form of help are unknown to the client system (Lippitt, *et al.*, 1958). Although I had talked with the staff members one time before I went to the unit as head nurse, I was a stranger to them. I found the staff members reluctant, once I took over the leadership, to share with me just what difficulties as nursing staff they actually perceived. There was a lot of pain centered around the relationships between staff and the unpleasantness of the unit's milieu, and this was perhaps the motivation of the staff for change to take place. Change theory talks about a subpart of the system as frequently benefitting from the status quo (Lippitt, *et al.*, 1958). A few of the nursing assistants had found favor with the social worker and were being stroked with more "therapeutic" responsibility from him (*e.g.*, being asked by him to attend his group when none of the nurses were allowed to do this). In return for this, these staff members were sabotaging any efforts by nursing staff to oppose the control by the social workers over the unit. With all this resistance, I found it very difficult, initially, to establish a relationship with the nursing staff as a change agent.

Definition of the Problem, Alternatives, and Goals for the Change

Lippitt, *et al.* (1958) identified several problem areas which could occur within the client system including: a faulty internal distribution of power which may be exerted in harmful or ineffective ways, a problem channeling and mobilizing energy in other than nonproductive ways, and the existence of defective patterns of communication. The change agent might obtain information about the problem by direct questioning or observation in the client's system, or by seeking information from other systems with which it interacts.

It was clear that the nursing staff on the locked unit was struggling with a faulty distribution of power, both within the nursing group, itself, and between the nursing staff and another system, that of the social worker and those he could manipulate. As a direct observer in the client's system, I noticed that one nursing assistant routinely made all the assignments for his peers, and the nurses did not take any responsibility or control of this. The nursing assistant had an esoteric system for the way he went about his duties, and he withheld information from the nurses about interventions he made with clients. This secrecy added to his control of the situation. In exchange for this power, he spared the nurses the need to coordinate and make decisions about direct client care.

The powerlessness the nurses felt in the multidisciplinary units where I had students was expressed in their lack of opposition or questions to me or the students about our proposed group (Wilson, 1980). As was noted in Chapter Ten, the nursing staff had very little ascribed status with the other disciplines on the units. I constantly observed the nurses not responding to a psychiatrist's question to them for their opinion about interventions for particular clients. Even when offered, they hesitated to assume any position of status within the multidisciplinary team.

My spoken goal was to provide a learning experience for students. My covert goal was to provide, through observational experiences and dialogue with staff who would visit our group, an exposure to how nurses could, through use of their knowledge base, make a unique contribution to the client's care. Although I was not direct with my entire agenda for change, I did indicate I wanted to make a change in the treatment program by having complete control of a learning experience for students, something the nursing staff never felt comfortable in doing or articulating to the other disciplines. It was my judgment that openly showing my goals for change would be too overwhelming for staff. By giving me permission to try the group, I felt the nursing staff was expressing some hope that nursing could be a more visible discipline on the units. The staff did not seem to know how to go about doing this.

In initiating change, one may directly support the client system through consultation, enter into the client's system as an active team member, or act as a mediary between a larger client system and its subpart (Lippitt, *et al.*, 1958). As I stepped in to initiate a change in the unit's treatment program, I was entering the client system.

Resistance by the nursing staff as well as the multidisciplinary staff to my efforts towards change has been discussed in Chapter Ten. Lippitt, *et al.* (1958) noted that resistance gives the change agent information about difficulties within the client system. In this case, resistance by various nurses to my getting female clients for our group gave me some insight into the disorganized power structure of the nursing staff.

In Example 1, as expected, resistance by both the nursing assistants and interference by the social worker intensified as I moved into the nursing staff system and began to exert some control. However, I was supported by the nursing supervisor and some very competent staff that she was moving onto the unit. They agreed that their goal should be one of active, direct participation in a multidisciplinary treatment program with direct control over those interventions that fell within the realm of nursing actions.

Generalizing and Stabilizing Change

When the change effort is given visibility, and information about the consequences of the change is allowed to disseminate throughout the client system and neighboring systems, this tends to stabilize the change (Lippitt, *et al.*, 1958). In Example 2, as nursing staff observed our group in action and then stayed to discuss group process with the students and me afterwards, our rapport increased tremendously. Staff gave students positive feedback, began to ask questions about nursing interventions, and started chatting about personal issues with the students and myself. "Recognition by the agency that we were accepted as a viable group doing credible work with clients came when one of the social workers asked us to lead a group for her in her absence." (Wilson, 1980, p.364.). Although the change had not reached the proportion I had wanted it to in opening up more power for the nursing staff in their relationship within the multidisciplinary team, I feel the groundwork had been set. Nursing was being more recognized as a discipline with viable treatment approaches.

In Example 1, visibility for the changes occurring with the nursing staff on the locked unit was quite visible. The controlling nursing assistant was assigned to a unit with an established nursing power structure which allowed him to use his skill at organizing nursing tasks without controlling his peers. I had some direct confrontations with the social worker about his use of my office, and he eventually retreated to an office off the unit. When the new ward chief established himself, the two of us requested another social worker and eventually got one. The nursing staff began regular nursing care conferences, inviting the clients to discuss with us their needs in a planned meeting. As a multidisciplinary staff, we established some unit policies for accepting clients from throughout the hospital who needed some intensive mental health interventions. Other units responded to our guidelines.

Achieving a Terminal Relationship

As the change agent works on terminating with the client system, a method for incorporating the change agent's role into the system needs to be established. This may be done through establishing a permanent group observer within the client system; planning for regular periodic checkups with the client system, and teaching the client system when and how to ask for further interventions (Lippitt, *et al.*, 1958). After a period of being head nurse, I moved into a clinical specialist position, working on the locked unit. I found this to be awkward for both the new head nurse and myself. I had a difficult time being an impartial observer, and the staff had difficulty allowing me to be. When I began working with several other units, I found I was still welcomed on the locked unit, but I noticed that one of the other clinical specialists became more involved on the unit. She became the new group observer and consultant, and I pulled away. I believe she was a more impartial observer than I was and, therefore, a more appropriate person to have available for any further change work that might require the help of a consultant.

The change as I had envisioned it was never completed on the units where I had nursing students. Our student group existed for a total of four years, and it served to make the nursing staff more aware of their opportunities for developing a treatment program for clients. Our group was only a very small part of the business of the units, and since we were only there two days a week during the school year and not at all during the summer, I am surprised we could pick up practically where we had left off when we came back each year. It gradually became easier to get clients, and we even started getting some referrals from nursing staff. This indicated that the staff did have some sense of taking the initiative for a treatment portion of the client's care. Since the change was not complete, either from my viewpoint or from nursing service's, I believe another change agent was needed. A new chief nurse with strong beliefs in providing an environment more conducive to independent nursing practices moved in and took over as a change agent. Since she had been the assistant chief nurse and an inservice director well-liked by the staff, she already had their respect. Although I did not stay to see more change occur, I believe it was possible. The process was underway.

Change for the Client: Preparing for a Group Experience

The detailed discussion of the change relationship is just as applicable to individual clients or to a group of clients as it is to the systems that affect the client's care. Reviewing some of the theory cited in previous chapters, one can see a parallel between group process and the steps in change theory. Every group meets with a certain focus, goal, or purpose in mind as a client system describing a need or desire for change. The change relationship has to do with the developing relationship between the group members and the group leader as the group talks about norms and about the executive structure or the power relationships in the group. Resistance in the form of avoiding self-disclosure or of actively opposing the group leadership occurs in most groups. The change process becomes most active during the working stage of the group's development and is stabilized as the group moves toward termination. Determining how to maintain the change outside of the group's existence is part of termination. The nurse who functions as a group leader is most definitely a change agent.

Selecting Clients for a Group

The nurse leader may not have the luxury of selecting those clients most appropriate for the type of group the nurse is doing. Frequently in inpatient settings, there is a client population that is to have group as part of their treatment program, and the group members are, therefore, the clients that happen to be on the unit at the time. Since most of the groups I have done have been of this type, I cannot fully imagine what selecting the group membership would be like.

Yalom (1975) listed extensive exclusion criteria when selecting group members. Among those that probably would not do well in a group he included: those that are high somaticizers; those that have problems with being too intimate (maladaptive self-disclosure) or too withdrawn; those with high denial as a defense mechanism; those that are paranoid, brain damaged, acutely psychotic, suicidal, addicted to drugs or alcohol, and so forth. This last group of clients listed in terms of a clinical diagnosis are on Yalom's list as not being appropriate for outpatient intensive group therapy. Obviously, an inpatient group made up of drug abusers would have different goals than an intensive psychotherapy group. The groups the students and I did with clients demonstrating psychotic behaviors, dependency on alcohol, and suicidal behaviors, among others, offered clients a chance to interact more intimately with one another than in the maze of confusion existing out on the unit. Those that were withdrawn began to address their group peers and offer them some feedback or an idea of what they were feeling. I have learned to determine group goals according to the capacity of those with whom I am working in a particular group. If an acutely psychotic client demonstrates some awareness of reality, I am very pleased. A support group can tolerate more client deviancy than an intensive psychotherapy group. A didactic teaching group does best with members who are able to reality-test. The nurse group leader will have to determine the appropriate client membership for the type of group he or she is leading.

Prior to selection, Yalom (1975) suggested a screening interview. The kinds of questions one would ask a client should relate to the type of group the client will attend (Yalom, 1975; Marvin, 1982). For an intensive psychotherapy group, Yalom suggested process-focused questions such as how the prospective member experienced the interview or interviewer, what particular areas of discomfort or anxiety the client felt, and so forth. He also suggested that one should ask the client about interpersonal relationships, degree of intimacy with both sexes, prior group history with various types of groups, and other questions related to the proposed group experience. For a support group, the leader might ask a prospective member how comfortable it is for that person to self-disclose or to listen to others do this. Another question might relate to the expectation the member has about the group. A support group is not a psychotherapy group, and a client expecting to work on personal problems not related to coping around the crisis the group members are sharing will be disappointed with the group. In a teaching group, the members can expect to learn from one another as well as the group facilitator. For clients who would find this difficult to accept, group teaching might not be appropriate.

An alternative to the individual interview is to observe the prospective members in a group situation similar to the one they would be attending (Marvin, 1982). Yalom (1975) noted that the greatest predictor for the behavior of a prospective member in a group is related to performance in a similar group in the past. Asking about previous group experiences would provide some information about this. It may be difficult for the nurse leader to either question or observe some prospective group members. Families of hospitalized clients attending a support group may meet the nurse for the first time at the initial group meeting. I have never held pregroup interviews, and often I have met members at the first meeting. I have had good experiences with groups, but I am also realistic about the expectations I have. Sometimes the members, because of their inexperience with groups, do not terminate with all or even some of the goals the group was designed to meet. However, most members at least find a sense of belonging and may increase their degree of interpersonal relatedness. These are also excellent goals and relate to the curative factors of a group experience which we will discuss in a later section.

A pregroup interview may be used to impart some information to the clients about the group: the purpose/goals for the group, the difference between a group experience and an individual experience, and technical aspects about the group, such as meeting time, place, length of meetings, and duration of the group (Yalom, 1975; Marvin 1982). If it is not feasible to meet with clients prior to the first official meeting, this information may be discussed at the initial group session. If the clients are not preselected for a group, a way of notifying prospective members about an initial group meeting needs to be initiated. A personal invitation or phone call is certainly more inviting than a letter. Frequently, the nurse may visit with the client's family during visiting hours and ask the family to a support group meeting at that time.

There has been much discussion about heterogeneity vs. homogeneity with regard to the group population (Yalom, 1975; Marvin, 1982). One theory of dissonance supports heterogeneity, since the mixture of differences among the group members would lead to some disappointment within each member and an increase in anxiety leading to searching for and trying out new behaviors to alleviate this. Marvin noted that members who are very similar or homogeneous still come from very different experiences and have different methods of coping. Some homogeneity provides for group cohesiveness. Yalom suggested pairing for members to prevent one member from feeling very different from the rest of the group. Differences in age, race, sex, occupational level, educational level, and so forth, may cause some anxiety if one member deviates greatly from the rest of the group in these characteristics. Group size should be between five and fifteen members. Yalom suggested that the optimal number of members vary according to the duration of the group. A group meeting over a long period of time could take more members and still provide for a positive group experience. Some members drop out, and this means one may start out with a few more members than is optimal. Obviously, the type of group will dictate the number of members. A teaching/support group could take more members than an intensive psychotherapy group.

The Structure of the Group

The length of sessions and duration of the group's life relate to the type of group and its goals (Marvin, 1982). A psychotherapy group often meets once or twice a week for an hour over a period of a year or more. A group of clients meeting to learn about their illness might meet everyday for thirty or forty minutes for a period of a few weeks. Sometimes, such a group then might have follow-up sessions once a month for several months for support and questions once the client returns home. A support group might meet once a week for an hour as an open-ended group for members to leave as their stress becomes manageable with new members being free to join at anytime. Closed groups finish at a planned time which is known to the members ahead of time. Most teaching groups are close-ended. Groups where the individual's growth is more important than the group's goals are usually open-ended to allow for individual differences in rate of growth. Open-ended groups must absorb new members as others leave.

Selection of a theoretical framework to facilitate the group depends on the training and expertise of the leaders in particular frameworks as well as the group composition, duration of the group, and purpose of the group (Marvin, 1982). Part One of this book presented several frameworks for group practice. The nurse who plans to use one of these frameworks needs specialized training to facilitate a group. A psychotherapy group lends itself to a variety of frameworks. A support group is less intense and could operate very nicely on a basic group dynamics framework. It is my bias that all group leaders should understand communications theory and the concept of how the group may be looked at as a system made up of a group of smaller systems, the group members. Leading a group with the knowledge of how to observe and facilitate process, even if the leader chooses not to ask the group members to look at their own process, would seem to be an essential for a group facilitator.

Group goals should always be shared with the group members in a way that allows both members and the leader to measure their accomplishment. The group goals as well as terms of the group's existence, frequency of meetings, and other aspects of the structure that affect the therapeutic goals constitute the group contract (Marvin, 1982). Groups focusing on individual growth will often have individual contracts describing personal goals that fit with the group's goals.

Curative Factors from a Group Experience

Yalom (1975) identified several values inherent in group membership apart from the goals designated for accomplishment through the particular type of group of which the individual is a member. The process of belonging to a group is itself a healing experience. Although Yalom based these curative factors on membership in a psychotherapy group, I find some of them applicable for the support group experience in which nurse leaders would most likely be involved. The following are described according to Yalom's definitions and will then be put in the context of a supportive group learning experience.

1) Universality. The belief by clients that their problems are unique tends to result from social isolation and not sharing with others. In a group, clients are able to talk about their problems and find that they are common to many other group members.

2) Altruism. Once common problems are shared, members find they receive support and suggestions from their peers. Yalom noted that clients frequently trust the reactions and comments of peer members more than they do the leaders' comments. Altruism helps members move outside themselves and think about others.

3) The Development of Socialization Techniques. Roleplaying and other exercises allow clients to practice those skills which they find stressful or difficult to do. Group members are able to give each other feedback immediately about interactional skills.

4) Group Cohesiveness. Yalom used this term to include several other outcomes from group membership that require the cohesiveness of the group to be successful. Recall that cohesiveness is the felt attractiveness by the members towards remaining in the group. The member with feelings of low self-esteem who is highly regarded by a cohesive group will tend to reexamine his own self-perceptions in relation to the public esteem he feels from others. In a cohesive group, there is increased acceptance and understanding between members and a tendency to be open about one's conflicts with another group member. This is helpful in conflict resolution.

5) Didactic Instruction. Cognitive explanations often decrease members' anxiety, particularly around their illness, whether it is more emotional in nature or due to a physical condition. Yalom found explanation and clarification to be curative processes and an initial binding force for a group.

6) Catharsis. With this process, the client shares concerns that may have been difficult to say out loud. Ventilation produces relief and also support and acceptance by the other group members.

Universality, altruism, and catharsis all further the development of group cohesiveness. In a cohesive group, altruism and catharsis, as well as conflict resolution, are more likely to occur. In a support group, there are interventions the leader might use to further these processes. Members need to be addressed by their preferred name. A warm-up exercise, such as some of the ones suggested in Chapter Nine, would help group members learn about each other and what each person desires as identity in the group. Names develop a person's uniqueness in the group and allow the leader to recognize individual contributions of members. It is much easier for group members to give each other feedback when they are comfortable with each other's preferred name. The nurse leader should not forget that well-timed experiential exercises can increase trust, promote self-disclosure, and help members get a sense of their oneness as a group. The support group is one that counts on the universality of the member's crisis and the member's altruism in wanting to share ways of dealing with this crisis to make the group a healing one. The leader needs to look for similarities between members' experiences and reinforce these within the group.

Catharsis and conflict resolution take a different focus in a support group than they do in a psychotherapy group. Catharsis is a central goal in a psychotherapy group, and the therapist purposely allows a member to experience a certain amount of discomfort/anxiety in order to further the individual's realization that he or she must deal with the pain by working out loud with it in the group. In a support group, the anxiety is reduced for members to allow the group to become a haven from the daily stresses that the members are feeling. Catharsis in such a group relates to the group allowing members to cry, share feelings of stress, and talk about those experiences of each day that have made them most stressed. Spilling all this in the group is a way of finally getting rid of it and then feeling accepted by the group in a place where this letting go is appropriate. The group leader needs to help members understand that such a process is healing for each of them.

Most often, conflicts between group members are not purposely brought to the group's attention unless they are disturbing the group's work or are preventing one or two members from reaching their individual group goals. Chapter Eight described the origin of interpersonal conflict. The group leader in a support group will more readily move in to resolve a conflictual situation than will the therapist of a psychotherapy group who may see the value of the two clients attempting to resolve their own conflict at their point of readiness. A long-lasting conflict within a support group might be very devastating for the members. One method of conflict resolution is to have the two members roleplay being in the other person's "shoes." Each member would assume the philosophical stance of the other in order to understand the other's position. A role reversal allows both parties to get some distance from their own emotions. I would have the members try a role reversal if I thought the conflict was one which other members of the group may have felt and which might relate to the stresses with which the group was trying to deal. Since the members of a support group are not contracting for therapy, an in-depth analysis of the motives and feelings underlying a person's anger towards another is not appropriate. I would attempt to move away from the conflictual situation as a problem with two people and instead look at it as a group problem and learning experience. I might make such comments as:

"I wonder if this interaction is related to some of the stress you have been feeling about your illness? ... Perhaps others in the group can relate to getting angry or losing your temper with a friend or family member?"

"What you and Jim seem to be doing is picking on each other's weak points. This is something I see happen quite frequently in this group. How does what you're experiencing right now with your child's illness relate to this irritability I see with you two?"

For the group members to know that feeling less than adequate in dealing with conflict is something that might happen when one is in a crisis, gives members permission to share their experiences with conflict in the group. This can be very appropriate learning. I often use group occurrences to teach didactically about crisis, stress, and any disease process that affects one's emotions.

Certainly, it is also appropriate to plan some didactic learning not based on something happening in the group but on information that the group should have to understand a family member's disease or their own illness. Information on anatomy and physiology, medications, treatments, or the process of a disease are frequently chosen topics. It is important to reinforce the exchange of accurate information between members and to clarify incorrect information. Problem-solving skills are appropriate to practice in the group and to relate to specific problems members are having. Group members often can teach each other some ways they have learned to handle living with a certain disease.

Roleplaying to improve interactions in a certain area may include such situations as how a parent asks a doctor about his child's illness or goes about seeking a second opinion. How one moves back into social circulation after losing a limb or suffering another disfiguring operation are topics that could lend themselves to both discussion and roleplaying. Individuals need to be desensitized to their limitations and to know how to handle other's reactions to them. Cancer has been such a frightening word to say or to discuss with friends or family. AIDS is fast becoming easily as sensitive a subject for its victims to handle. Giving group members back some confidence in their ability to interact socially with others is a very important skill on which to focus in the group.

The support group is a rich area for client teaching and "healing." Facilitating such a group can be a significant contribution to the care of many clients.

REFERENCES

Berne, E. *Principles of Group Treatment*. New York: Grove Press, Inc., 1966.

LeSor, B. and J. Phanidis. " 'Bring Those Outside Observers In,' " *Perspectives in Psychiatric Care*, 20, no. 1 (Jan.-Mar., 1982), 13, 45–46.

Lippitt, R., J. Watson, and B. Westley. *The Dynamics of Planned Change*. New York: Harcourt, Brace, and World, Inc., 1958.

Loomis, M. *Group Process for Nurses*. St. Louis: C.V. Mosby Co., 1979.

Marvin, L. "Group Organization: Selection Criteria, Member Preparation, Contractual Issues," in *Life Cycle Group Work in Nursing*, eds. E. Janosik and L. Phipps. Monterey, CA: Wadsworth Health Sciences Division, 1982.

Phipps, L. "Group Dynamics: Leadership Roles and Functions," in *Life Cycle Group Work in Nursing*, eds. E. Janosik and L. Phipps. Monterey, CA: Wadsworth Health Sciences Division, 1982.

Wilson, M. "Negotiating Group Process Experiences," *Nursing Outlook*, 28, no. 6 (Jun., 1980), 360–364.

Wilson, H. and C. Kneisl. *Psychiatric Nursing* (2nd ed.) Menlo Park, CA: Addison-Wesley Publishing Co., 1983.

Yalom, I. *The Theory and Practice of Group Psychotherapy* (2nd ed.). New York: Basic Books, Inc., 1975.

TABLE 11.1 STEPS IN THE CHANGE PROCESS

Step	Actions Needed	Responsible Agent
1. Problem awareness of the need for change	1. Analysis of power structure within the existing system(s) 2. Description of interpersonal system(s) needing to be changed 3. Decision re: which system will become the client system for change	Initiated by: a) the client system; b) a participant-observer outside the client system; or c) a change agent
2. Establishment of the change relationship	1. Dialogue with client system about areas needed for change 2. Assessment of capacity and motivation to accept change agent's help 3. Assessment of areas of resistance	The change agent: a) outside the client system; or b) as an autonomous subpart of the client system
3. Definition of the problem, alternatives, and goals for change	1. Gathering of information about the problem by direct questioning or observation of the client system or by seeking information from other systems with which the client interacts 2. Formation of goals acceptable to the client system and based on problem definition 3. Initiation of change through: a) consultation; b) as an active part of the client system; c) as a mediary between the client system and a subpart 4. Assessment of resistance and continual evaluation of the defined problem based on reaction of the client system to active change	Change agent

TABLE 11.1 STEPS IN THE CHANGE PROCESS (Continued)

4. Generalization and stabilization of the change	1. Making visible the change actions and results 2. Disseminating information about the consequences of the change	Change agent and subparts of the client system
5. Achieving a terminal relationship	1. Evaluation of change completed and any further work needed 2. Establishment of a method for incorporating the change agent's role into the client system through: a) establishing a permanent group observer; b) planning periodic check-ups with the client system; c) teaching the client system the process of asking for further change	Change agent and client system

SOURCE

R. Lippitt, J. Watson, and B. Westley. *The Dynamics of Planned Change.* (New York: Harcourt, Brace and World, Inc., 1958).

The Client Support Group: Teaching and Supportive Elements 12

Introduction

The nurse in almost any setting will eventually encounter a set of clients who would benefit from some increased knowledge of their disease process, the treatments or medications they are receiving, or some help with the adaptation required status postsurgery, a myocardial infarction, or other medical procedure that has changed their lifestyle. Many clients must learn to live with chronic pain and severe physical limitations. In seeing the client at both birth and death and in the many life crises in between these two milestones, such as parenthood and midlife, the nurse has the opportunity to make such maturational crises tolerable and even growth-enhancing. Particular emphasis in our society is now on aging and the needs of the geriatric client. Support groups for dealing with the natural losses encountered with aging and with the tasks that the aging person needs to do to prepare for death are becoming as important as groups to help new parents or the adolescent client.

For the purposes of this book, the group which focuses on the learning needs of its members who are experiencing stress related to a particular developmental period in their lives or to an illness of their own or of someone close to them is labeled a support group with teaching elements. One way to relieve someone's anxiety is to give that person some control over what is happening to him. If a client understands the disease process that is ravaging his body, he is able to control runaway fears that would lead him to support any myths related to the disease. Cancer is a prime example of how myths about the disease can frighten families of clients as well as the individual who is ill. Accurate knowledge about an emotional subject given in an understanding way is helpful for clients and their loved ones. Inherent in the function of the support group are the expectations that one needs to know about coping skills and how stress can be translated into physical symptoms as well as emotional ones. Therefore, this chapter talks about the support group as offering both emotional coping and teaching elements.

Peer Support

In a group setting, both teaching and emotional supports come from the group leader as well as the individual members. Although some teaching is best done on an individual basis, either because of the client's inability to tolerate a group learning experience or because the information is very personalized to the client's need, most health teaching is appropriate for a group. The advantages of the members' sharing their experiences with one another adds another dimension to learning and is very helpful in dealing with the crisis of an illness or with a new experience in life, such as the birth of a child. One's peers are often the most significant part of a group experience for members. It has been pointed out that Yalom's beliefs about group psychotherapy focus on the importance of the members to one another in obtaining positive results in therapy (Grunebaum and Solomon, 1980). The support group is no different. Recall that the initial stage of the group's development is characterized by a belief in the perfection of the leader to meet all the members' needs. Initially, members do not see themselves as effective agents for help within the group. It is up to the group leader to reinforce every member-to-member response that facilitates the group's work. When the nurse leader sees an opportunity to use a member rather than him or herself to teach or offer emotional support, the process of peer facilitators is reinforced. A basic result of such interactions is an increased feeling of self-esteem for the member that does participate in this way.

The Support Group

In the following sections, the client support group is discussed as it relates to both developmental and situational crises. A crisis occurs when one's normal coping skills are no longer adequate to meet the problem situation that is occurring. (See Chapter One for review of crisis theory.) A developmental crisis occurs as one attempts to respond to the stresses of some maturational event. Since all humans move through specific periods of development and must deal with their transition from one developmental stage to another, everyone experiences developmental crises (Wilson and Kneisl, 1983). They happen with regularity but affect individuals with varying degrees of severity. Historically, one's adolescence is a time of trauma, but some people respond with deviant behaviors while others remain relatively free of real difficulties. It has only been in the last several years that literature abounds with writings about the midlife crisis experienced between the ages of thirty-five and forty-five (Wilson and Kneisel, 1983). A movie, "Middle Age Crazy," depicts a man caught in such a crisis. The other period that has captured a great deal of attention lately is the period of old age. Much of this chapter will look at support groups for the aging client.

The situational crisis occurs in response to an anticipated or unanticipated external traumatic event. While one realizes that developmental crises will occur and can anticipate these, the situational crisis often comes without warning (Wilson and Kneisl, 1983). The death of a child or a serious illness are examples of an unanticipated situational crisis. Anticipated situational crises involve some participation by the person in the event, such as a marriage, a change in jobs, or a move to a foreign country. Victim crises are also situational in nature since they have to do with an external traumatic event. A natural disaster or a man-made one, such as war or crime, are victim crises (Wilson and Kneisl, 1983). In this chapter, we will focus on the unanticipated situational crisis as being most apt to generate the need for a support group in which the staff nurse would become involved. As the reader will recall, the support group meets the needs of those clients who are experiencing stress related to their life situation. A particular member may or may not be in an actual crisis. However, the support group is not designed to resolve an individual member's particular crisis but to provide a setting for effective problem-solving and sharing of those experiences common to all the group members. The support group is often open-ended, whereas the crisis group lasts only for the defined crisis period of six weeks.

A support group may be considered a means of intervening to prevent a fully developed crisis situation.

The Elements of Stress and Anxiety

Hans Selye (1980, p.127) defined stress as "the nonspecific response of the body to any demand." He noted that stress cannot be completely avoided or one would be dead, since the body is always demanding energy to maintain life. He concluded that the way people handled life situations made a difference in the amount of stress the body experienced. Certainly illness may be considered a situation which results in extra stress on the body. Studies have also shown that stress, although not necessarily causing illness, does lead individuals to use "illness behavior" as a way of coping with the stress (Minter and Kimball, 1980, p.204). In sociological theory, stress is believed to occur when the individual's support systems fail (Simpson, 1980). Simpson believed that social support as an intervention for stress works best when done face-to-face as opposed to a telephone hotline or other less personal mode.

Anxiety has been defined "as a mildly pathological way of reacting to stress." (Selye, 1980, p.141). An anxiety response seems to be related to the personality of the individual responding to stress. Those that have an anxiety trait tend to respond with anxiety whenever stress is felt. However, acute anxiety occurs only in specific situations and is a feeling of tension and apprehension associated with activation of the autonomic nervous system (Simpson, 1980). Education to improve both one's problem-solving ability and coping skills may lead to less stress and less anxiety (Simpson, 1980). It seems, therefore, that a support group designed to both educate and offer face-to-face social support is a helpful nursing intervention with those clients experiencing stress and anxiety from illness or other situations that make excess demands on one's body.

The Support Group and Client Populations

The rest of Chapter Twelve will explore the content and, to some degree, the process of particular support groups with which the nurse leader might be working. Some theory on normal growth and development throughout the lifespan will be included, since this is a significant factor when working with a specific developmental age-related client population. Since groups for children dealing with the stress of illness, a parent's death, or other tragic events require the leader to have extensive knowledge in theories of child emotional development, the nurse leader should have preparation on the masters level to be an effective facilitator. Such theory is too specialized for purposes of this book.

Developmental Stages of the Client-Impact on the Support Group

In this section of the chapter, we will explore the support group as it relates to a client population experiencing a particular developmental stage and the stresses that accompany this stage of growth.

The Adolescent Client

The nurse will encounter opportunities to structure an adolescent group on an in-patient or outpatient unit and should consider doing a group with an experienced coleader who has preparation at the masters level in adolescent theory. The group most appropriate for the beginning facilitator would probably center around educational needs of the adolescent client, such as parenting for young teenage mothers, weight reduction and nutrition, diabetes mellitis and its management, and so forth.

Erik Erikson (1968) identified several graphic characteristics of the healthy adolescent. He talked about the identity confusion of the adolescent as a developmental crisis manifested in faddish, delinquent-like, and psychotic-like behaviors, along with creative moments and movements related to specific idealistic causes. The many new dance steps, dress styles, and even the style of talking the adolescent group initiates is an example of this creativity. The adolescent tends to be clannish and intolerant of others who are different in dress, aspects of gesture, and even language use. Erikson postulated that the adolescent's need to form a clique and exclude others not fitting a particular stereotype was part of the way adolescents as a group handled their discomfort of this age.

The importance of the peer group to the adolescent has particular significance for the use of the group as an intervention strategy. Griffith (1982) noted that maturational crises of adolescence are often more treatable within an individual or family intervention pattern; whereas, a situational crisis for the adolescent is best treated in a group setting. The adolescent's developmental struggling may have adversely affected the family system, or the adolescent may be experiencing more of a crisis as a result of something occurring within the family that made this period excessively stressful for the adolescent member. The young person who ends up being hospitalized on a mental health unit may be the identified patient from an unhealthy family system, or at best, from a family in crisis. It has been postulated that the adolescent with anorexia nervosa may be reacting to a dysfunctional family system. The anorexia serves to draw attention away from the interactional problems within the family system (Stein and Davis, 1982). The nurse not working in a mental health setting will be more likely to see the adolescent who has been hospitalized for a physical illness or who is going to an outpatient clinic for prenatal care, treatment of a chronic illness, birth control, weight reduction, and so forth.

The adolescent population tends to be resistant initially to being in a support group. He may worry about what he will or will not say in the group and if, in fact, he will even fit in with his peers. Depending upon the age of the adolescent, there may be different responses to the adult group leader. The younger adolescent tends to engage in hero worship and to define certain adults, other than one's parents, as "heroes." However, the older adolescent focuses more on the disillusionment he finds with the world and, in particular, with adults who have failed to make his world a place with which he is pleased (Levin, 1982). It is important for the group leader to initiate a specific contract, often in written form, with the members to make clear what the leader's and member's responsibilities are and facilitate trust between them. A contract may also include the group objectives and the length of time the group will meet (Griffith, 1982; Langford, 1981).

Most adolescent groups are time-limited. Since ending the group means the adolescent must terminate with peers with whom he or she has identified and formed relationships, the group leader should carefully plan termination to minimize the feelings of loss for members. The adolescent may react to the loss of the group with irritability, disruptive behaviors, or other actions that signify the importance of the group and the inability of the clients in this developmental phase to deal with loss easily (Griffith, 1982).

The lack of verbal skills makes groups with adolescent clients more difficult. It is sometimes necessary to restate feelings for the member who may not be able to put her feelings into words. Adolescents have some difficulty transferring from one situation to another unless they can see themselves in the particular situation (Stein and Davis, 1982). Using the group member as an example, the group leader might want to then suggest ways that what is being talked about in the group can fit with the member's own situation outside of the group, such as at home. Roleplaying helps the young person rehearse social skills that are not yet comfortable for the individual. Audiotaping and videotaping can provide instant feedback with regard to the skill level that has been developed. For specialized group techniques see Chapter Nine, particularly the content on games and psychodrama, which are very comfortable means of expression for the adolescent client.

Some specialized groups for the adolescent client are described in the following paragraphs. These groups are typical of what the nurse leader might find as needs with the adolescent population with whom he or she is working.

The obese adolescent is especially sensitive about her appearance and is most likely lacking a positive self-concept, a situation that is true for many adolescents who see their appearance as less than desirable. The literature on weight reduction focuses on groups for adolescent girls. Generally, such groups emphasize one's overall self-concept, grooming, and social skills rather than just weight loss (Langford, 1981; Stein and Davis, 1982). In keeping with the importance of the peer group for the adolescent, a common peer activity centers around eating at odd times, in fast-food places, and eating fattening, faddish food items. One's socializing as an adolescent frequently takes place around food. A focus on nutrition rather than dieting is helpful in the adolescent group as well as some suggestions for how to eat less and still partake of the adolescent social scene. Some weight reduction groups have a planned activity time, such as bowling, swimming, or learning a new dance step, which helps teach healthy physical habits, increase caloric expenditure, and contribute to socialization between the group members. Hair styling, dating, clothes, and other personal topics also add to the group's topics for discussion. Generally, group members are told to weigh only once a week, and the weight loss is not a central part of the discussion (Langford, 1981; Stein and Davis, 1982).

Pregnant teens not only face the stresses of adolescence but the anticipated situational crisis of motherhood. Medically, this group is at high risk perinatally, and they need, therefore, a lot of health teaching and emotional support (Griffith, 1982). The fact that the adolescent may need to face a decision of whether or not to keep the baby adds more stress to this time and suggests another topic on which a support group may speak. In a group, the role of parent and the parenting process should be presented along with information about abortion, contraception, sex, the physiology of pregnancy, delivery, and the postpartum period, and some discussion on relationships (Griffith, 1982). It is very important for the nurse leader to remember that underlying all this group content is the process of the peer adolescent group with interactions that may include a great lability of emotion, silliness, withdrawal, and other behaviors typical of the adolescent. Instead of being able to explain their feelings, group members may respond more to the leader suggesting feelings that might relate to the situation they are experiencing, *e.g.*:

"I guess I might be feeling really sad right now, Kim, if I had to think about not even seeing what my baby looked like. From the way you're sitting so curled up in the chair it looks like you just want someone to put her arms around you and take care of you like you want to do to your baby."

The dialogue incorporated observations of the client's body posture which frequently gives cues to what the individual is feeling. According to Gestalt theory, a person frequently does to themselves what they wish others would do to them. Kim's position could be associated with the fetal, curled-up position of her unborn baby. As an adolescent, she may wish for some return to the protection and comfort of early childhood, and her facing motherhood brings this all the more into focus. Even if this is not what Kim is feeling, she may welcome this caring message from the group leader.

A parenting group for new teenage mothers or for both spouses is another group that may be offered by the nurse leader. My bias is to include the father as well. The teenage father is also coping with the developmental crisis of adolescence and the situational crises of marriage and parenthood. A group co-led by a male and female set of facilitators offers the opportunity for learning through observation of modeling behaviors and also the chance to occasionally split the group and have the male coleader meet with the fathers and the female with the mothers in the group. The relationship between the leaders and the adolescent members is particularly important, since the adolescent will frequently distrust adults and be wary of their interventions. Hands-on tasks for new parents, such as the holding, feeding, bathing, and diapering of the baby provide for less focus initially on the interpersonal process occurring in the group. Teaching a skill that the adolescent member can learn easily increases the adolescent's self-concept and reduces the stress that would accompany a demand to verbally interact with the group leaders and other members. It is important to remember that the adolescent group members are still interested in those activities in which their nonparent peers are involved. Encouraging some social activities for the group while problem-solving with regard to baby-sitting may be very helpful for new parents who might be feeling cheated out of their time to have fun.

The Young Adult

The nurse group leader interfaces with the young adult client when he or she is the victim of a debilitating, chronic, or terminal disease, when the client has an ill child or parent, or when the client is a parent for the first time. Although all these events are classified either as anticipated or unanticipated situational crises rather than developmental crises, one may argue that marriage and parenthood, as well as the process of choosing to remain single, are really part of one's development. The nurse may be quite helpful in facilitating these processes which are anticipated and planned for in one's life. To facilitate a couples group, the content of which may include communication between the spouses, sexual function and dysfunction, or parenting the children as this relates to the interactional dynamics between the couple, the nurse should have specialized training at the graduate level. A group for couples that focuses on skills needed for parenting or on didactic information about contraception has as its focus support/teaching elements rather than the more psychotherapeutic focus of the former group. This group is appropriate for leadership by a beginning nurse leader.

A group for parents with children who have been hospitalized for mental health problems is an example of the kind of parental support needed when a child has an illness that may not be well-understood by others, even the family members. The goals of such a group are to provide support for the parents and effect a better method of communicating with and disciplining the children in the family (Ferguson, 1979). Very often, one child is the identified patient within the family system, but the other children are also at risk for emotional problems related to the dynamics between the parents, children, and spouses. For families that may need some help as a unit but resist this, the support group is a good alternative. The support group will not work on family dynamics but may help parents and children to gain a better understanding of each other's needs. Certainly, not all families need family therapy because their child has been hospitalized. As a leader in a support group, the nurse may refer families for more intensive therapy. Often, the nurse can help families to be less frightened of seeking the additional help they need.

The particular group that Ferguson (1979) described met for twenty-one weeks (the average length of the child's hospitalization) for one-and-a-half to two-hour sessions. Some of the specifics which the group worked on were making parents aware of their child's normal growth and development patterns and having the parents compare this to memories of their own developmental history. The parents roleplayed specific communication and discipline problems they were having with their child and received feedback from other members and the leader. Ferguson (1979) described a technique originated by Yalom to take the power out of "secrets." Each member writes on a slip of paper something that would be hard to share in a group. The papers are anonymous and are redistributed so that each member reads aloud someone else's secret and talks about how it would feel to have that particular secret. This helped the parent group deal with feelings of guilt and isolation. Ferguson (1979) suggested that this same group format could be used for groups of parents having children with cerebral palsy, cardiac problems, digestive problems, and other overwhelming and chronic or debilitating diseases that require the parent to gain more understanding of their child's expected pattern of development.

Johnson (1982) discussed similar goals for a group experience for parents of the chronically ill child. Such a group would help the parents: understand the illness and its treatment; increase acceptance of the ill child; become more aware of their fears, isolation, and feelings of helplessness and how to handle them; decrease feelings of guilt related to having a child with a genetically transmitted disease; and recognize the resources available both within themselves and in the health care community. Groups for parents of the chronically ill may be coordinated with the child's clinic visits. It is important that parents understand they do have control over their personal relationship with the child although they may not have control over the child's disease process.

The young adult client may also be a member of a support/teaching group for expectant parents, for new parents, for stepparents and their spouses, or for parents of adopted children. A group for the parents of a dying child is documented later in the chapter in the section dealing with loss. The young adult who acquires a chronic disease will also have to deal with the dynamic of loss in relationship to lost future goals, lost physical functions, and other occurrences that one would not expect at such an early stage in life.

The Person of Middle Age

This period of life spans a wide range of years anywhere from the middle thirties to age seventy. Those elements which generally characterize one's entrance into middle age include such events as: the children leaving home; being passed over for a promotion; experiencing an increase in illness; losing one's spouse through death; or entering retirement. This is a time when the individual may have reached specific career goals and finds that these accomplishments are no longer as satisfying as they used to be. Some events that occur in middle age are unpredictable, such as unemployment prior to a planned retirement, the unexpected death of a child, or divorce after many years of marriage (Chiriboga, 1981). Several clients with whom I have worked have experienced severe depression over losing a son or daughter. Most prominent are feelings of anger and helplessness and the question of why God's order for things seems to have been altered. I find my own experience as a parent allows me to empathize more easily with these clients, but it is also hard to keep my subjective feelings of sadness separated from my work as a clinician. It seems that a support group is a most appropriate intervention to allow members to care for and comfort one another.

Middle age differs from those previous developmental periods where there were specific events and roles for one to look forward to in the future. Although the individual may feel fulfilled in a career or with a family, the only sure future is old age and, eventually, death (Chiriboga, 1981). Instead of counting age from one's birth, the number of years left has more significance. Those who have not met particular goals they had for their productive years must now accept that these will never be met. As one's children prepare for marriage or other events in life, it is difficult to not feel some jealousy at their opportunities. This age is also a time when one's parents may need to be taken care of, and the reversal of roles may be difficult to accept. Facing a retirement income and possible increased expenses for illness adds to the uncertainty of middle age (Goin and Burgoyne, 1981). The death of a spouse requires one to deal with a devastating loss.

The empty nest syndrome has been frequently cited as a problem for the mother when the last child leaves home. However, more is now being written about the father's experience with this same situation (Roberts and Lewis, 1981). Those fathers most likely to experience this are older men who have had fewer children and those who have had children later in life; who are not supported with understanding wives and a positive marriage experience; and who find their family needs less of their financial support or nurturing than it once did. The trend that has been developing for the man to take on more of the responsibility and nurturing of his children may make the empty nest syndrome more prevalent for fathers in the future (Roberts and Lewis, 1981).

Other factors involved in the postparental adjustment period include the mixture of role messages which parents receive from their married children. "In-law" jokes are very prevalent as are the admonishments to be good grandparents. Children may still be paying off financial education debts to parents, or they may remain in the home longer than expected because of financial problems or lack of direction for their own life. Children remaining too long in the family of origin or leaving home unexpectedly early cause stress for the parents (Roberts and Lewis, 1981). One client I worked with individually had two children who chose to remain at home because they were unable to find jobs and had little success in completing their education in a satisfactory manner. The father continued to feel the need to nurture by allowing the son to drop classes at a local college with a promise that he would do better the next class period. The wife wished to "kick" the son out to force him to be self-supporting. The couple had agreed to disagree about this matter. Although the husband was retired on disability, his wife continued to work and to put most of her energy into that endeavor. My client had refused the role of house husband, but he had not developed any other interests to pass the time. My focus with this man was to help him develop some new roles for himself independent of his wife's functioning but compatible with their relationship. His skills as a teacher in a volunteer capacity would allow him to function as an active member in the community but within the limitations of his problems with anxiety. Some of his need to nurture the son could be transferred to the nurturing of others outside the home.

Roberts and Lewis (1981) suggested treatment for the empty nest syndrome to include both remedial work and preventive education to help clients develop new social roles or more adequate ones that would also meet the need for intimacy. Anticipating change in one's role before it occurs is helpful in preventing problems, especially if the individual is then able to develop substitute roles or invest more energy in those activities that are already very fulfilling. These years are frequently a time when people find more hours for community work, as a volunteer or paid worker. Many of our legislators have been middle-aged when they entered politics for the first time. Accepting a political appointment on a local or state committee during this stage of life is another way to become involved in a satisfying way. Consciousness-raising groups may be helpful in preparing men and women to find new roles that will prevent the feelings of loss created by the children leaving home (Roberts and Lewis, 1981). I suggest that the nurse explore this as a topic of concern in any support group he or she might be leading with clients at this stage of life. The opportunity to form such a group might occur as the result of either parent wanting support with the experience of hospitalizing a parent of his or her own. The nurse who works with elderly persons with middle-aged children who are looking for some way of handling their parent's illness may find such a group very helpful.

Not much has been written on the support group for the middle-aged client. Those persons who experience the death of a spouse during this time would find a group for widows or widowers to be helpful in the long grieving process. Since the empty nest syndrome is an important factor for both men and women, some education as well as emotional support may be helpful. Very often, teaching groups for clients experiencing debilitating physical illnesses in middle age, such as cardiac problems, diabetes mellitus, hypertension, and so forth, may also offer the members emotional support. The nurse leader needs to look at what is occurring in the members' lives other than the physical disability and to offer both education and support for any such emotional stresses.

The climacteric is certainly a factor in one adjusting to the physical changes that occur at middle age. The term "climacteric" comes from a word related to "ladder" and refers to having reached the top where the only way to go is down from that point (Henker, 1981). In both males and females, there is some reference to a diminished sexual interest at this time and a change in the hormonal balance with a decrease in the production of the sexual hormones. However, authors seem to agree that this time is most stressful because of the environmental factors which we have listed previously about middle age, such as the children leaving home, the death of a spouse, and the personal realization that one is looking at more of his or her life having gone by than is left (Henker, 1981; Ballinger, 1981). Ballinger noted that the menopause has received the brunt of a multitude of symptoms blamed on it which are not necessarily related to the female climacteric. Those emotional symptoms claimed by women relate more to the children leaving home than to the physical changes caused by the menopause. Therefore, it seems appropriate not to give the climacteric power by suggesting it as a reason that someone is having difficulty during this period of his or her life. It is appropriate for the nurse to consider this as one of many changes the middle-aged client is experiencing and to note that the emotional effects of the climacteric may be related to how individuals are perceiving this change in their lives. Certainly, it is important to educate persons to the myth of the power of this change while being sensitive to its effect on some individuals. Didactic information may be quite helpful to clients, particularly in a group setting where members might share their questions, experiences, and concerns with one another.

The Elderly Client

As if growing old with its multitude of physical and emotional stresses is not enough, the process of aging has also been very much maligned in our youth-oriented culture. The Gray Panthers special interest group calls attention to the need in our society for someone to take up the cause of the aging individuals, and it has been their own group that has been one of the first to demand some recognition as persons that still have much to offer to the world. The abundance of senior citizen discounts has been one type of recognition that has come to this population group. However, I believe the aging person wants to be considered as someone with cognitive abilities and contributions to make that go beyond mere recognition that this group deserves monetary discounts because of their age and limited incomes. The term *ageism* refers to an uneasiness by the young and middle-aged of the process of growing old and a perception of this as being a time that is quite distasteful because of disease, disability, powerlessness, and uselessness leading one to eventual and certain death (Settin, 1982). Settin cited an example of ageism in the belief that exists that reality orientation is the therapy of choice for the hospitalized aging client because of lost cognitive powers. However, most aging clients have not, in fact, lost such cognitive abilities. The following paragraphs will explore some of the realistic occurrences in the process of aging.

Settin (1982) maintained that a group for clients who are experiencing the process of aging but who are not cognitively impaired should focus on problem-sharing and solving, should be primarily verbal rather than activity-focused, and should allow for confidentiality and the opportunity for catharsis of negative feelings. My own experience with the aging client in a group setting has been the reminiscing group another colleague and I have co-led. Although the focus is reminiscing, which we will discuss as a particular process which promotes the developmental tasks of aging, the group members demonstrate a broad range of interactions that facilitate a "here-and-now" process. The group has become quite cohesive, and the members talk about their feelings of depression, thoughts about suicide, relationships with family members, and the importance of the group in their lives as a place where they feel comfortable and supported. Most of the group members did not have any positive history for mental health problems but found themselves becoming depressed as some of the environmental stresses associated with aging impacted on them. Although I did not expect the group to be as functional in focusing on an insight-oriented process, I am so pleased that my coleader and I did not limit the group to reminiscing exercises only. As I recall my initial thoughts about the group, I see that I underestimated their capabilities. My attitude is a perfect example of the ageism of which Settin was speaking!

Although reminiscing is a process not reserved just for the elderly, since it begins in the middle childhood years, it is done with greater frequency and with more vivid imaginations in the aging individual (Donahue, 1982; Blackman, 1980). Reminiscing is a calling to mind of past events, people, and feelings in a purposeful or spontaneous manner. These thoughts may be kept to oneself or shared verbally or through writing, such as in an autobiography (Donahue, 1982; Burnside, 1981). Burnside noted that reminiscing helped the individual cope with the loss of life-long social roles and cherished physical objects as well as with the feelings of boredom and isolation.

Reminiscing helps one with the process of the life review, which Butler (1963) described as an internal process exclusive to the aging person that promotes the resolution of those conflicts experienced in life that have affected one's self-concept, especially in a negative way. Being able to satisfactorily resolve those aspects of one's life that have felt unsettled or in conflict with the perception of the way life was supposed to be, helps prepare the individual for death. The life review, being an intrapsychic activity, is not readily observed except through the results of the process. The outward signs of the person's involvement in the life review could include isolation, depression, suicide, or such positive behaviors as increased adaptation to aging, autonomy, and statements of self-worth (Blackman, 1980; Burnside, 1981).

To promote the process of the life review for the aging client, one needs to stimulate the elderly person to recount life events. Listening is an important part of promoting reminiscing (McMordie and Blom, 1979). I have noticed I need to purposely make myself keep silent or say only a few words that might encourage more reminiscing when I am coleading the senior group. If I am patient, very often even the quietest member will contribute to a discussion about familiar battles or towns prominent in the battlefronts of World War II. Since all of these clients are veterans, the war is a shared experience for the group. At times, I am tempted to think that such discussions do not lead to much important "here-and-now" process between the group members. Even though the content of a past event is most prominent, I can switch to the present by asking the group to look at what it is like to talk about the war or to not have anything to contribute to the discussion. These questions elicit process. I do not have any data on how the reminiscing affects each member's life review process, but I know some members get more depressed when talking about the War, and some members find it exhilarating. I can gather data about how reminiscing affects the members' relationships with one another, and this process helps me assess the group's cohesiveness, sociability level, etc.

Forming a reminiscing group allows members to focus on this process to promote their own life review while gaining some of the benefits of a supportive group experience. The size of the group should be between four and eight people, with six being ideal (McMordie and Blom, 1979). This is a little smaller than the usual support group, but each member is expected to need some time to verbalize, and probably take up more of the group's time than the support group where only a few of the members share extensively. McMordie and Blom (1979) suggested that the group's population could include those with brain damage, physiological regression, blindness, and even expressive aphasia or mutism, because these persons could profit from the reminiscing experiences of other group members. The fact that reminiscing taps into the brain-damaged client's strongest cognitive asset, that of remote memory, allows these persons to participate.

Techniques to promote reminiscing offer the group some structure. Props such as recordings of old songs, picture albums, or pictures of past events may be used as well as cherished objects the members might like to share (McMordie and Blom, 1979). Burnside (1981) suggested topics such as one's earliest memory, the most exciting moment in history, or an exciting personal event for the subject of a group discussion. It is important for the group leaders to make each member aware of his or her identity of person to help with the process of the life review as well as to increase the awareness of group members for each other. Using members' preferred names, noting to the group any absent members, and using touch as a means of promoting intimacy are important interventions (Blackman, 1980).

Groups for the elderly may serve the purpose of normalizing the aging process. Treating aging as an inevitable yet adaptable part of life means that group members are encouraged to try out ways of getting around physical problems and to look for new interests and activities with which to become involved. Those members with hearing problems may be seated in the group where it is most conducive for hearing. Because of such physical disabilities, the group circle may need to be made smaller with members sitting closer to one another while not violating each other's space. However, touching or hugging as comfort permits should be part of the interpersonal closeness between members and the leaders (Britnell and Mitchell, 1981). I find the elderly client responsive to touching when I am comfortable with it and do it spontaneously. Important considerations that Britnell and Mitchell noted when doing groups with elderly clients have to do with the difference in response pattern for persons of this age. Storytelling is frequently a way of reducing tension for the elderly as well as being part of the process of reminiscing. The older client is not conversant in the psychological jargon which has become popular in the last few years. These individuals also have difficulty sharing very personal matters with one another. The openness with personal problems that is so natural for many of us is quite foreign and improper for the aging client. However, a support group is still an important intervention for clients who are hospitalized, in senior day-care centers, or in other agencies where physical limitations and other processes related to aging have created some stress. One does not need to share deeply personal data in order to give and receive support with the difficulties of aging.

With those who are institutionalized, the problem of loss of control over one's environment, freedom of movement, and so forth, makes the process of giving some of this control back to the aging person even more important (Tappen and Touhy, 1983; Britnell and Mitchell, 1981). "The use of group work with the institutionalized older adults can be an effective approach to counteracting some of the negative aspects of institutionalized life." (Tappen and Touhy, 1983, p.36).

Tappen and Touhy discussed the *spread phenomenon* as a concept that might be evident with some staff members who tend to think that a client with one type of deficit, such as a loss of hearing or sight, may have multiple deficits, such as psychological problems or total physical degeneration. This leads to overprotectiveness of the institutionalized client and a loss of control for this person. Staff members need to watch a tendency to infanticize the elderly client with scolding, baby talk, the use of pet names, overexplaining, or the withholding of information on the impression that the person is unable to understand. Staff need to give clients a choice of group activities and a choice of even whether to participate in group, as well as making sure that child-like activities, such as cutting or pasting, are initiated by the clients rather than the staff (Tappen and Touhy, 1983). If these points are followed, the elderly, institutionalized adult will feel more in control and maintain a sense of personal esteem.

Multiple Losses and Grief

With the process of aging comes the reality that one is losing both loved ones and loved objects and, to varying degrees, one's faculties and physical attributes. Although aging is a process that all of us experience daily, the elderly client is confronted with physical aging at an accelerated rate and with a loss of some mobility. Almost everything about our bodies works less well as they get older. Senses, such as hearing and sight, are often weaker, and it becomes more difficult and painful to engage in sexual intercourse. Very often, the elderly person has lost his or her life-long sexual partner. The aging person is often on a fixed income and must deal with a loss of financial security. Illness may force a person into a strange environment, such as a nursing care facility, a retirement home, or some other place that is not "home." Even staying with a relative does not allow the same freedom of movement and independence as being in one's own home. The individual may not be able to hold on to some prized material possessions. Clients in our senior group talked about the pain in losing their ability to be useful, to work. The group also spoke about missing what they felt was a simpler time of life. One member noted that after World War I, which was "the war to end all wars," no one worried about a future war as they do now. Even though that was a time when the world may have buried its face in the sand, this attitude resulted in less anxiety about the future. He really missed that freedom from anxiety.

All of the losses described above create a grief reaction in the aging individual. Certainly, the ultimate loss is that of one's spouse. This is not peculiar to the elderly client but is more likely to happen, of course, to those of an advanced age. Chances are that one or more people with whom the elderly person relates with varying degrees of intimacy will also be lost through death. The loss of a loved one results in a specific grief reaction studied by Lindemann (1944). Symptoms of this include somatic complaints, guilt feelings over possible neglect or negligence with the deceased, and a preoccupation with the image of the person who has died. Some hostility may exist for the health professionals who cared for the loved one (Huston, 1967; Goin and Burgoyne, 1981). The acute stage of grief lasts for four to six weeks, but delayed grief can occur from months to years after a death. This happens particularly if triggered by events or times, such as an anniversary, that remind one of the deceased (Huston, 1967; Kolb, 1973). Especially devastating for the widow or widower is the loss of shared activities with the partner and even the sharing of one's day that most often is part of such an intimate relationship. Research has shown that the bereaved spouse tends to hide the continuing pain of the loss from others who have not experienced this and so would not understand. The bereaved share mostly with each other (Goin and Burgoyne, 1981). Part of bereavement theory describes a stage of reorganization and redefinition of one's roles. This would seem to be especially necessary for a widow or widower. Widows need both personal contact and structured direction that would take the place of that given by the deceased spouse. It has been shown that the most effective person to do this is another widow (McWhorter, 1980). A grief reaction or mourning process also occurs when one experiences other losses. Somatic difficulties, preoccupation about the lost object, hostility towards those connected with the loss, and so forth can occur in the person.

Grief therapy groups are one way the health professional might help the aging person deal with the grief associated with loss (Burnside, 1981). The group leader should be a therapist trained in grief work. However, a support group for the aging client may also be helpful as a way of validating that this time of life is filled with the pain of multiple losses and that grief is an appropriate response to such losses. The actual grief work may need to be done on an individual basis, depending on the severity of the losses. Grief work may proceed quite naturally in the person who has good ego strength and who is not overwhelmed by multiple losses. We are not doing grief work in our senior group, but we have given the group time and encouragement to talk about loss and may refer some members for individual work.

The Chronic Client

Chronic illness has its rise during the middle of one's life and will add to the expected stresses of middle and old age. Any chronic illness requires a change in lifestyle for the person as well as a demand to learn new ways of taking care of personal needs, and frequently leads to social isolation due to the stigma of whatever the illness might be. Physical readjustments may lead to a loss of autonomy and an increase in dependence on others (Schmitt, 1982). In the following sections, we will discuss chronicity as it impacts on the mental health of both the elderly client and the younger client. The chronicity of physical illness is included in the last section of the chapter.

The Elderly Regressed Client

For those persons who have experienced either a loss of cognitive abilities or a loss of reality-testing ability that has led to a marked regression in being able to maintain oneself, an institutional placement usually results. The client often isolates himself, behaves bizarrely, or becomes overwhelmingly depressed or hostile. "The leader for group work with regressed aged must have the patience of Job, the perseverance of a nag, the stamina of an Olympic athlete, and an abundance of empathy.'' (Burnside, 1981, p.222). Important considerations for the group leader include moving more slowly as a precaution for those clients who have been physically mistreated in the past and who might become fearful of any rapid movements toward them. Burnside (1981) suggested the leader speak to the client while moving towards the person or touching him. She noted that the psychiatrically impaired client is often isolated from human touch. The use of props to provide sensory stimulation, such as strong pleasant odors of food, perfume, and shaving lotion, as well as pictures, music, and different textures provide structure for group activities and eliminate the sterility of the institutionalized environment. Burnside (1981) cautioned that choices of stimuli are important, since some pictures (nakedness, for example) and other props might be upsetting or repulsive or even frightening. Since clients are used to being in silence most of the day, a group leader needs to be comfortable with a more active orientation of breaking up silences as well as actively participating with the clients in activities (Burnside, 1981). On a visit to a closed unit for psychotic elderly clients, I observed a group community meeting. The social worker led the group in morning exercises, which the clients could do while remaining seated. She participated with them and consistently allowed only a few seconds of silence to go by before initiating some conversation. When clients who were called on to introduce themselves or offer comments declined to speak, she would ask other group members to comment on their interactions with that person or speculate about what the individual was feeling. She would suggest that the group would have to guess about the person's well-being if he or she were not going to speak to the group.

Yalom and Terrazas (1968) offered some similar interventions for group leaders working with the psychotic elderly. Interpretive feedback based on nonverbal cues from a silent or delusional member provides an opening for that member to speak to correct the leader's or group's perception. Since it is impossible to dislodge a delusional thought, the leader needs to look for ways to include the delusional member in the group with something that member has in common with the others. It is important to include rather than to further isolate the elderly clients from one another. I sometimes suggest a feeling that I think the delusional client may be expressing through her delusion. If the delusion relates to her dying of some poison or dread disease, this person may be frightened by a lack of trust from others in her environment or feel out of control about her own destiny. I might suggest these feelings, especially if they relate to what others have talked about in a more reality-based manner. With members who are displaying bizarre or disruptive behaviors, the leader might ask another group member to say how this behavior is affecting him or how he interprets what the person is trying to express. The leader may then give the disruptive client a chance to comment on the reactions by other group members. It is important for the leader to respond in a way that will enhance the client's ego strengths. This means looking for the reality in the communications and behaviors that occur in the group (Yalom and Terrazas, 1968). A member who is complaining about the food she is served being spoiled needs to be stroked for using the group as a place to bring up ''community'' issues. The food may or may not be spoiled, but the process of bringing the issue up is an appropriate behavior.

The institutional population may be included in groups for stress reduction, ego strengthening, and decreasing isolation unless clients are unable to comprehend the group conversation or cannot identify fellow group members. If a client is mute, very often this person gives nonverbal cues that he or she is receiving some input from the group. It is probably too difficult if the group has to absorb more than two very hostile paranoid clients (Yalom and Terrazas, 1968).

The regressed elderly client who may have either a problem with recent memory and orientation due to cognitive impairment or who may be emotionally withdrawn and socially isolated due to a psychiatric disability may benefit from groups designed to deal with these problems. Two such groups, the remotivation group and the reality orientation group, are both highly structured and have specific goals. The leader is usually very directive and controlling (Tappen and Touhy, 1983).

The remotivation group is designed to stimulate thinking and task performance in areas of daily living, to stimulate mental processes towards greater alertness, and to prevent further deterioration or withdrawal. Those that attend a remotivation group need to be fairly well-oriented; be able to use their senses for sight, smell, vision, and so forth; and not be preoccupied with hallucinatory stimuli. The group is process-oriented in that the goal of the group is not to reach a certain specific outcome but, rather, increased participation of the members in responding to the stimuli within the group. Since the focus is not on individual problem-solving or insight, the group may function well with up to fifteen members. A topic is selected by the group, usually at the previous meeting, and this is discussed for about fifteen minutes. Sensory aids, such as music, pictures, smells, food, or poetry, are then used to expand on the topic. Finally, the topic is applied to the personal experiences of members. It is important, however, that personal data be restricted to their application to the topic under discussion. The leader needs to be very directive with this. At the close of the group, a topic is selected for the following week, and the group members are thanked for their participation (Janosik and Miller, 1982; Needler and Baer, 1982). Topics might be current events, holidays, different countries or cultures, community sights, and so forth. Since the group members will be selecting the topic, the group leader does not have total control over this. However, the leader may offer suggestions and provide tools to help with selection, such as newspapers, pictorial books, and calendars.

A reality orientation group focuses on basic exercises that help the cognitively impaired aging person be more aware of the time of day, the day of the week, the time of the year, the place where he or she resides, the way to find the bathroom or bedroom, and one's age, name, role and so forth. Obviously, the structure is one of repetition with multiple visual aids, such as calendars, pictures, and maps. Structure tends to offer security for those that are cognitively impaired (Tappen and Touhy, 1983). The reality orientation group offers the client less autonomy in a group setting than a support or a remotivation group, thus mimicking the institutional control over the client's actions. However, the cognitively impaired client has fewer options and will, hopefully, gain something from the awareness that the reality orientation group offers. Perhaps, the members might be given the chance to make some choices about what occurs in the group. These could be such things as deciding on the type of refreshments served during or after group or making a choice of whether to meet outside or inside. It is probably wise to meet as often as possible in the same room to stabilize the group's "place" of meeting. The group leader needs to find ways to give clients in this group as much autonomy as possible.

Chronicity and the Mental Health Client

For outpatient mental health clients, many of whom have problems reality-testing, interacting socially, or finding activities to occupy their day or to help them feel worthwhile, the support group is helpful. Many clients with chronic mental illness are still in their young adult years and demonstrate social behaviors usually seen in adolescents. This adds to the problems these clients encounter in trying to relate in the community in which they live as outpatients. Some of the time spent in a support group may be to discuss the problems of having to take psychotropic medications. Serving refreshments may help to focus on social interaction and give clients some opportunity to practice this. Discussing reactions of family members and the community at large is helpful to promote problem-solving. The group may offer didactic information on such things as how to manage one's funds, acquire an identification card, or interview for a job.

Group experiences that focus on activities of daily living, such as cooking, shopping, and banking, are helpful for the chronic mental health client. A process outcome of the resocialization activities occurs when members begin to recognize their own maladaptive behaviors by observing them in others. As the group discusses how to change these behaviors, members learn from each other while maintaining some "OK-ness" as a person. Reading aloud from well-known literature or other documents promotes verbalizing without the threat to members of having to reveal feelings in the group (Lancaster, 1980).

For clients who may be so depressed that it is hard to get them participating in their environment at all, the use of music with an option of just listening or moving about may be helpful. Teaching relaxation exercises to music is quite nonthreatening for even very withdrawn clients. Members do not have to interact but focus only on themselves and their breathing (Wadeson, 1982). Drawing is another nonthreatening medium that allows nonverbal clients to begin to express themselves. Although art therapy is often part of an outpatient mental health program and is led by a trained art therapist, a nurse might use art media as a basis for an activity and impetus for some discussion later (Lancaster, 1980). A nonthreatening sharing between clients of what they are depicting in their drawings serves to strengthen the reality base for the group members.

Groups for chronic clients who are taking psychotropic medications are structured in a support framework to give both didactic information about medications and their importance in promoting mental health and to help clients cope with the side effects and other problems of taking medications. The nurse who is frequently involved in health teaching is an important source for leadership in this type of group. Compliance with medications is one of the most important ways of keeping one's emotional illness in remission and remaining out of the hospital. Yet it is also a problem, since the psychotropic medications have some very unpleasant side effects. In a group co-led by a nurse and a psychiatrist, client advocacy was one of the important outcomes of the sessions (Cohen and Amdur, 1981). Teaching clients how to talk to their doctor about medications, ask intelligent questions, and discuss untoward effects helped clients maintain medication compliance and feel more in control of their treatment. Realistic ways of handling side-effects were discussed as well as the need to tolerate an unpleasant effect for a short period of time during an acute treatment phase. For those clients who wanted to stop their medication, they were encouraged to discuss this with their psychiatrist first. Another important focus for the group was the unrealistic expectations some members had about what their medication might do for them *i.e.,* make their life happy. Encouraging the members to take responsibility for those things in their life which they wanted to change became a goal for the group leaders. A group for very disorganized mental health clients needs a structured didactic approach (Cohen and Amdur, 1981). A group described by Volkmar, *et al.* (1981) had a more interactional "here-and-now" focus but was for clients with a bipolar affective disorder who had difficulty with lithium compliance. Besides much sharing about lithium, the members discussed the impact of their mental illness on their families, employment, and other aspects of daily life. Their sensitivity and support of one another was a positive outcome in this group experience.

There is certainly a variety of groups that are possible with a chronic mental health population. It is not the intent of this book to teach the reader to lead a psychotherapeutic group for mental health clients. Observable group behaviors which include verbal withdrawal, physical or verbal aggression, poor impulse control, psychotic manifestations, disordered and autistic communications, restlessness, narcissistic demands for attention, and so forth, require that the group leader be a skilled therapist with extensive training. Although staff members without training attempt to lead such a group, my bias is that this is not nearly as effective for either the clients or the staff. The beginning mental health nurse may have many opportunities to observe a psychotherapeutic group and engage in dialogue with the leaders about specific interventions. This is certainly helpful for learning.

A family support group is a very helpful intervention for the families of mental health clients. Those groups that provide for a discussion of coping measures helpful to the family but that do not focus on the interactional dynamics of individual families or their members keep the group supportive rather than psychotherapeutic. Community resources, books, and other didactic information may be helpful for group members. The experience by members that they are not alone is a positive outcome from the support group (Harris and Tarbutton, 1983). Several self-help groups operate for families of the emotionally ill client. Parents of Adult Schizophrenics is a group that has become quite active in some areas of the country. A psychotherapeutic focus based on a systems model is another type of group offered for families of the mental health client. Very often, the client is also included. The leaders of this group are trained family therapists and may see a group of families together or individually.

—— The Support Group for a Client with an Acute —— or Chronic Physical Illness

In discussing physical illness and its effects on the individual, the theme of loss and grief again becomes a factor. The loss of mobility, of the role as a provider or care-taker, of a particular body part or physical identity, of independence or autonomy, and of one's life are all possible with illness. It is important to consider some of the theory we have not yet talked about in relationship to loss, that of terminal illness and of the disturbances of body image.

For most terminally ill clients, their death is something others have more difficulty discussing than they do. The dying client wants to talk about impending death and will not hesitate to use the word as a signal that he or she is comfortable with the subject (Bowen, 1976). Often, a support group for clients that have a disease that may be terminal, such as cancer, deals directly with the subject of death, both for the client and for the client's loved ones. Members may work through very personal feelings about dying while helping a peer to face the same prospect. If a group member dies while the group is still in existence, other members are then less able to ignore their finiteness. A support group for the families of terminally ill relatives may be led by a nurse. Staff may also find themselves asking for a support group to help them deal with caring for the terminally ill. Part of the difficulty we have in helping the dying client are our own personal thoughts about our death. It would seem that the more death can be talked about by staff, the significant others, and the client, the less formidable it becomes. The nurse who plans to do a support group for clients with a terminal illness needs to be willing to confront personal feelings about dying.

In disturbances of body image, the family or significant others as well as the client need help in grieving the change in image. The parents of a deformed child may react with sadness, guilt, depression, or even humiliation. They may be jealous of others with healthy babies (Kolb, 1959). Certainly the degree of emotional health within the family system affects the family's response to a deformed or disabled child. The birth of such a child creates a crisis for the family, and depending on the needs within the family, crisis intervention or a support group with other families experiencing a similar crisis is appropriate (Bowers, 1982). The healthier the family, the less need there might be for crisis intervention. A support group may be helpful for some ongoing problems and anticipation of particularly stressful periods. The reactions of others, community resources, sibling jealousy, the couple's needs, and parenting are topics appropriate for a support group (Bowers, 1982). The disabled or deformed child who is also dying presents added stress for the family. The child's life needs to be as normal as possible while the rest of the family also experiences some normalcy. Anticipatory grief is part of preparing for the death of a significant other. A support group organized for families with the dying children of the same age allows the group leader to focus on that period of development (Bowers, 1982). A special need in this group is to help the family understand the child's perception of death at that age.

The sensation of the phantom limb, which amputees experience and which paraplegics experience in a similar way, maintains the original, intact body image of the person. The phantom limb is a healthy, expected response, but this must not keep the client from discussing the disfigurement or paralysis. Some body parts carry a lot more significance for the individual, such as the breast or uterus of the woman. Loss of one's body image or a body part is similar to the loss of a significant other in impact upon the person (Kolb, 1959). Grief theory is quite applicable to these situations. Preparation of the client and family members prior to disfiguring surgery is important. Support groups for the client or significant others are generally formed after surgery or after the loss has occurred. Didactic information about what to expect with the healing process, with prostheses, or possible rehabilitation are important supportive elements to discuss in a group.

Cancer is a specific disease that can cause disfigurement, a change of body image, a great deal of pain, and death in its terminal form. For this reason, support groups for cancer clients may need to focus on many aspects of loss, and group leaders need to be prepared to facilitate and deal with the grief response. Cancer treatments, including chemotherapy, radiation, and other interventions, may be very frightening for clients and lend themselves to some didactic teaching to allay some needless fears and give clients more control over the treatments they receive. One group for clients was organized as a formal class to teach chemotherapy to outpatients and their families, but a mental health clinical nurse specialist acted as an observer and offered feedback (Krumm, *et al.,* 1979). Another cancer support group limited their membership to outpatients and their families, primarily because inpatients already had supportive staff around them and focused more on current physical crises rather than ongoing daily needs. The group leaders also screened out potential members with excessive denial or other defenses that would keep them from directly confronting the problems of living with cancer each day. Content of group sessions included: a focus on loneliness as an acute problem once the client leaves the hospital; the reactions of family and friends and how to deal with this; the physical weakness that saps much of the enjoyment of life; and the lack of information available about living with cancer (Kelly and Ashby, 1979). It has been noted that clients in a cancer group tend to control anxiety by containing their feelings. Sometimes this is done by discussing "safe" subjects or by displacing anger onto the staff (Whitman, *et al.* 1979). Commenting on the process, including nonverbal behaviors, may be helpful for gently uncovering feelings.

Another physical illness which leads to a change in body image and to many losses, including loss of mobility, of one's independence, and even of sensory awareness, is the cerebral vascular accident. The client sees his usefulness within the family system diminish, and he may fear he will lose his family entirely. One support group for stroke victims and their families attempted to focus on the resolution of loss that both clients and their families were feeling. Members were asked to share how things had been before the stroke as a means of facing the loss directly and adapting later to a realistic assessment of the client's level of functioning. Families were encouraged to look for community supports and resources (D'Afflitti and Weitz, 1979).

Another group for clients who had experienced a cerebral vascular accident was made up of members who had been hospitalized for extended periods of time, were still inpatients, and had become isolated because of various sequelae from their strokes (Puppolo, 1980). One member was blind, one an amputee, one had expressive aphasia, and some had paralysis that limited their mobility. The coleaders were quite creative in their interventions with the group members. The blind client received verbal feedback about who was talking, who came late to group, and so forth. The aphasic client was given a pad to record comments and questions which were read aloud by the person next to her. However, she was also encouraged to speak out loud at a rate she could manage. The coleaders encouraged both the client and other group members to talk about the frustrations of experiencing aphasia. A member with a paralyzed hand was given an assignment to practice writing a letter with the other hand. Positive feedback from the group was incorporated in the meetings to encourage clients in their physical rehabilitation. Teaching the group to refrain from doing too much for a paralyzed person was modeled by the coleaders giving examples from their own impulses to reach out and help a member. Other problems which the leaders dealt with were memory loss and uncontrollable labile emotions. Members were given written notes and verbal reminders of the meetings. They were also reassured that their emotional outbursts were cues that something was wrong, and they were encouraged to try and verbalize that. This group was truly one of multifaceted supports and much growth and learning for the members.

Some important considerations for nurse leaders who might be attempting support groups for clients or families experiencing difficult losses is that the readiness to deal out loud with the pain may vary from member to member. The nurse leader needs to confront his or her own fears about emotional expression and how to deal with this (McHugh, *et al.* 1979). McHugh, *et al.,* talked about a support group for families of burn victims. Since body image and other losses are also part of this physical problem, both clients and their families need to work on grief reactions. In any such group, the leader tries to be alert to verbal as well as nonverbal cues that indicate some readiness to discuss pain. Sometimes clients are vague or impersonal and should be asked how what they are saying applies personally to them. Casual comments about "heavy" subjects or an opposite reaction, such as choking back tears, all may mean the member needs to get in touch with some feelings (McHugh, *et al.,* 1979). I find it important to not assume something about what the client might be feeling. Generally, I will share my observation as a way of opening up an opportunity for the person to share if this is that I think the cues have meant.

The possible client populations for a support group are as many as there are illnesses that present problems in coping for the client and their significant others. Since illness is a state that demands new or revised coping skills at times, the value of a support group cannot be underestimated. The nurse, as a group leader, is an important intervenor in this process.

REFERENCES

Ballinger, B. "The Menopause and Its Syndromes," in *Modern Perspectives in the Psychiatry of Middle Age,* ed. J. Howell. New York: Brunner/Mazel, Inc., 1981.

Blackman, J. "Group Work in the Community: Experiences with Reminiscence," in *Psychosocial Nursing Care of The Aged* (2nd ed.), ed. I. Burnside. New York: McGraw-Hill Book Co., Inc., 1980.

Bowen, M. "Family Reaction to Death," in *Family Therapy: Theory and Practice,* ed. P. Guerin. New York: Gardner Press, Inc., 1976.

Bowers, J. "Group Work with Couples and Families," in *Life Cycle Group Work in Nursing,* eds. E. Janosik and L. Phipps. Monterey, CA: Wadsworth Health Sciences Division, 1982.

Britnell, J. and K. Mitchell. "Inpatient Group Psychotherapy for the Elderly," *Journal of Psychiatric Nursing and Mental Health Services,* 19, no. 5 (May, 1981), 19-24.

Burnside, I. *Nursing and the Aged.* New York: McGraw-Hill, Inc., 1981.

Butler, R. "The Life Review: An Interpretation of Reminiscence in the Aged," *Psychiatry,* 26, no. 1 (Feb., 1963), 65-76.

Chiriboga, D. "The Developmental Psychology of Middle Age," in *Modern Perspectives in the Psychiatry of Middle Age,* ed. J. Howell. New York: Brunner/Mazel, Inc., 1981.

Cohen, M. and M. Amdur. "Medication Group for Psychiatric Patients," *American Journal of Nursing,* 81, no. 2 (Feb., 1981), 343-345.

D'Afflitti, J. and G. Weitz. "Rehabilitating the Stroke Patient Through Patient-Family

Groups," in *Stress and Survival: The Emotional Realities of Life-Threatening Illness,* ed. C. Garfield. St. Louis: The C.V. Mosby Co., 1979.

Donahue, E. "Preserving History Through Oral History Reflections," *Journal of Gerontological Nursing,* 8, no. 5 (May, 1982), 272–278.

Erikson, E. *Identity: Youth and Crisis.* New York: W.W. Norton and Co., 1968.

Ferguson, B. "A Parent's Group," in *Journal of Psychiatric Nursing and Mental Health Services,* 17, no. 12 (Dec., 1979), 24–27.

Goin, M. and R. Burgoyne. "Psychology of the Widow and Widower," in *Modern Perspectives in the Psychiatry of Middle Age,* ed. J. Howell. New York: Brunner/Mazel, Inc., 1981.

Griffith, L. "Group Work with Children and Adolescents," in *Life Cycle Group Work in Nursing,* eds. E. Janosik and L. Phipps. Monterey, CA: Wadsworth Health Sciences Division, 1982.

Grunebaum, H. and L. Solomon. "Toward a Peer Theory of Group Psychotherapy, I: On the Developmental Significance of Peers and Play," *International Journal of Group Psychotherapy,* 30, no. 1 (Jan., 1980), 23–49.

Harris, P. and G. Tarbutton. "Support Groups: The Family Connection," *Free Association,* 10, no. 2 (Mar.-Apr., 1983), 1–4.

Henker, F. "Male Climacteric," in *Modern Perspectives in the Psychiatry of Middle Age,* ed. J. Howell. New York: Brunner/Mazel, Inc., 1981.

Huston, P. "Psychotic Depressive Reaction," in *Comprehensive Textbook of Psychiatry,* eds. A. Freedman and H. Kaplan. Baltimore: The Williams and Wilkins Co., 1967.

Janosik, E. and J. Miller. "Group Work with the Elderly," in *Life Cycle Group Work in Nursing,* eds. E. Janosik and L. Phipps. Monterey, CA: Wadsworth Health Sciences Division, 1982.

Johnson, M. "Support Groups for Parents of Chronically Ill Children," *Pediatric Nursing,* 8, no. 3 (May-Jun., 1982), 160–163.

Kelly, P. and G. Ashby. "Group Approaches for Cancer Patients: Establishing a Group," *American Journal of Nursing,* 79, no. 5 (May, 1979), 914–915.

Kolb, L. "Disturbances of Body Image," in *American Handbook of Psychiatry,* ed. S. Arieti. New York: Basic Books, Inc., 1959.

Kolb, L. *Modern Clinical Psychiatry* (8th ed.). Philadelphia: W.B. Saunders Co., 1973.

Krumm, S., P. Vannatta, and J. Sanders. "Group Approach for Cancer Patients: A Group for Teaching Chemotherapy," *American Journal of Nursing,* 79, no. 5 (May, 1979), 916.

Lancaster, J. *Community Mental Health Nursing: An Ecological Perspective.* St. Louis: The C.V. Mosby Co., 1980.

Langford, R. "Teenagers and Obesity," in *American Journal of Nursing,* 81, no. 3 (Mar., 1981), 556–559.

Levin, S. "The Adolescent Group as Transitional Object," *International Journal of Group Psychotherapy,* 32, no. 2 (Apr., 1982), 217–232.

Lindemann, E. "Symptomatology and Management of Acute Grief," in *American Journal of Psychiatry,* 101, (Sept. 1944), 141–148.

McHugh, M., K. Dimitroff, and N. Davis. "Family Support Group in a Burn Unit," *American Journal of Nursing,* 79, no. 2 (Dec., 1979), 2148–2150.

McMordie, W. and S. Bloom. "Life Review Therapy: Psychotherapy for the Elderly," in *Perspectives in Psychiatric Care,* 17, no. 4 (Jul.-Aug., 1979), 162–166.

McWhorter, J. "Group Therapy for High Utilizers of Clinic Facilities," in *Psychosocial Care of the Aged* (2nd ed.), ed. I. Burnside. New York: McGraw-Hill Book Co., 1980.

Minter, R. and C. Kimball. "Life Events, Personality Traits, and Illness," in *Handbook on Stress and Anxiety,* eds. I. Kutash and L. Schlesinger. San Francisco: Jossey-Bass Publishers, 1980.

Needler, W. and M.A. Baer. "Movement, Music, and Remotivation with the Regressed

Elderly,'' *Journal of Gerontological Nursing,* 8, no. 9 (Sept., 1982), 497–503.

Puppolo, D. "Co-leadership with a Group of Stroke Patients," in *Psychosocial Nursing Care of the Aged* (2nd ed.), ed. I. Burnside. New York: McGraw-Hill Book Co., 1980.

Roberts, C. and R. Lewis. "The Empty Nest Syndrome," in *Modern Perspectives in the Psychiatry of Middle Age,* ed. J. Howell. New York: Brunner/Mazel, Inc., 1981.

Schmitt, M. "Groups for the Chronically Ill," in *Life Cycle Group Work in Nursing,* eds. E. Janosik and L. Phipps. Monterey, CA: Wadsworth Health Sciences Division, 1982.

Selye, H. "The Stress Concept Today," in *Handbook on Stress and Anxiety,* eds. I. Kutash and L. Schlesinger. San Francisco: Jossey-Bass Publishers, 1980.

Settin, J. "Overcoming Ageism in Long-Term Care: A Solution in Group Therapy," *Journal of Gerontological Nursing,* 8, no. 10 (Oct., 1982), 565–567.

Simpson, M. "Societal Support and Education," in *Handbook on Stress and Anxiety,* eds. I. Kutash and L. Schlesinger. San Francisco: Jossey-Bass Publishers, 1980.

Stein, M. and J.K. Davis. *Therapies for Adolescents.* San Francisco: Jossey-Bass Publishers, 1982.

Tappen, R. and T. Touhy. "Group Leader—Are You a Controller?" *Journal of Gerontological Nursing,* 9, no. 1 (Jan., 1983), 34–38, 44, 59.

Volkmar, F., S. Bacon, S. Shakir, and A. Pfefferbaum. "Group Therapy in the Management of Manic-Depressive Illness," in *American Journal of Psychotherapy,* 35, no. 2 (April, 1981), 226–234.

Wadeson, H. "Combining Expressive Therapies in an Effort to Survive on a Depressive Ward," in *Helping Through Action: Action-Oriented Therapies,* eds. E. Nickerson and K. O'Laughlin. Amherst, MA: Human Resource Development Press, 1982.

Whitman, H., J. Gustafson, and F. Coleman. "Group Approaches for Cancer Patients," *American Journal of Nursing,* 79, no. 5 (May, 1979), 910–913.

Wilson, H. and C. Kneisl. *Psychiatric Nursing* (2nd ed.). Menlo Park, CA: Addison-Wesley Publishing Co., 1983.

Yalom, I. and F. Terrazas. "Group Therapy for Psychotic Elderly Patients," *American Journal of Nursing,* 68, no. 8 (Aug., 1968), 1690–1694.

Supplemental Learning Activities

9-12

1. Choose a specific client population for which you might lead a support group. Note those areas of importance related to both the developmental stage of the clients and the specific problem area around which the group is structured. Decide on the size of the group membership and how you would select the members. What specific interventions would you make to prepare the members for their group experience? Identify the theoretical framework you would use to facilitate the group. Create an experiential exercise to use in either one of the three stages of the group's development. Identify the goals for the exercise and anticipate a variety of outcomes based upon the client population of the group.

2. What belief does your agency or staff have about group as a therapeutic modality? If it is negative, identify the steps you would use to go about changing this view. If it is positive, what factors have contributed to this viewpoint?

3. In those task groups to which you belong, how is the power within the group distributed? Note any difference in goal production between the task groups that value either achieved status or ascribed status more highly.

4. Compare the composition and functioning of a specific nursing task group and a multidisciplinary task group using the following chart. Use two groups in which you have membership or to which you are acquainted as an observer. Speculate on each group's probable degree of functioning (*i.e.,* task accomplishment).

	Nursing Staff	Multidisciplinary Staff
Membership		
Size		
Characteristics		
Defined Task of Group		
Power Structure		
Communication Channels		

Analysis of task accomplishment:

Section Two

Advanced Group Practice Skills

Process Illumination 13

Introduction

Since process is the "meat" of the work that goes on in most groups, too much time cannot be spent on this phenomenon. Although the psychotherapeutic group defines itself as process focused with the facilitation of process being the central work of the group, the movement in other groups is greatly enhanced from the identification and use of process. The developing relationship between the group members and between the members and leader affect all other aspects of the group's activity. Group leaders will greatly enrich their own group experience by understanding process. The leader who is aware of process may then choose whether to share this awareness with the group members or simply store it away as information that will add to the leader's understanding of the events in the group. Nurses need not be group leaders to use process in nursing interventions with clients. This chapter will give the reader an in-depth look at process and some of the unique tools for illuminating its presence. Facilitating a psychotherapy group requires a strong theoretical background and understanding along with many clinical hours of practice. It is recommended that nurses leading psychotherapy groups have at least masters-level educational preparation. For a complete discussion of process, Yalom's book, *The Theory and Practice of Group Psychotherapy* (2nd ed.), 1975, is an excellent resource.

Coleadership is a specific method of interventions that facilitates process illumination. Coleadership is effective, because the relationship of the coleaders with each other has a specific impact on the process that occurs in the group. A brief description of the coleadership process was presented in Chapter Eleven. This chapter will provide the group leader with a detailed discussion of the roles and purposes for coleadership.

Process Interventions

Yalom (1975) suggested that the effectiveness of an intervention could be judged by how well it helped the group to focus on itself. His ideas about focusing, or discovering process, are discussed in the following paragraphs.

Questions to Ask Oneself to Illuminate Process

I find that my main task in leading a group is to constantly observe what the group members are doing. I do not pay nearly as much attention to the content of what is being said but ask myself questions about why it is being said (i.e., what stimulated the response?). I also ask myself questions about the origin and meaning of nonverbal behavior, and I wrestle with how to make a content issue "here-and-now" process. In attempting to grab onto process, the group leader may observe a particular behavior but will not necessarily come up with an answer about its meaning, especially if it is in the early stages of the group's development. It is also possible that the leader may infer something that is not correct. If the group leader is unsure about an interpretation of process, she may wait for more data or share the observation with the group and ask the members to look at its occurrence in relation to their present feelings and awareness. Sharing process inferences is a powerful intervention. Yalom (1975) noted that the leader does not have to be correct if the intervention leads the group to focusing on the "here-and-now." It is important, however, to not state an inference as fact but as merely a question that the group might want to consider. Descriptive observations are facts and are helpful process interventions. Notice the difference between these two interventions:

Intervention 1: "I noticed you haven't said anything in the group today. How come you don't like being here?"

Intervention 2: "I noticed you haven't said anything in group today. That's different from your usual high level of participation. How might what is happening in the group right now relate to your silence?"

In the first intervention, the facilitator has come to a conclusion based on very little objective data. It could be that the member does not like being in group, but there may be many other reasons for her silence. This intervention could affect the group in several ways. The leader might be seen as unfeeling and presumptuous. Other group members may come to the rescue of the member that was confronted by the facilitator. The member could become angry with the leader and express this and/or walk out of group. The rest of the group may decide not to talk for fear of having their behavior interpreted out loud. The possibilities are many.

Many possible outcomes also exist for the second process intervention. However, there is probably less chance that the member or the rest of the group would react defensively with the leader. The member may not know what her silence means, but she is more apt to search for some awareness, because the facilitator has pinpointed her behavior as being significant and has expressed interest in understanding her behavior as it relates to her presence in the group. The leader has also suggested that the group has a definite impact on the individual's behavior and that behavior does not occur in isolation. This is a major point that a group facilitator wants a group to understand. There would be no purpose for having any group unless the collective presence of the members had an impact on each individual participant. It is important to note, also, that once the leader says or does something, he or she becomes part of the process of the group. Not intervening is also a process and may serve to silently sanction whatever is occurring in the group at the time.

Some of the questions which a group leader should ask himself to illuminate process include:

1) How do a member's nonverbal behaviors relate to events occurring in the group? (Notice any nonverbal behaviors as well as the timing of behaviors.) EXAMPLE: Perhaps Ben turns around in his chair and stares at the wall while Dan is talking. Does Ben's behavior relate to the fact that Dan, rather than another group member, is talking, or does it have to do with the content of what Dan is saying? Is Ben saying something about his relationship with Dan or how Dan's communication affects him? The fact that Ben chose to make an unusual move just as Dan was speaking most likely means that he is reacting to something about Dan or his message. There are times when a client's actions are delayed, and it is more difficult to tell what stimulated the behavior. There are also times when even an unusual behavior has little to do with the group process. The member may be responding to some personal internal stimulus that has caused him to laugh or look around. Since nonverbal behaviors are so difficult to control and to hide, I trust that there is generally some significance to them.

2) How does the timing of a member's statement relate to the events going on in the group? EXAMPLE: It is five minutes until group is over, and Betty tells the group that this is her last session and she wants to say "good-bye." The group had done some problem-solving with a member who had just been diagnosed as having an inoperable tumor. Although this took up much of the group's time, the last ten minutes had been spent discussing a light news article about the birth of a panda at the zoo. Betty had not said anything during this time. There had been three different brief silent periods in which she could have spoken during that last ten minutes. Does the timing of her statement mean that she really does not want the group to discuss this? Is her intention to leave the members puzzling about why she is not returning to the group? Did the discussion earlier with the member who just learned about her tumor have some effect on the reason Betty hesitated so long before speaking? How controlling is Betty's statement? (*e.g.*, Does she want to engage the leader in a power struggle over who will determine when the members will leave?) Was Betty just afraid to tell the group she was leaving, so she waited until the last minute? Did she feel that her leaving was not as important as what the other member was working on? These are not all the questions that could be asked about this example but should give the reader more of an idea about how one elicits process information.

3) How does conversation about the past relate to the "here-and-now" process in the group? EXAMPLE: The members have been discussing how comfortable they feel with each other and how free they feel to share personal kinds of information. Nancy recalls a secret club she and her girlfriends had when she was about ten. She remembers that this made her feel very special because only the club members had the secret password, and other girls would do favors for her in hopes of getting her to let them in the club or, at least, reveal the password. Everyone in the group seems to enjoy listening to Nancy and are content to let her continue talking. For several minutes, she keeps the group involved telling them of her adventures. At this point, the group leader needs to ask Nancy to look at how what she is saying relates to what she is feeling about the group at the moment. It may be that Nancy has not been feeling as close to the other group members who have said how wonderful it is to be so intimate with one another and to share. She has decided to recall a time when she had been intimate with a group, special, and not left out, which contrasts with her current feelings in the present group meeting. Taking over the conversation also allows her to change the subject from present relationships to what had been important relationships in the past. She can then control how the conversation goes and perhaps earn the group's love by letting them in on the story of her secret club. Only Nancy can really identify how what she said about the past relates to how she was feeling at the moment. If the member is not able to answer this question, the group leader may have to make some objective observations to help her become more aware of her feelings. Sample dialogue follows:

a) "Nancy, I noticed you really sounded pressured and intense when you were telling us this story. It seemed to hold a lot of meaning and emotion for you; more, perhaps, than I would expect with someone just telling a story about something that occurred so long ago. What is that emotion you're showing us?"

b) "Nancy, you seemed really quiet during the discussion we just had about the group giving people a feeling of closeness. I'm guessing that your need to change the subject and talk about an important childhood memory related to how you're feeling in the group today, especially about the closeness and how you fit in with that.''

There may be times when a member will deny any relationship between the past and what she is feeling at the moment. The leader makes observations but should not lead the member toward an interpretation that may not be valid. This can be a good time to just store the observations away for future use, especially if this member continues to want to run away from the present. The leader also has the option of being authoritarian and strongly suggesting that the most helpful part of group is when members talk about their present feelings and thoughts and notice how they are reacting to other members and the leader. This enforces a norm that the leader feels is important.

4) How does a leader make a member's outside issues part of the group process? EXAMPLE: Vincent is having difficulty with a neighbor who keeps borrowing money from him. Vincent has difficulty saying ''no'' to him but comes to the group meeting very angry with himself and the neighbor and uses a lot of the group's time to discuss this. Since a member will tend to demonstrate the same interactional pattern inside the group as in his outside relationships, the two most often are connected. The leader could ask Vincent if he has ever felt anger in response to an incident that occurred in the group. Direct feedback is also helpful, such as observations of his nonassertiveness with group members and the resultant irritation or anger with himself. It might be that he is feeling nonassertive or powerless at that moment in the group and would be able to identify that if asked to look at his anger as it related to something that just happened in the group. A general sense of powerlessness with the other group members or leader may trigger a memory of the outside incident. It could be that he dreads coming to the group for this reason. He comes, but with some anger that he may also wish to address to the group. If the member denies his behavior as being important or significant in relation to how he feels in the group, the leader might suggest that the anger is so obvious and takes up so much of the group's time week after week that it needs to be dealt with in the group. If the member still resists, he may need to do this as a way of maintaining some sense of control or power for himself.

5) What does a member's behavior towards a group leader say about his relationship with the leader and the rest of the group as well as with significant others in his or her life? Since the group is a system and the members are a part of that system and of other systems including their family, work group, and so forth, the rules for living systems apply to the process that occurs in the group. Recall that a change in one part of a system will affect the rest of the system in a variety of ways, both the subparts and the whole. Interactions are dynamic; once they occur between two or more people, the relationship between these individuals is never quite the same. The process between the group members and the leader constantly redefines relationships in the group. A change in the way two members relate to each other will, most likely, alter other relationships in the group. The presence of leftover feelings toward signficant others in one's life that affects the way one interacts in current relationships, which Sullivan called parataxic distortion (see Chapter Two), can be seen in a member's relationships in a group. This is especially true when one of those in the interaction is the group leader. The leader has a unique position, being seen by each member as an important person who may contribute to that member's adaptation or growth. This is particularly true in the initial stage of the group where the leader is seen as omniscient. Certainly, the way a member behaves towards the group leader has the attention of the rest of the group members and will affect their perception of the relationship they have with the leader. It is in this context that we look at the process unfolding as a member interacts with the group leader.

EXAMPLE: Jo Ann, a member of a support group for families of terminally ill young adults, is treating the group leader as if he were her son. He is about the same age as her son who has terminal cancer. She has often talked in group about feeling like she neglected this son, her third child, and she is quite protective of the leader, asking him about his health, bringing him vitamins, and jumping on any member who disagrees with him. The group leader has tried to be as objective as possible, making process comments such as:

"Jo Ann, sometimes I feel very special and singled out when you bring me presents in group. I'm concerned about how this relates to your feelings toward your son right now."

"It seems that you're having a lot of difficulty coping right now, Jo Ann, because you are needing to take a lot of the group's time. I also notice you are spending a lot of time talking with me. I'd like you to listen to what some of the other members are experiencing. I think several of them have had similar feelings towards their children that you seem to have toward your son. This is the kind of group where other members can really share their way of getting through these difficult times."

The group leader is not overly confrontive with Jo Ann. He does not want to make her any more anxious but hopes to increase her ability to cope and, thereby, handle her son's illness less pathologically. He also recognizes how detrimental her interactions with him could be to the rest of the group. If Jo Ann gets to have a special relationship with the group leader, the other members will have more difficulty using the group leader as a teacher and sounding board for their needs. The leader will have a hard time maintaining his credibility with the rest of the group members. The leader also needs to be aware of how other members may start reacting to Jo Ann if they feel she is monopolizing the leader's time and expertise. If she is seeking out the leader for emotional support, she probably has not found it comfortable to engage the help of other group members. The leader has triggered a parataxic response, and this may have helped to isolate her from the emotional support of the rest of the members. In the last sample dialogue, the leader both validates the other members' worth and lets them know indirectly that he expects them to make an effort to understand Jo Ann and support her. His authority with Jo Ann is unquestioned. Therefore, his speech to her, to allow the other members to help her, will probably be heeded. Finally, he has made a statement about the purpose of the support group that everyone in the group has had an opportunity to hear.

Other Clues to Process

Yalom (1975) noted that process is often clarified if the group leader watches for obvious omissions in topics which the group addresses or for omissions in behaviors that would normally be expected to occur in the group. If a group of terminally ill clients never talks about death, this is a definite clue to their strong feelings about this topic and its pain or fear for them. The leader needs to share her awareness that this topic has been left out, perhaps with an open-ended question to the group asking the members to take a look at this group behavior and what it means for each of them. If one father in a support group for parents of severely handicapped children is the only member who does not identify any difficulties in coping with this problem, he is probably highly defended around this. The leader does not want to increase his anxiety by taking away that defense, but he might gently offer some support to the whole family, including father in the discussion. He could support the wife's attempt to find a special day center where the child can go periodically to give the family some relief and sense of normalcy. The father does not have to admit to a difficulty in coping to get the benefits of some community supports.

A clue to the role each member plays in the group is often highlighted by the process of the rest of the group when the member is absent (Yalom, 1975). A member that is always vying for control with the leader will be the source of a lot of tension in the group created by this conflict. When this member is not in group, the emotional climate will probably be less intense. If the leader has been dealing with the absent member's need to control by well-timed process comments (*e.g.*, when the member succeeds in responding in the role of therapist, the leader asks the rest of the group how it feels to have the member interacting in that way), the group is going to be sensitized to this process. This time, the group may look at what it feels like not to have "two leaders." Members less able to identify the dynamics occurring in the group, such as in a support or task group, will show their response to the absent member by acting out their feelings rather than verbalizing them. A less controversial leader may emerge, or several members may perform some leadership activities. If the absent member's behavior had contributed to an avoidance of self-disclosure in the group, one may see more self-disclosure occurring. A task group may proceed with their task more efficiently with only one leader to direct them.

In another example, a member who has taken on a role of peacemaker will greatly affect the group by his absence unless another member assumes that role. Conflict will be expressed more openly, and the members will feel more anxious and unsettled. This may be very good for the group that has avoided some honest confrontations with one another. The leader may then help the members look at the process of their avoidance and their fear of conflict. In a psychotherapy group, the leader wants to sensitize the members to what process is and have them become aware of their own process and how that affects the others. Most likely, the other members' fears have facilitated the peacemaker maintaining his role.

Group members who are able to make some self-observations and come to some conclusions about how they relate to the rest of the group may be good facilitators of process themselves. The leader, through the process comments he or she makes, offers some modeling behaviors that members may pick up. Feeding back to one another observable behaviors or interactions between them is very helpful if it is done in a nonjudgmental, matter-of-fact fashion. Very often, members listen to each other better and with less anxiety than if the leader were to tell them the same thing. Some leaders begin to feel threatened if they see their ultimate power, their knowledge and use of process comments, being taken from them. It is most often the novice, insecure leader that wants to maintain that sense of power over the group. I stroke members for process observations, and I find that I may do a better job of facilitating a group if the members understand process. Each member will still be very subjective with his or her own process, and I will, hopefully, remain as an observer of the total process. When my student group leaders started to understand process and use it in both the client groups they led and in our postgroup review sessions, I was really excited. Maybe I associated their new-found skill and increased enthusiasm and respect for group therapy as a compliment to my teaching ability. I imagine a similar feeling could exist for group leaders when the members become more skilled in process and more involved in the group.

Coleadership

A Definition of Coleadership

Process illumination may be facilitated through the potency of the coleadership relationship. Once the two group facilitators have truly become "coleaders" or have reached the stage of "stabilization" in their relationship, they are able to focus their energies almost entirely on process illumination. The development of the coleadership role, however, takes much time and work on the coleaders' own process.

Cotherapy involves a "mature," "open," and "playful" relationship between the two group facilitators. "The crucial element of cotherapy lies in the relationship established between the cotherapists." (Hannum, 1980, p.161). The significance of the relationship is seen in its comparison to marriage. Although closeness is not an essential element early in the partnership, open communications and problem-solving are crucial for the long-term productivity and well-being of both marriage and cotherapy. The partners must be aware of each other's growth and need to grow, must work on helping each other with this process, and must be willing to look at their own personal problem areas with each other (Dick, 1980). Yalom (1975) described coleadership as a complementary relationship in which the partners were dissimilar but could feel close to each other. Such descriptions of the role indicate the importance of the selection process between coleaders. Trainees often have less opportunity to choose their partner. One of the techniques I used with nursing students was to have them do a coleadership inventory prior to their work together. I made sure that I did not pair a very verbal student with one who was intimidated by this. It seemed to work well to have either two verbal or two less-verbal students work together. Since the students had been together for three years, much of this in intense nursing situations and had to self-disclose in small groups in my class, they had begun the process of openness and intimacy with one another, to varying degrees. This was helpful in their attempting a coleadership role. Potential coleaders definitely need a preliminary time of relating to each other prior to their facilitating a group together.

Stages of Development in the Coleadership Role

The coleadership role is only as strong as the quality of the relationship between the two leaders. The development of this relationship can be identified as specific stages of growth (Dick, 1980). Dick noted that not all stages are reached by each pair of coleaders, nor is each stage necessarily completed before the group leaders move into another phase of development. The stages of development of the coleadership relationship may be compared with the stages of group movement that characterize its development. Both need a beginning period of getting acquainted before the actual process of working together can proceed effectively. In the middle stages of development, the coleaders work on specific issues about their relationship, much as the group members work on issues that, when solved, will move the group towards its goal. Following are the stages of coleadership development as identified by Dick (1980).

1) Formation. Getting acquainted requires the potential coleaders to share treatment philosophies, particular personal habits related to their interactional style, their communication activity level (*e.g.*, an active, commanding style of verbalizing, a low-keyed, "lay-back" sparse style), and so forth. At this beginning stage, the leaders are more sensitive about their personal weaknesses, both in their professional skills and in their personal lives. This is a time where much contact outside of the group session is spent on talking together about their feelings and relationship. Depending on their level of expertise, they may require ongoing supervision or periodic meetings with a peer supervisor. Energy must be spent on organizational issues with the group, adding to the complexity of this formation stage. Dick notes that during this period the cotherapists are not functioning as one, multifaceted therapist, although this is the ultimate goal.

I have found it helpful to facilitate the developing relationship between student coleaders by having them use a tool created by Wilson and Kneisl (1979). *The Co-leader's Self Inventory* is in a short-answer format which I adapted to the particular learning needs of my students. It includes a question on the individual's philosophy of group as a source of help for the client, the expectations one has about the co-leadership process (fears and wishes), and some possible personal responses to particular group incidents that might develop. There is also a question about behaviors one would not tolerate in a coleader. I had students complete these forms individually and then verbally share their responses with one another. They each then wrote a summary of their discussion together, highlighting areas of concern and compatibility. Although the tool varied in its value to particular dyads, I felt it always served to sensitize the students to the complexities and importance of the coleadership relationship. I was not as concerned about the specific content of their responses as much as the process of their relationship with one another which was highlighted as they worked on the inventory. Throughout their time as coleaders, the students were asked to do a number of exercises together that focused on both their process with each other and that of the group.

2) Development. As the coleaders move into a working mode, the focus is on processing the issues between them to allow the dyad to move toward a complementary relationship which allows them to function better as a team than they would as group leaders working separately. The focus in supervision is on the quality of the coleaders' working relationship. It is important for the coleaders to learn each other's strengths and deficits (Dick, 1980). Certainly, it is helpful if these strengths and deficits are different for each leader and if one coleader's strengths bolster the other coleader's deficits and vice-versa. This is ideal and not possible to meet very often, but the awareness of each other's skills and problem areas allows for problem-solving between the coleaders. The process of problem-solving facilitates the growth of the relationship between the dyad, regardless of whether they solve all the specific deficits in their pairing.

Among the student dyads doing coleading, a pair would frequently find they both felt very insecure about making a particular kind of intervention in the group. For example, one pair of student coleaders did not feel comfortable interrupting a member or refocusing the group. In a coleader dyad where one of the leaders is willing to attempt a variety of interventions once the group has gotten on a nonproductive tangent, the other coleader may observe for the effects of an intervention on the process of the group and its members. If neither coleader feels comfortable refocusing the group, they need to plan some strategy to deal with this. The coleaders might plan to have a dialogue between them about the process they are observing and the difficulties of interrupting members. In order to speak with one another, they will be interrupting the process but not directly confronting a member. The members listen to a description of their behavior and observe the coleaders problem-solving. In the following dialogue, Chris and Susan are the coleaders.

"Chris, I don't know if the group is getting much done right now. I've noticed that when Richard starts talking about his time in the service, he speaks more quickly, and most everyone else looks real involved in their own thoughts. I wonder what keeps people from telling Richard how they feel?"

"I find it really hard to interrupt Richard when he gets going. I even feel like just tuning him out and letting my own thoughts take over. I'm uncomfortable when I catch myself doing this. I suppose it is a good escape for others to just let Richard talk on and on."

"I don't know if others are afraid to interrupt Richard or if they just would rather make us do that. And I guess right now I'm wondering what Richard is feeling since I did interrupt him?"

The coleaders have done several very effective things in this set of statements. They have stopped a nonproductive process by identifying that process for the rest of the group. They have avoided directly interrupting a member by, instead, talking to one another. Although the effect is the same, the dialogue with each other allows the group to hear about the process, and Richard is given some feedback about how controlling he is and how cooperative the group is in letting him be this way. Saying this out loud takes away some of the power of this process, because now when Richard takes over the group with his nonthreatening war stories, both he and the other members have been identified as having a responsibility in this behavior. In this example, the coleaders are still struggling about how much responsibility they should take for seeing that the group works. It seems that Susan puts this decision "on hold" by drawing Richard directly into the process. If he and the group will now hash this over, Susan and Chris do not have to directly intervene, and the members may learn something about their fears and their ability to deal directly with each other.

If Chris had decided that he wanted to be more directive and refocus the group when he had observed a reasonable amount of time go by, then Susan could be an observer of the process. Susan may not like to directly interrupt and confront others. If the group is in the initial stage, this directive intervention might be necessary, since group members may be hesitant to take on any leadership roles themselves. Susan could then ask the members how they felt when Chris interrupted, and she might even talk out loud about how uncomfortable or embarrassing being interrupted can be, thereby modeling identification and expression of feelings and giving Richard some support. The possibilities for work with the process are endless, regardless of how comfortable either coleader is with a certain intervention. As the group leaders work together, they find ways to support each other. Chris' and Susan's dialogue is a result of many hours of behind-the-scenes discussions between the two of them.

When coleaders find a particular personality or communication style exhibited by group members that neither coleader feels comfortable or skilled at handling, they may still discover a way to support each other if this process comes up in the group. For example, if neither coleader is effective against a very dependent, whining individual, both first need to acknowledge this as an area in which they must be creative. Just noting this as a weakness of their coleadership style allows the dyad to be more observant of each other's reactions to such a member. Tracy may find herself being sympathetic with a dependent member's many insurmountable problems, and she becomes so much a part of the process between them that she is ineffective in helping the member problem-solve. Jim, however, becomes impatient with the same member whose dependence leaves him feeling irritated and a little guilty for reacting with such impatience. What Tracy and Jim need to do is to try not to both react in their typical ways at the same time with this member. If both get caught up in the process, it becomes more difficult for either to be therapeutic. If Tracy notices Jim becoming angry with the member, Tracy might try to break this nonproductive process by questioning her coleader about how he feels. If she were to engage the member instead, she might also get caught in the process. The following is a sample dialogue:

"Jim, you really sound angry with Bob (the dependent member). I don't know if he would understand what you're reacting to. What is it that you're feeling?"

"I know I'm feeling impatient with Bob. I find myself feeling like this every time he acts very helpless about his job, as if he were not responsible for trying to do anything to help himself. I guess I'm a person that really believes in trying to make things happen for me. I don't see Bob doing that."

"I don't know what Bob wants from the group, but I think it's important for him to know how his behavior affects others. Maybe Bob needs to hear from the rest of the group."

"Okay, why don't we see if someone wants to comment right now."

Tracy was still learning about Jim and decided to make the focus a group problem. This allowed her coleader to regain his composure and to let the group members become involved in interacting with each other. Tracy was able to validate for the rest of the group that they were correctly perceiving anger from her coleader. Often, the group members hesitate to check out their perceptions of a leader's reaction or comment, especially in the initial stage of group development where the leaders are seen as omniscient. She and Jim will need to talk about this incident in supervision or consultation. It could be that Jim was pleased to have Tracy jump in, or he may feel that she was not supportive enough of him. Once the coleaders become more secure in their individual skills as well as in their trust with one another, each can tolerate being a model of humanness and fallibility. If the group members see that the coleader relationship is not destroyed by an honest exchange of feelings between the two leaders, they will be more likely to take risks to self-disclose more with each other.

3) Stabilization. This stage of mutual trust between the coleaders allows the dyad to focus their energies on interacting with the members. Any conflicts or misunderstandings between them should have greatly diminished or are easily handled. The process of running the group now becomes automatic, and the coleaders can begin to experiment with some new ways to be more effective as a team. Dick (1980) noted that reaching this stage means the coleaders' effect on the group is both therapeutic and economical, even though two therapists are putting their energies into one group. The quality of the work they do more than compensates for the increased use of manpower. Supervision is not as necessary, since the coleaders are able to monitor their relationship with more insight and ease. There are times, when depending on their personal stresses, the coleader relationship may falter and slip back into stage one or two for awhile (Dick, 1980). Certainly, any close relationship is subject to these same stresses.

The balancing functions between coleaders serve to facilitate the group process in a very effective way, often more successfully than if one leader were trying to do the same thing. The most functional pattern for this activity between coleaders is for one coleader to be an active participant while the other observes the process (Hannum, 1980). In our senior group, my coleader or I are frequently caught up in the content of a member's reminiscing. Since reminiscing is a significant part of the group, content frequently becomes the main focus. I find it valuable to have one of us sitting back trying to think beyond the content to what individual or group process may be occurring. One member tends to tell stories, but so impersonally, that nothing about his connection with the story is evident. My coleader had become involved in the dialogue in the group, which was about ships, diving, and decompression chambers. The member, who remains very objective, was telling several stories but had not identified any personal data. I shared with him that I found his stories interesting, but that I did not understand how they affected him personally. After a pause he said he felt very frustrated because he had loved diving so much and he could no longer do it. His storytelling made up for his being unable to dive anymore, but his failure to personalize his loss had kept him from dealing with it. I doubt that I would have noticed his disengagement if I had not been sitting back just observing while the dialogue was going on. Very often, the coleader involved in the content does not notice nonverbal cues. One member might be physically withdrawing from the group. If one coleader is talking with another group member at the time, he or she will probably not notice the member's withdrawal. During a pause in the conversation, the other leader may share these observations with the group.

It is important that the coleaders exchange roles of observer and participant frequently to keep a balance in their verbal activity level in the group and prevent the members from identifying one coleader as having a particular function or being the senior leader. The observer may choose to do one of a number of things with the process he or she is observing. The coleader who notices one member withdrawing from the group might want to speak directly to that person about his observations. He is then becoming the active coleader beginning a dialogue with a member, and the other leader might now become the observer. Although the dialogue will be process-focused, *i.e.*, the coleader will be commenting on the nonverbal he had observed and saying something about this member's relationship to the rest of the group at that moment, it is important for the other coleader to continue to observe for more process. The silent leader might look for reactions from the rest of the group or watch her colleague if she thinks her partner may have some personal process that will affect the outcome of the dialogue with the member. In a family group, it is very easy for one coleader to identify some personal family issues and act these out while trying to work with one or more family members. It is important for the observer part of the leader dyad to look for ways that his or her partner may be preventing the family from changing because of some personal issue to which he is reacting (Hannum, 1980). The observer alters or facilitates the course of the group's process. This coleader becomes active when his partner overlooks something important, when there is an impasse in the process, or if there is a need to support or contrast the partner's behavior (Hannum, 1980).

Often there is a balance with the one coleader focusing on individual content or process and the other coleader focusing on mass group process or the group theme. As I was listening to the member in our senior group tell stories, I was asking myself several questions about what I was observing and where I should put my energies, *e.g.*: with the personal process going on with the member while my coleader focused on the group's overt theme; in searching for a covert theme which would also identify the mass group process; or with any personal process occurring with my coleader or with another group member not involved in the conversation. I did not see the latter occurring, and the covert theme was escaping me, so I focused on the member who was the most verbal and the process he was communicating. I felt that the way he was choosing to identify himself in the group was an important issue to address. Part of the process which he never acknowledged, nor did I, was that his manner of relating to the group was to act as the expert and titillate his audience with what was to come next. I did not have enough data to suggest this as an observation, and I was not sure his ego strength or sense of self-esteem could tolerate this awareness. I was also not convinced that uncovering this would be helpful to the member or the group. This is a support group and not a psychotherapy group. My goal is to help the members achieve some peace in dealing with aging. Since the life review is a healing process, old business that has not been resolved is dealt with at this time. However, new, negative material only stirs up excess anxiety, and the elderly client is not able to assimilate this data about himself in a way that can facilitate growth and change at this period of his life. Group leaders need to consider the purpose and outcome of every intervention.

Another balancing function is that of one coleader playing a ''bad guy'' or the confronter, while the partner is the ''good guy'' or the supportive person. Obviously, it is important for the coleaders to switch roles to prevent the group from seeing one coleader as harsh and unfeeling and the other as the more compassionate person. The following dialogue demonstrates this process. Matt is a member who has attended a support group for outpatient cancer clients for several months but who continues to maintain that he does not need this group and only comes because of his family's wishes. The coleaders have decided that Matt's denial is not preparing him to deal with his cancer.

''Matt, I don't believe you. I think you're scared and that you want something from this group, but I'm tired of having you take up space here if you're not going to offer anything to the others or do anything for yourself.''

At this point, the rest of the group says nothing but appears surprised at Coleader A's comments. Matt, also, remains silent.

"Being quiet isn't the way to take care of your fear, Matt. I'm beginning to wonder if you have any feelings."

Matt is now becoming more restless. He appears close to tears but is able to hold them back. The rest of the group sits quietly, but the members are all avoiding each other's gaze. Finally, Coleader B addresses Matt.

"Matt, you're really getting it today. Jim is being pretty hard on you, and I'd be quite upset with him (Coleader A). I don't agree with Jim. I think you are showing a lot of feeling right now. It looks like you are close to tears. I know you don't want to show your feelings in the group, but I don't mind if that happens. I'm seeing a different, more sensitive side of you right now, and I'm glad you feel safe about showing that."

Although Coleader A and B appear to be at odds with one another, one has been able to take Matt to the point of expressing feelings by confrontation while the other then identifies the process for both Matt and the group in order to validate what the group has just witnessed. Coleader B then tries to enhance Matt's readiness to identify and express feelings by empathizing and giving him permission to let the pain out. The coleaders count on Matt's readiness to accept Coleader B's sensitivity and encouragement to self-disclose after he, most likely, has felt deserted by Coleader A. In a future group session, Coleader B should be the "bad guy."

In some group situations, the coleaders might help each other get across a particular point to a member or members by saying the same thing in two different ways. If one of the partners asks a member how he copes with his wife's frequent hospitalizations, he may not respond because he is not thinking about the process he goes through when his wife is in the hospital as "coping." The other coleader could then clarify this question:

"I think Colleen noticed that you have some overwhelming pressure on you when your wife goes into the hospital, yet you are always here for group and you talk about getting the children to school on time and yourself to work. Colleen is wondering what you do to reduce the stress all this pressure must create for you. What do you do to keep functioning so well?"

As illustrated in earlier examples, the coleaders may dialogue with one another to discuss the process out loud for the rest of the group to hear, particularly if talking directly to a member or members would create a defensive response or further a disruptive process. If one member is monopolizing the group, the coleaders might discuss his behavior, speculate on the reasons for it, and discuss how it affects the group and what they might do about it. The member who is monopolizing and has heard the coleaders talk about her behavior has a chance to validate their perceptions. She is also getting some attention from them, and she hears how it affects others. Often, a monopolizer's behaviors work to stymie the group's movement because other group members welcome the opportunity to avoid any meaningful work. By discussing the group's part in this, the coleaders comment on the mass group process and take some of the burden away from the monopolizer. They also stop a process that has not been helpful when they interrupt the group to dialogue with each other. If the group has become nonproductive in its interactions, the dialogue between the coleaders stops this cold. The coleaders' interaction may not necessarily solve a particular behavioral problem immediately, but it does stop nonproductive process and give members a chance to hear what they have been doing. Occasionally, the coleaders will notice a particularly productive process by the whole group or with an individual. They may reinforce this by waiting until the process is concluded and then commenting on it out loud to each other. This might be in addition to offering positive comments directly to the individual group members. All of the functions we have discussed are possible when the coleaders have reached a point of stabilization in their relationship.

4) Refreshment. This stage is reached only for brief periods and is characterized by effortless cotherapy and creative innovations by the dyad. This stage, and even the stage of stabilization, may not be reached until the coleaders have worked together for two to three years (Dick, 1980). The importance of the cotherapy role is seen in its most sophisticated applications in working with families. In a systems approach, the family therapist wants to intervene in the pathological system that the family is maintaining and change this to make it a more adaptive way for the family to operate. Often, the therapist must make brief supportive alliances with individual members but continue to be seen as a neutral person by the family. This is very difficult if one therapist is working alone (Hannum, 1980). Cotherapists, however, may facilitate this process quite easily. For example, one partner may support a parent and one, the child. Other uses of the cotherapy role with families include the following (Hannum, 1980).

One cotherapist notices that his partner has become another "parent" in talking with a child member of the family. He may make a process comment to his partner, commenting on this observation, or he may switch the focus to another level to take his partner out of the position of being part of the family system. If he chooses the former, a second part of this intervention is to work on how the family interactions elicited this "parent" response from the coleader.

One partner may exaggerate the behaviors/interactions of a family member, even to the point of adopting the nonverbal style of that member. The coleader taking on this role gets an indepth feeling for the effects of the system on the particular member he is playing. The other coleader may observe the interactions and then attempt some changes with the process.

Both cotherapists may choose to mirror an interactional pattern they have observed in the family that serves to continue maladaptive family responses. They may exaggerate its effects, and then introduce some different, more adaptive ways of responding to the pattern. This is a form of modeling.

If one person in the family is keeping two other family members from being adaptive with each other, one cotherapist may sit beside that person and ask that he or she observe the interaction but not say anything until it is time to discuss it in the group. The close physical proximity of the therapist and, if necessary, a gentle restraining touch may keep the family member from interrupting the observed conversation. During this time, the second cotherapist is actively involved with the other two family members in working through their interactional difficulties.

The above interventions require an indepth knowledge of family systems theory and its clinical application and a coleadership relationship that is approaching the refreshment stage. The creative possibilities are endless given the large amount of process with which to work and the skills of the cotherapists.

Modeling and Role-Taking

Modeling various behaviors and taking on a variety of roles, such as the "good guy/bad guy," allow for innovative interventions by cotherapists. These interventions will probably work best for cotherapists in the third or fourth stage of their relationship. A combination of modeling and role-taking may be done when a male and female cotherapist lead a group. If the group is focusing on issues between couples, the coleaders may model positive, adaptive communications between couples, including conflict resolution. I have found that I need to have a genuine issue to work on with my male coleader to make the conflict resolution process ring true and be effective. It helps the group members to see that my partner and I are not devastated, nor does our relationship dissolve if we disagree with each other. Obviously, we need to have a strong cotherapy relationship to allow for effective modeling of conflict resolution. The roles of mother and father may also be done with the male/female coleadership pairing. This is particularly effective in an adolescent group where the members need to experience some positive transference from the leaders to replace the negative interactions they remember from their real parents. A group that does not have any terribly burning issues about their parents will still find it helpful to redo some old interactional patterns or practice trying out new ways to interact with their parents. Finally, another advantage of the male/female coleader partnership is to model an assertive, nondominant male-female relationship. This allows couples to observe the results of this process and try out some new ways of interacting with each other.

Other Points About Coleading

With modeling and other coleadership interventions, it is probably best for the leader dyad to separate themselves physically from each other in the group. This distributes the leadership power within the group and does not overwhelm any one or two members that may be physically caught in chairs in between the powerful coleaders. The authority figures, as members sometimes see the leaders, are also then dispersed within the group (Puppolo, 1980). I find it much more convenient to look across to my coleader to exchange nonverbal glances, get her attention, and observe her more easily. It is awkward if I must crane my neck to see my partner. Each of us is able to observe more easily a different set of clients. We may not observe the same ones every group period, but we try to station ourselves to complement our observations.

When coleaders are doing a staff support group, it is often helpful for one of the leaders to be an outsider to the staff group. This brings an objective person into the group who is not used to the nonproductive interactional patterns between staff. The more "inside" leader, such as the unit's clinical specialist, understands the demands made on the staff group, the lines of authority, and so forth (Scully, 1981). This can be a very productive partnership in which to colead a staff group.

Problems with the Coleadership Role

If one coleader is more experienced than the other, both the group members and the coleaders may be adversely affected. The pairing that results in the junior/senior partnership is helpful for training as the senior leader may role-model effective interventions and guide her junior partner. However, group members will frequently place the senior person in authority and direct much of the interaction to this person, even though the junior person may be demonstrating some excellent group skills and closing the gap between herself and her senior partner. An inexperienced coleader may feel less competent and decline to take some risks to participate in a creative way with the senior coleader. At times, the two may feel at competition with one another (Hannum, 1980). This may be further compounded by the members' attempting to split the coleaders and feed upon their lack of trust with one another (Yalom, 1975). If the coleadership dyad is working on their relationship to move beyond the formation stage and if they have a supervisor helping them work on the problems with their relationship, the difficulties between them may be greatly reduced. Yalom (1975) noted that an attempted splitting of the coleaders should be examined in terms of the member's process. Frequently, a member is expressing his or her own need to split the authority in the group, much like the splitting of parental authority. If the coleaders remember to focus on whatever process occurs in the group, even if it is a splitting between them, they will most likely find they are mirroring some of the needs or problems of the group members. Families will often demonstrate system problems through their interactions with or effect upon the coleaders. The coleaders tend to act out in their dyad the family's or group's process with one another. If the problem has, however, arisen from the coleaders, and their process has affected the way the group members are interacting, it is important that a third person help the dyad look at this process. Coleaders still in the formation or development stage will have more relationship difficulties and will need more time with a line or peer supervisor.

The time involved before and after group may be a drawback to cotherapy. Since dialogue between the leader dyad is so important, the two must be prepared to spend many hours at this. The group's process is another commitment of time. Coleaders must plan interventions to deal with particular problems within the group or with an individual member. They also will be working on creative ways to facilitate learning for the group members. It seems that the coleader's relationship to one another and to the group members are so closely tied together that it is not easy to identify a particular time when the dyad is working just on one or the other. As their relationship with each other matures, they will need to spend less time outside of group on this. It is then that the real productive work with the group may proceed.

—— Other Specialized Techniques Highlight Process ——

Some specialized process techniques that work with either a single leader or a co-led group also serve to highlight process. The written summary requires a significant amount of the leader's time outside of group if it is to be done effectively. Videotaping is both a time-consuming group process and one which requires some special training. However, both these techniques are worth developing by the advanced nurse group leader.

The Group Summary

The written group summary is a technique developed by Yalom *et al.* (1975) to promote "recent trends toward demystification of the psychotherapy experience" and "an egalitarian collaborative therapist-patient relationship" (p.605). It initially was developed for use in groups with alcoholic clients where an intensive interactional structure, necessary to help clients look at how their personal process contributed to their alcoholism, actually caused many members to return to drinking due to the anxiety this aroused. The summary, appropriate for use in any psychotherapeutic group, decreases the member's anxiety and offers many very valuable curative effects as well. These effects will be discussed in detail and illustrated with a sample group summary.

The format for the written summary is a narrative account of both the content and the process of the previous group meeting. Added to this are comments by the therapists about the process that has been noted in the narrative. In the following example of this format, Kay and Tom are two group members. The therapist's comments are in italics. Note that these are *process* comments about the group's process.

The meeting was late getting started today, with several members drifting in about five minutes after the hour. When I commented on the lateness, everyone who had been late had very legitimate excuses. *I am wondering if the group does not yet feel comfortable in being angry with me directly.* (I am not surprised at the lateness since I was ill last week and failed to notify the members in time to keep them from having to make an unnecessary trip to the office). *Perhaps in the next few meetings someone will take the risk to tell me when they are irritated with what I am doing.*

Kay shared how hard this past week had been for her since she found out her grandmother was quite ill. She talked about the closeness she feels to her and her sadness at the thought that she might be dying. Tom interrupted her several times with his philosophy about dying and how it was important to be strong and concentrate on the living. Eventually, Kay told him she did not find his comments helpful and asked him to be quiet. *It was good to see Kay attempt an assertive comment. I don't recall her ever giving someone in the group negative feedback.*

The group summary is most effective if mailed out to members prior to the next group session to allow members to read it in the privacy of their home and when they are less defensive and more objective about the events of the previous meeting. The group leaders may also view the meeting's events with more objectivity after the meeting than during it, and their comments in the summary serve as an aid in illuminating process without having to interrupt important interactions that were occurring in the group at the time of the meeting. However, the summary is not meant to take the place of the therapist's process comments, interpretations, and so forth, that should be made during the group meeting (Yalom, *et al.*, 1975). The following are a list of the functions which the written group summary may serve. These were identified as reinforcing many of the tasks the group leader has in facilitating the psychotherapeutic process (Yalom, *et al.*, 1975).

1) Facilitates the Importance of the Group Sessions for the Members. The group summary is a reminder to the members of the importance of this hour or hour-and-a-half a week in their lives. They get a special reminder of what occurred at the last meeting and some reinforcement for attending the next session. The members also get a second chance to view their own process. As a participant and then an observer of their process, the members may more fully integrate the events that occurred with them in the meeting. Because some of these events are quite complex and emotional, it is possible that a member will not understand the full impact of the experience at the time it is happening. Only after reflection and even asking some questions of the therapist or members at the next meeting will the member gain some understanding of very complicated processes (Yalom *et al.*, 1975).

It is important to note that the summary, itself, becomes an event in the group. How the member accepts the summary, chooses to respond to it or comment on it at the next meeting, and how it highlights or helps uncover other parts of the member's personal dynamics are all important (Yalom, *et al.*, 1975). The group leader needs to allow the summary to have a place in the evolving process at the next meeting and to give the members a chance to question, argue, or reinforce any aspect of the written account.

The summary also serves to clarify for members the group norms and highlights behaviors by members that were helpful to others in the group. The therapist often strokes members through the medium of the summary. The group is able to see what processes the therapist had questions about, and members may more readily learn what behaviors are not helpful in the group. During the group meeting, the leader may not have been able to focus on some of this information that needs to be imparted to the members.

2) Provides the Leader with Another Structure for Highlighting Important Processes. The leader benefits from the chance to reinforce already existing norms that the members may or may not be keeping. If he notices the performance of a norm, he can reinforce this. He may suggest new norms for the group or comment on the ineffectiveness of a norm that has resulted in a negative outcome for the group. Sometimes the group may be encouraged to take action on changing an existing norm that is not helpful for the group's task.

In looking at the process of individual members, the therapist may repeat in the summary a significant event in that client's work toward change. He also might remind the individual of a personal goal and how the member's behavior in the group relates to accomplishing or not accomplishing this goal. Continuing to avoid self-disclosure or suddenly taking the risk and doing it in the meeting is an example of avoidance or progress towards a personal goal.

The group summary may be a forum for the leader to reflect on parts of the process he did not fully understand during the meeting. If he has come to an "aha" about these, he can now share this in the summary. He may also comment on a process that he did not wish to comment on during the meeting. In the example of the group summary with Kay and Tom, the leader may have felt his suggestion that the members were afraid to confront him with their anger directly would have been met with defensiveness during the meeting, since their lateness was such an indirect expression of this anger. He also may have felt that the group was not quite ready to consider this. This would be especially true of a group still in the initial stage of development. Perhaps the members needed to experience their anger to a greater degree first. There may be many reasons for the leader to withhold a comment until the group summary.

It is helpful if the leader can put into a time perspective the events that have occurred in the growth of the members as a group (Yalom, *et al.*, 1975). The summary is a way to disseminate this kind of historical information. Individual members may not see much growth occurring and may find it encouraging to hear that the therapist has observed changes. Repetitive events that have meaning for the group are also important in this perspective.

In meeting the goal of demystifying the psychotherapeutic process, the therapist will sometimes choose to self-disclose through the group summary. This would involve describing a bit of strategy or theory to the group members (Yalom, *et al.*, 1975). In the example of the group summary with Tom and Kay, the leader could have discussed why she did not intervene when Tom kept interrupting Kay:

I was trying to decide if I should step in and rescue Kay since I knew she was genuinely upset, and I did not want Tom to derail her from being able to get these painful feelings out. As it turned out, she was able to take care of this herself and to also share her hurt with the group. I'm glad I hesitated.

Recall that self-disclosure can be helpful in modeling appropriate behaviors and in making the therapist more real. The above example not only gives some insight into the process of intervening, but shows the therapist as fallible and unsure of himself at times.

3) Provides a Method for Facilitating the Entrance of a New Member into the Group and for Catching up Absent Members on the Events of the Meeting. This allows for reintegration of the absent member and quicker integration of the new member into the group. An open-ended group must constantly deal with new members. Since the group summary is such a complete account of the group, its history, its norms, and its members, the written account offers much help to an orienting member. Certainly, a summary does not take the place of an individual meeting with the group leaders prior to a member's first group meeting. Nor should the summary mean that members do not have to be as regular in their attendance. If a member is frequently absent, this process needs to be discussed in the group as well as in the summary.

The group summary is a multifaceted tool for illuminating process and providing a solution to some of the logistics involved in holding a group. It is a great deal of work for the group leader but adds to the leader's undertanding of the group events as he or she reviews the previous meeting's process. It may help the group leader feel more relaxed and less controlling in group, knowing he has a second chance at facilitating process through the summary. It is also a helpful tool for group supervision. Novice therapists may write up summaries for their own and the supervisor's use (Yalom, *et al.*, 1975). Following is a sample group summary which highlights the functions described above. The therapist's comments illustrating these functions are in italics. I usually record the process and content of a group meeting before I add summary comments. With the group recreated before me, I find it easier to understand the meeting's events and to then add the summary comments. The group presented in this summary is a psychotherapeutically focused staff group:

My first thought is how come I was so involved in the group that I forgot what time it was supposed to end? I know I have a lot invested in this group (i.e., that I am committed to making this group a good learning experience for the staff and a fulfilling experience for me). Karen and Jack said they thought I was purposely letting group go on until someone said something. No one did. *I wonder how come everyone allowed this to happen? Perhaps others in the group also see this as a problem. I'd like to talk more about this at our next meeting.*

Jesse asked me to comment again on what I had said the last session about his process with others. He used the word "superficial," *which is not what I had said. Perhaps the idea of superficiality comes from some feelings Jesse has about himself.* We spent much of the group time talking with him, and many group members invested much energy in trying to get Jesse, once again, to not disengage himself from the process but take the risk to share some feelings. Jesse talked a little about his parents' divorce and the "love-hate" messages he felt. Fran empathized with Jesse's experiences with his parents and worked very hard to get Jesse to say more about the feelings inside of him. I shared with Jesse my feelings of sadness, helplessness, and hopelessness about his decision to not risk getting out what must be a lot of pain and hurt inside of him. Jesse continued to bait the group by not dropping the issue entirely, *and several times he "rehooked" us. I applaud the rest of the group for their initial try at helping Jesse self-disclose. I don't recall the group being this concerned about a peer before. That's growth!*

Arnie again asked the group for reassurance that he was performing his duties well on the staff team. *I like it that Arnie let us see a little of the conflict he must be feeling inside* when he shared how he was feeling more responsible in areas of his life that he never was before. Arnie thinks the new responsibilities of his position, however, are now creating doubts similar to those he had experienced in his personal life. *Arnie retreats a lot from looking at the turmoil I imagine he feels inside. I'd like to see him really make a commitment to himself to "work" on this. I hope he allows that part of him that wants to, to win out.*

Eugenia and Jesse argued about Eugenia's "time out" behavior in group. That led Jesse to accuse everyone in group of not dealing with feelings. This point was left unfinished. *I imagined no one wanted to touch such a "hot potato"!*

Videotaping

Videotaping is an excellent medium for teaching potential group leaders about their own process and that of the clients as well as for illuminating process in a group therapy session. In this chapter, we will talk about its use with clients and, in the last chapter, focus on its use as a teaching tool.

Therapeutic Goals

Since a member is able to view himself on a videotape as others see him, taping allows the individual to more realistically perceive who he really is and to believe more readily the feedback that other group members may have been giving him about his behaviors, particularly his nonverbal. The member's self-image may change as early as the first playback session. In later sessions, the individual begins to focus more on his interactions with others. Videotaping, therefore, is a powerful tool for the group leader to use, and he is at an advantage with this, since most often the leader has become familiar with his or her own self-concept on tape while the members are still feeling quite hesitant about this medium (Wachtel, *et al.*, 1979; Yalom, 1975). The group leader is able to comment on process while she and the members are viewing the playback. One might think of this almost as an instant group summary.

"Viewing the videotape produces a visual and auditory confrontation of one's self-perception and perception of others outside the realm of a normal intervention, which is a purely verbal statement.'' (Wachtel, *et al.*, 1979, p.81). The person's defenses are less effective with such a direct confrontation, and the result is generally a willingness by the member to be more open after this (Yalom, 1975). As a member becomes desensitized to being on tape, she may be more objective in how she sees herself.

The Logistics

All videotaping must be done with the permission of the group members. This is usually obtained in writing. The members need to know what the taping will be used for, who will see it, and what will happen to it. If videotaping is used for training purposes, and others whom the members do not know will be viewing it, permission is especially important.

The amount of the session to be videotaped needs to be decided upon as well as when the playback will be. If there is another therapist just to do the videotaping, this leaves the second therapist free to concentrate on what is occurring in the meeting. I have found this the most workable set-up. I seem to even forget the videotaping is going on, and sometimes the group members might also, allowing the taping to be more natural. It is important to time the videotaping with the period of the group's development where it would be most valuable. Probably the initial stage is too early. The group members need to be working well together and ready for some self-disclosure. It is also important to not videotape without specific goals in mind (Wachtel, *et al.*, 1979). I share the goals I have in general terms with the group. There are many options for viewing the tape: taping half a meeting and then viewing the rest of the time; taping the entire meeting and viewing at an extra session during the week; or viewing at the next regularly scheduled meeting (Yalom, 1975). Viewing later in the week or at the next meeting allows members to have a more objective view of themselves and the process, much as the group summary does. However, it seems that some of the energy in the interaction is lost through the week. If the group leader wants to keep a member's anxiety heightened to facilitate some changes, an immediate playback would probably do this more effectively.

Seating becomes a problem if there is only one camera. Yalom (1975) recommended a horseshoe seating in this case. However, this is not as effective therapeutically as the circle. If the cameras are permanently stationed in the ceiling or wall, much of the mechanics will be eliminated. It is important that the group leaders who will be doing videotaping get some practice in using the cameras and in seeing themselves on the tape. We will talk more about this in the next chapter. There are many sophisticated uses with videotaping. Although the logistics are sometimes troublesome to work out, videotaping is an excellent way to extend the illumination of process.

Since process is such a complex part of the group and the center of its work, it is important for the leader to know many different ways for highlighting its presence in the group.

REFERENCES

Dick, B., K. Lessler, and J. Whiteside. ''A Developmental Framework for Cotherapy,'' *International Journal of Group Psychotherapy,* 30, no. 3 (Jul., 1980), 273-285.

Hannum, J. "Some Cotherapy Techniques with Families," *Family Process*, 19, no. 2 (Jun., 1980), 161–168.

Puppolo, D. "Co-leadership with a Group of Stroke Patients," in *Psychosocial Nursing Care of the Aged* (2nd ed.), ed. I. Burnside. New York: McGraw-Hill Book Co., 1980.

Scully, R. "Staff Support Group: Helping Nurses to Help Themselves," *Journal of Nursing Administration* 11, no. 3 (Mar., 1981), 48–51.

Wachtel, A., A. Stern, and M. Baldinger. "Dynamic Implications of Videotape Recording and Playback in Analytic Group Psychotherapy: Paradoxical Effect on Transference Resistance," *International Journal of Group Psychotherapy*, 29, no. 1 (Jan., 1979), 67–85.

Wilson, H. and C. Kneisl. *Learning Activities*. Menlo Park, CA: Addison-Wesley Publishing Co., 1979.

Yalom, I. *The Theory and Practice of Group Psychotherapy* (2nd ed.). New York: Basic Books, Inc., 1975.

Yalom, I., S. Brown, and S. Bloch. "The Written Summary as a Group Psychotherapy Technique," *Archives of General Psychiatry*, 32 (May, 1975), 605–613.

The Nurse as a Supervisor, Consultant, and Teacher of Group Process

14

Introduction

The roles of the supervisor and the consultant have been mentioned briefly in Chapter Thirteen in the discussion of the coleadership process. Supervision of group leaders is a process engaged in between two or more persons, one of whom is an expert in group dynamics and process and the others' learning the practice of group leadership. The consultant as an expert is an advisor on the coleadership process for nurses who already have a good understanding of group leadership skills. As an expert on group process, a masters-prepared clinical nurse specialist may be asked to serve as a supervisor or consultant.

A supervisor should have extensive clinical experience with the type of group he or she is supervising. Most often, the supervisor is a senior member of the same profession as the supervisees (Caplan, 1970). The supervisor initiates the process with the group trainees and takes on the responsibility for evaluating their work while seeing that the group members' needs are not compromised (Caplan, 1970; Gallessich, 1982). The supervising process with group leader trainees includes an understanding that each supervisee's personal process with the members and the supervisor is important data for discussion. Supervision may be for group leaders who have had little or no experience with groups, or it may be for leaders who have not had experience in a particular modality of group practice in which the supervisor is an expert.

Although I had been a group leader for a considerable length of time and had supervised other nurses leading support groups, I had little experience working with families when I began an internship in family therapy. I had as a supervisor a family therapist who happened to be a psychiatrist. The unit trainees and supervisees came from a variety of disciplines and crossed disciplines frequently for supervision. This type of supervision is what Caplan (1970) identified as resembling consultation, since it pulls in outside staff for inservice training. However, the multidisciplinary supervisors, most with private practices, still engaged in all the behaviors of a supervisor but had little administrative authority in the agency.

The consultant nurse works with a group of professionals needing education in a particular topic, problem-solving, a list of resources, or other help for a client-centered problem or an internal system-related problem. Nurses are often consultees, receiving input from a variety of experts in other disciplines as well as from other nurses. The nurse consultee may be a head nurse asking for help with his or her management skills, or the consultee might be a nurse administrator retaining a budget analyst, or a personnel recruiter, and so forth. This chapter will focus on the process of consultation from the nurse consultant's point of view. Although the nurse consultant may fit the traditional consultation model as described by Caplan (1970), as a nurse consulting to nonnurses, she may more often consult within her own discipline. The masters-prepared nurse may also engage in a consultation-like process, peer supervision, which has both consultative and supervisory aspects. Each of these roles will be described as it relates to the use of group process skills.

As a teacher of group process, I have found it necessary in my own experience with students to blend a didactic approach with a strong experiential component to promote the student's awareness of group process, a necessary tool for all practicing nurses. It is this model which I will discuss in the latter part of the chapter. The use of videotaping as an adjunct to teaching will also be presented.

Although this information is very specific to the nurse in a supervision, teaching, or consultative role, I feel it is valuable for all nurses to have an awareness of these processes. Most nurses have many opportunities for exposure to consultation when partaking of a group-focused consultation session. They also have a chance to provide suggestions for inservice education and more in-depth training of whatever skills they feel they are needing in the work setting. Perhaps this chapter will serve as a resource for the type of training and consultation available from nurses to nurses.

——— The Process of Supervision In Coleadership ———

Since there is so much data coming from any group, group therapy supervision requires much more processing than supervision for individual client work. The supervisor and trainee leaders need to be selective in their focus to not become lost in the multiple layers of process (Yalom, 1975). It is best to form a contract between the supervisor and supervisees to prevent any misunderstandings about the process or the expectations of either party. Included in the contract should be at least the following:

1) an agreement that the supervisor will explore the coleaders' relationship and each coleader's individual process that impacts on the coleadership relationship;
2) the length of the supervision process, including hours per week (generally one hour per hour of group) and the method for determining the time and way of terminating supervision (*e.g.*, at the end of so many weeks, when the coleaders have reached a certain stage of development, with a gradual tapering of time with the supervisor);
3) the coleaders' goals;
4) the method of observing the coleaders' group (audiotape, videotape, one-way mirror, process recordings or other written reports, and so forth); and
5) the logistics of the process (*e.g.*, location of meetings, coleadership assignments, confidentiality agreements).

The supervisor takes particular notice of the process that occurs between himself and the coleaders, for this is a "microcosm" of the group process between the co-leaders and members (Yalom, 1975, p.507). Such observations as the level of trust between the supervisor and coleaders, the presence of any competition for his attention, and the presence of tension in the supervisory session give cues to the process that may be occurring in the group (Yalom, 1975). This adds another dimension to the data regarding the coleaders' process with one another. It is important for the supervisor to be aware of any time he may be reacting because of his own unfinished business with others. This countertransference will adversely affect supervision. I encourage supervisees to point out to me any response from me that they are not understanding. I find it important to facilitate a freedom for three-way feedback with training coleaders.

Yalom (1975) suggested that the coleaders make postgroup notes that include observations and conclusions about major group themes, the transition between themes, each member's contribution to the meeting, feelings about each member and the group meeting, and reactions to interventions made by each coleader. In my work with nursing students learning coleadership, I had them conduct a postsession meeting with the student observers and me. They were to identify their strengths and weaknesses as group leaders with particular focus on their relationship as coleaders. The way they interacted with each other in the postgroup meeting often highlighted problems they had during the group meeting with the clients. I found I spent much time helping them identify subjective feelings they had towards group members or each other (Wilson, 1980). There were also times when particular behaviors by clients had demonstrated some transference that the coleaders had not noticed. We talked about how to handle this in subsequent meetings.

—— Supervision For the Individual Group Leader ——

The supervision process and contract with one leader is essentially the same as with coleadership except for the missing focus on the coleadership relationship. The relationship between the supervisor and group leader continues to be a rich source of data, and the supervisor needs to use observations about the leader's response to him as a clue to his process with the group members. The supervisor should be aware of countertransference responses to the group leader that will color the assessment of the supervisee's process with others. The same openness to feedback is necessary whether working with one training group leader or with a dyad.

Supervision is a rewarding process for both the supervisor and supervisees. I have found it enhances my own learning when I must closely examine the work of others. Supervision is absolutely essential for beginning coleaders who are novices in the group leadership process, and it can provide growth to those leaders who want to expand their repertoire of group skills.

—— Supervision and Consultation Contrasted ——

In comparing the consultation process and supervision, a most glaring difference is the amount of personal intrusiveness each process allows. Recall that supervision in the coleadership process necessitates a close look at the coleaders' process with one another and with the supervisor. Much of the growth in supervision comes from exploring the supervisee's intrapsychic and interpersonal dynamics. The way a group leader trainee reacts to a member may be the result of parataxic distortion or of some internal conflict with which the supervisor is not aware. Supervisees may find this process very uncomfortable, but they are given very little choice about this aspect of supervision. Certainly, a trainee could resist this process, either openly or with defensive behaviors, but unless this resistance eventually is resolved into a personal learning experience for the supervisee and new insights for his work with clients, resistance could mean this person is not suited for such work. Since a supervisor is presumed to be the expert in the therapeutic process under his supervision, and the trainees are only novices in this process, it is not possible for a peer, egalitarian relationship to exist between the supervisor and supervisees. This is quite different from the relationship between consultant and consultees.

The consultant cannot completely ignore the personal process which a consultee brings to the relationship. However, the only time this is allowed to be part of the consultative process is when it is affecting the problem for which the consultation has been requested. For example, a nurse consultant who is an expert in group process might be asked by a manufacturing company's senior management staff to identify the reason for the poor morale among the junior executives and to problem-solve with the senior group a way to correct the situation. If, in the process of his analysis of the dynamics within this group, the consultant finds that one of the junior executives is a marginally functioning person due to a high degree of family stresses and poorly developed coping skills, the nurse must use this data to assess the effect it has on the senior team. The impact of the executive's stress behaviors shows itself in how the senior executive staff handles this person in relation to the rest of the junior staff. Some of the senior executives react in a protective manner. Others feel his stresses should not be an excuse for poor work productivity. When allowances are made for him in the productivity and quality of his work that are not made for the others, this creates resentment and more competition among the other junior executives. The disagreement between the senior management team on how to handle him has caused confusion in the junior ranks. The nurse consultant's clients are the senior management staff that contracted with him. This means he will not directly intervene with the junior staff person's style of coping or with the particular personal responses to this behavior that several of the senior staff have made. It may be that some of the senior executives have very personal reasons for responding as they do to the junior staff person. To explore these dynamics is not appropriate in the consultation relationship, but the nurse might look at how he could educate the senior management staff in those principles of systems theory and group dynamics that would help the senior staff be more objective with their clients, the junior executive group.

By educating the senior staff, the nurse consultant is preparing them to deal with future problems by applying appropriate group theory rather than reacting very personally and subjectively. The junior group may perceive their bosses as weak leaders and their group as functioning with very few common norms that they can count on to be predictable ways of behaving in that system from day to day. Since personal interactional styles of particular senior executives are only explored in relation to how this affects the group process, the nurse consultant needs to generalize any intervention to the whole group to avoid an uncomfortable interpersonal situation. If a senior person has difficulty accepting negative feedback or allowing disagreement among the junior group, the nurse might do some desensitization with the whole senior group around this issue. The focus is on helping the senior group be more functional as leaders and not on the defensive responses of one member.

Peer supervision has qualities of both the consultation and the supervision process. As with traditional supervision, both parties are from the same discipline and the same agency, and the supervisor is considered an expert in the area of focus. However, a peer supervisor often does not have line administrative control over the supervisee or his work, although the supervisor's input is generally accepted and used by the trainee. Often the supervisee seeks out the supervisor with specific requests for the focus for their work together. The freedom the supervisee has to structure his learning is more consistent with the consultation process. A clinical nurse specialist frequently supervises staff nurses in a peer relationship. Since the clinical specialist is not in a line authority position over the staff nurse, she may provide a more non-threatening atmosphere for the supervision relationship. This facilitates the personal self-disclosure by the supervisee so important in supervision. For a comparison of the various types of supervision and consultation see Table 14.1, p.278.

The Consultative Process

Major Concepts

Consultation occurs between two or more professionals, one professional being the consultant and the others being the consultees. Consultation becomes an indirect service to clients, since the consultee is seeking guidance on a specific aspect of his professional work with clients but will retain control of how he uses this knowledge in his case load, agency, and so forth. It is assumed that the consultee's learning in the affective, behavioral, cognitive, or attitudinal domains will be incorporated in future work of the same kind. Thus, consultation has a snowballing effect in which many people as well as the consultee eventually benefit (Caplan, 1970; Gallessich, 1982). Even if the consultee is not working directly with clients, such as in the case of a hospital administrator seeking help to deal with poor morale and retention problems within the nursing service, the outcome of these problems directly impacts upon the client's care.

In the traditional consultation model, the consultant is an outsider not employed by the agency or connected with the group seeking consultation. The relationship between consultant and consultee is a temporary one. It is also egalitarian, the consultant and the consultee both being full professionals whose areas of expertise and responsibility are usually not the same. Finally, the relationship is a voluntary one between the two parties, and both retain control over the amount of involvement they wish to have in the relationship. The consultee may define what kind of help he or she needs, and the consultant can expect to receive the information necessary from the consultee to formulate an understanding of the presenting problem. It is then up to the consultee to decide how, or even whether, to use the consultant's recommended actions (Caplan, 1970; Gallessich, 1982).

The Consultation Contract

Caplan (1970) recommended a written agreement be executed between the consultant and consultees. Although this does not have to be a formal document, it is helpful if some written exchange takes place between the two parties. The purpose of the written contract is not to legally bind the process but to clarify the consultee's requests and the specific services the consultant has to offer. Each party's role in the relationship is specified as well as any stipulations about confidentiality, particularly since the consultee's clients may be discussed in the course of the consultation process. The consultant's fee would also be agreed upon at this time.

Group Consultation

Consultation frequently takes place in a group, because the process of consultation often involves several consultees who work together in an agency and who have identified a particular need for a consultant's services. Very often, these professionals share the work of a client load or interface with administrative responsibilities and common problems. Group consultation can occur over a period of time with group meetings or in one time-intensive process (Gallessich, 1982). Consultee groups may work best if the consultant initially directs the group with some informal teaching or structured presentations while the members of the group become more comfortable with one another and with the consultant. Such a group goes through the stages of development that any group experiences. The initial stage is characterized by some anxiety about the process, and some mistrust of the leader (the consultant) and of each other, especially if the consultees have not worked together for any length of time or with any depth of interpersonal interaction (Gallessich, 1982). Case-centered consultation sessions work well in a group and facilitate the interpersonal process between the consultees as well as an increased understanding of the management of a particular client group. The consultees may take turns serving as co-consultants with their peers (Gallessich, 1982). In this role, they would experience the process of facilitating the interactions of others in a group and of having to meet the learning needs of their peers.

A very valuable experience for me was a period of about six consultation sessions with the clinical specialists with whom I worked and with a psychiatrist as our consultant. The focus was case presentation which was rotated among us. Some of my learning resulted from observing the consultant help a peer define exactly what information she needed and determine how to answer her own questions with the information she had. We were free to participate in the discussion and to apply this process to clients with whom we were each working. I felt I was learning a new method for analyzing both the client's process and my own. The consultant did not pursue our individual personal dynamics but encouraged us to explore these as part of the information we needed in defining the problem with a client. As a consultee, I also learned about the process of consultation through the experience of receiving a consultant's services. It seemed like the group approach to consultation offered us a richer view of our client and showed us how we could be more helpful to each other in our work with clients in the future.

The consultant who works in a group setting with consultees must identify and deal with group process, although he will most likely not discuss his assessment of the process with the consultees. Skills in group process and group dynamics are essential to his work (Gallessich, 1982; Lange, 1979). The consultant has both a task role and a socioemotional role similar to any leader of a group (Lange, 1979). The task has been identified in the contract between the parties. The socioemotional role is not discussed except to identify the boundaries of the consultant's involvement in the personal process of the consultees. Since this is generally limited, the consultant's role centers around what process the group members chose to deal with among themselves. However, the consultant is constantly aware of the possibilities for process development and tries to guide the group towards using that which fits with the problem the group is exploring. In our clinical specialist consultation group, the psychiatrist leader moved us into sharing a lot of personal process with one another as we explored the client's dynamics with whomever was presenting the case. He had assessed our interactions with one another and had most likely concluded that we were a close group that could handle exploring personal data together. How the group process is handled has much to do with how successful the consultation group turns out to be. The group process is a pervasive factor in group consultation.

The Nurse Consultant

The consultation process has been compared to both the steps in problem-solving and the nursing process (Lange, 1979). Although the traditional consultation model describes the consultant as a professional from another discipline, nurse-to-nurse consultation allows a professional rapport to more easily develop between the consultant nurse and the nurse consultees (Fife, 1983). The nurse consultant is a catalyst for problem-solving among the members of his or her profession. With the myriad of problems in nursing, such as the conflict over the entry level into practice, the certification of nurses, and the issues around peer review, nurses consulting with nurses can be of great value in facilitating the resolution of these problems.

The nurse who becomes a consultant to a non-nursing group will need to feel comfortable asserting herself as an expert with other professionals in other disciplines. Some new roles for the nurse consultant may be in the school system as an expert in human sexuality, or in consciousness-raising classes, or in public relations and mass media where the role of the nurse needs to be more clearly defined to the public (Polk, 1980). A directory of nurse consultants who are experts in a particular area of nursing practice and who also have the necessary consultation skills is published annually by the *Journal of Nursing Administration*. Other sources for nurse consultants include universities, medical centers, professional nursing organizations, and health care consultation firms which have been started by nurses (Pati, 1980).

The Steps in the Consultation Process

The following discussion will describe consultation as the nurse consultant would approach the process with both nurse and non-nurse consultees. Although the latter represents the pure model for consultation between the members of two different disciplines, the nurse-to-nurse consultation process follows the traditional model in all other ways. The reader will notice a definite similarity with the steps in the problem-solving process. The first two steps are preliminary to the actual consultation contract which uses the problem-solving method and is designed to facilitate the relationship between the consultant and the consultee(s).

1) Identifying Specific Skills the Consultant Has to Offer. The following roles are those most often described by nurse consultants as the type of skills they have to offer (Pati, 1980). The nurse consultant may analyze and facilitate the consultees' ability to perform a particular task, to make a change in the work setting or within a health care delivery system, and so forth. The consultant is a new person who is objective and able to view the system within which the consultees work from a different perspective. This analysis is most helpful in diagnosing the problem area. As a facilitator, the nurse acts as a catalyst for the group that has engaged him. He must work with the group's dynamics and process to move the consultees to a productive level of problem-solving. There may be times when the consultant will provide more direct problem-solving through both facilitating a process and doing some teaching about what is needed, what is missing, or how things might work more efficiently a different way.

Education is also a function for the nurse consultant to those looking for new educational tools or techniques, or for an educational program for their agency. Finally, the nurse consultant serves as a resource person with his own expert knowledge and experience as well as with an awareness of where other information the consultee is seeking may be obtained.

It is important that both the consultant and consultees are clear about the qualifications and roles necessary to carry out the particular contract for which the consultant is being engaged. A mutual interviewing process is important prior to engaging a consultant (Pati, 1980). Both parties need to be comfortable with the anticipated relationship with one another.

2) Developing a Rapport with the Consumer. Non-nursing consumers of the consultant's skills would include management groups, multidisciplinary health care staff, school systems, clergy, and lay groups, such as self-help groups or parent groups. Any group that is looking for the skills the nurse consultant has to offer is a possible consultee.

Nurse consumers of the nurse consultant's skills include individual nurses, especially those in specialty positions that as a group would seek a consultant, and administrative nursing staff that frequently have problems or needs around quality assurance, staffing, career development, and other management issues (Pati, 1980).

Whether it be a nursing or non-nursing consumer of the consultant's services, rapport between the two parties develops after dialogue and a sense of the personal and professional credibility of the consultant (Pati, 1980). I feel the initial interview and the succeeding dialogue between the consultant and the consumer are important to get the correct "fit" between the two parties. Someone with extensive experience and expertise still may not be a comfortable match for the consultee(s). The preliminary time of dialogue needs to be used to decide on the potential for the two parties to be able to work together effectively and comfortably.

The next six steps discuss the actual process of consultation. Material already presented on the problem-solving approach and on change theory will provide further clarification for the reader.

3) Defining the Specific Need for Consultation. Defining the problem and the desired outcome according to the consumer's needs are important principles in consultation. Questioning the consultee and observing for clues to the problem situation provide data to the consultant (Polk, 1980). Information which is particularly important to the consultant's assessment of the situation would include: the consultee's perception of the problem; others' perceptions, such as other health care workers, departments, supervisors, and so forth; and specific approaches that have been tried and their degree of success. Problems that could be dealt with by a nurse consultant are generally in one of three different categories: client-care issues; interpersonal conflicts between individuals or groups or organizational or managerial issues (Fife, 1983). All of these categories may define a variety of needs for which a consultant could be used. Problem-solving, educating, providing resources, and the other activities requested of the consultant should be identified when defining the problem.

If the consultee is having difficulty identifying the problem, it is the consultant's responsibility to help with this process. Sometimes a consultant's greatest service is to define the problem in a way that makes it possible for the consultee(s) to work on it. I find it helpful to reflect back on what the consultee is saying to further encourage a dialogue about the problem. Interrupting, expressing one's own thoughts, and taking a very active role while being careful not to put the consultee on the spot with questions he could not answer further the process of problem identification (Gallessich, 1982). The nurse may discover that there is more than one problem with which the consultee and he could work. However, the consultee has requested a particular service and has contracted for that alone. The nurse consultant may share his observations with the consultee while remembering that it is the consultee's need that must be met rather than the consultant's need to fix everything! Sometimes it is difficult not to give the consumer more than what he asks for. For example, the nurse consultant may observe that several changes need to be made in the way staff are chosen for participation as coleaders in support groups on a particular unit. However, the head nurse has only asked for some client-focused conferences to further the application of nursing theory to the interventions the nursing staff members are doing. Some of these interventions involve support groups for clients. In dialoguing with the head nurse about the problem, the leadership of the support groups may have been discussed. Even though the consultant wishes to pursue the group leadership in more detail, this cannot be done without the head nurse's consent to this as part of the consultation contract.

Once the problem has been defined, the desired outcome is identified. It is important for the consultant and consultee to work together on this aspect of the problem, particularly to define an outcome that can be a realistic result of the consultation effort (Fife, 1983). As with the problem-solving process, outcomes are best stated in measurable terms. This helps with evaluation and allows specific plans to be formulated for reaching the measurable goals. The following are examples of measurable outcomes.

a) Identify the specific behaviors by staff that cause splitting in the client's care.

b) Identify staff-to-staff conflict that is the result of poor communications between the disciplines. Formulate a plan for correcting the communication problems.

c) Develop a method for covering the three shifts without disrupting the staff nurse's involvement with a particular treatment team.

4) Formulating a Contract with the Consumer. The consultant puts into writing those skills which he or she has agreed to offer the consultee(s) in a time-limited period. The boundaries of the consultant's involvement, as well as the complementary exchange of information between the two parties that will provide the data for the consultant's work should be clearly defined. It is here that any concerns about confidentiality may also be noted (Caplan, 1970). The contract may be renegotiated as agreed upon by both parties. Certainly, a written contract does not take the place of the personal rapport that should exist between the consultant and consultee(s). It would seem that, if the personal interactions are open and comfortable, the written contract will be seen as less impersonal and will cause little concern.

5) Collecting Data. Questioning and observing once again become important during this part of the process. A preliminary search for data has resulted in problem identification. If the consultant has established enough rapport to be able to move freely about the consultee's work area or system of operation and to be trusted to receive information that may originally have been withheld until trust could be established, the process of consultation can proceed more smoothly. I recall being initially very hesitant to share a lot of data with the psychiatrist that was consulting with our group of clinical specialists. It was helpful to have him "give" us something initially by talking about resistant clients to allow for time for our group to develop trust with him. It seems that the formal interactions between the consultant and consultees that occur at the beginning of the relationship often help to allow a natural readiness to develop for more openness later. Informal chats with unit staff often yield very important information about the system and its points of difficulty. Just sitting quietly and observing the process within the system that has requested the consultation may yield excellent data. As in the change process, being an observer in the consultee's routine activities may provide helpful insights. I find that the more open I can be to receiving information from a variety of resources, the more data I generally collect.

6) Deciding on the Methods of Meeting the Contract. One of the most familiar methods is case consultation in which a consultee presents a client for discussion (Caplan, 1970; Langman-Dorwart, 1979; Lambert and Lambert, 1981). This discussion may be supplemented by more active methods such as roleplaying and assertiveness training (Langman-Dorwart, 1979). Several times it may be appropriate to use experiential exercises to help facilitate awareness of how group dynamics and process can affect communication, task accomplishment, and so forth. Lecturing or other didactic forms of instruction are also appropriate methods used by the consultant, particularly early in the consultation relationship. As noted before, this may give the group of consultees time to develop trust in the consultant. The consultant is "giving" something to a group that feels "needy." Exercises for conflict resolution, including role reversals, are helpful tools for a group that needs to learn how to deal with conflict in an adaptive way. Any method used in the consultation process should be mutually agreed upon by both parties. The consultant, as the expert, offers those methods that are most appropriate for the goals decided upon by the consultation group. The consultees may decide to reject some of the methods as too threatening or difficult. Although this may interfere with reaching some of the goals, the consultee has the right to give this input, and the consultant needs to inform the consultee of the merits of using one method over another for goal achievement.

7) Meeting the Particular Goal(s) and Renegotiating as Needed. As discussed in Step Six, renegotiation may occur if either party is not satisfied with the method or the outcome. Another reason for renegotiation is to add new goals and expand on the consultant's contract, including the time spent with the consultee(s). This is the step where the actual method decided upon is carried out. It is interesting to note that there have been six preliminary steps prior to the action which the consultees look to as the process that will help them reach their goals. From the consultant's point of view, the preliminary steps are probably much more important in getting successful results. Much of the consultant's work may not be evident to the consultee.

8) Evaluating the Outcome. The measurable goals are used for an objective evaluation of whether or not the outcome has been met. If it has not been met, a look at what went wrong may be carried out by going through the steps again. Perhaps some data were missed, either due to the consultant's inability to collect the necessary data or due to resistance by the consultees. A faulty assessment of the data might have been made. At any time, a new contract may be negotiated, or the relationship between the two parties may be terminated. Occasionally, either the consultant or the consultees decide that their relationship is not working out. There may be more requests from the consultee if new information yields further work to be done or if the consultee wants to do more than originally planned. The consultant, however, is not bound to continue the relationship unless he or she wishes. Certainly, a continuing relationship with the consultant shortens the awkward step of developing rapport. Each time new requests are made and agreed upon, the problem-solving process of consultation starts over.

Teaching Group Process

A Model for Teaching Group Process

Both the supervisor and consultant roles provide the prospective supervisee and consultee with some new learning in group process awareness. Inherent in these two roles are both direct and indirect teaching. The supervisor shares insights about group process more directly than the consultant does. However, the consultant will, most likely, leave with the consultee a greater understanding of group process.

Whether one is teaching nursing students or graduate nurses in a continuing education class, or holding an informal discussion on process elements in a multidisciplinary group, it is most important to model sensitivity to process. In other words, teaching group process means living it with one's students. Although this is a bias which I feel about teaching this skill, several other educators support this approach. The therapeutic use of self as a model to teach other health care workers who also can be effective instruments in helping clients with their process is an important concept for teaching group process skills. The instructor who self-discloses with students and is free to be "human" promotes a greater desire within the students for sensitivity to their own process and to their clients. An instructor cannot teach affective responses if he or she does not experience these also (Hannon, 1980). Hannon (1980) talked about making a group process class a laboratory for students to experience this process themselves. In this model, activities were chosen to facilitate the growth of the students in a group setting. As a by-product, the students could use time in their groups to deal with some of the stresses which occur during a nursing student's experiences in class and clinical practice. Although the groups were not therapy groups, the outcome was therapeutic for the students.

A group experience for graduate nurses was described by Lammert (1981) as a way to combat burnout that nurses sometimes feel and to teach group process. If a group experience could bring about closer relationships with staff while allowing staff members to use the group as a comfortable place to receive emotional and social support, this would be an effective intervention for the stress that leads to burnout. Increasing awareness of oneself and how to take care of one's needs are by-products of a group learning experience. The idea that one feels more positive towards clients when relationships with peers are supportive certainly makes sense. Interpersonal skills increase one's ability to be open and free to ask for support from others (Lammert, 1981). Lammert's model for teaching group process skills is very similar to the one I used with students and which will be described in the following sections. Since nurses spend so much of their professional time as members or leaders of groups and are increasingly being expected to function competently in groups, teaching group process to nurses is an important role for the clinical specialist or nurse educator. Immersing the nurse in a group process laboratory results in the translation of abstract principles of group process into concrete experiences that describe what the concepts feel like (Lammert, 1981). The following quote sums up the rich connection between understanding one's own process and being competent in the use of group process with clients:

"To learn about group process and the possibilities of meaningful experiences in groups, one must be intimately aware of and familiar with one's own feelings, reactions, biases, values to know where the boundary is between those feelings, biases, etc. that are one's own and those that belong to others in the group." (Lammert, 1981, p.45).

An ideal setting for teaching group process is one which allows the student to experience both membership and leadership in a process-oriented group, such as a self-awareness or growth group. In my own experience with students, I found that the clinical laboratory where the students coled a group for mental health inpatients (see Chapters Ten and Eleven) provided a rich group process experience. Clinical conferences, process recordings of a dyad relationship between the student and an individual client, and a personal journal of the student's clinical experiences and subjective reactions are other tools to facilitate understanding of process. In the clinical group, students were observing process firsthand, and I could point it out to them in our postgroup sessions. They also began to analyze each other's process as they became more comfortable as a peer group (Wilson, 1980).

A personal journal that is used as a tool to teach process awareness, particularly awareness of one's own process, should include a brief objective description of a group event, an experiential exercise, or an interactional encounter. The rest of the entry for that particular experience should be the student's subjective reaction to the event. I reinforce this subjective account by asking students to turn their journals in to me for comment. I then circle, underline, and give extensive feedback to those parts of the journal that are subjective in nature. I self-disclose when something a student has said sparks an affective response within me.

I find that this self-disclosure models the appropriate subjective response that I am looking for from the students. Any instructor who is uncomfortable with self-disclosure should probably not attempt this type of activity. My personal comments all relate to the student's experience and are not, therefore, an attempt to solve my own unfinished business. This caution is an important one if an instructor is considering using self-disclosure governed by the same rules that define self-disclosure for the leader of a group. If used appropriately, both clients and students can profit from this intervention. If used inappropriately for one's own personal need, the outcome can be devastating for both students and instructor. Students cannot be made to share personal feelings, but an explanation of the goal for such an exercise and a testimony to the positive outcome will be helpful in convincing students to try this.

Probably the most valuable group process teaching involves some didactics with regard to theory and group dynamics while the student is experiencing group process as a member or leader of a group. One way to structure such an experience would be to have the students participate as group members with their peers. Groups of four to six students can be organized during an early class. Often, didactic teaching is planned to correlate with process learning. For example, students may have a group assignment such as an experiential exercise, a group dynamics activity, or a group project. If the didactic material is focusing on the leadership structure in a group, the group activity might be an experience with different leadership styles in one's group. An experiential activity of self-disclosure with one's group members could occur during the same week as a discussion on the way self-disclosure facilitates the group's process.

Group process activities are most helpful if used as the laboratory for an analysis of the student's own group experience. Each time the group members must organize themselves to do a group activity, they experience the leadership process, the development of interpersonal relationships between members, perhaps some conflict or power struggles, and other processes that identify the group's movement. If the group members keep notes, both as individuals and as a collective body, these written records establish the pattern of interventions occurring within the group. Oftentimes, a group activity will illuminate process elements that tend to be kept hidden by group members when the group is told to focus on its own process. For example, the group might be assigned the task of planning a teaching group session for newly diagnosed diabetic clients. During the process of working on this project, group members will be less likely to analyze their process, thereby allowing the process to unfold more naturally. After the project has been completed, the group might be asked to write a paper analyzing the group's structure and movement and dynamic interactions with one another. I have used this method of teaching with nursing students and have found it to be a rich learning experience. If the group must construct one collective paper, the process of completing this is, in itself, very enlightening. I have had some groups which were unable to do the paper collectively but whose members turned in individual analyses. Table 14.2 gives a suggested outline for a collective group paper.

Group Process Curriculum Sample from the Literature

Lammert (1981) described a group experience for both undergraduate nursing students in their junior year and graduate nurses. Nurses were put in groups of five to seven members and were assigned a group task to prepare a presentation for their peers on an aspect of group process or structure. These projects were to be evaluated on how the group worked together as demonstrated through their project. An hour each week was spent working in their groups on this task and then another hour or so was spent as a large class with didactic instruction. Experiential exercises promoted process development for individuals and the groups. A representative from each group also met with the instructor to talk about their group project. Each member had to write an individual analysis of their process in the group and the group's development. An interesting additional learning experience was the process of having each group observed by several peers from other groups. This occurred during the time the group was meeting for task work, and the data could be used as material for the members' individual analysis of the group process. Lammert's ideas allow for a more in-depth study and experience in process than those experiences which I created for students. However, our methods of illuminating and teaching process seem quite similar.

If the group process learning time is much less than several weeks in length, a "here-and-now" group for students is not possible. Teaching in a workshop setting needs to focus on material that gives the students a feel for what process actually is and how it affects the development of a group. Exercises that allow a group of people to experience competition, a variety of leadership styles, and the completion of a group task are examples of activities that would serve to point out process. Individual students could then be instructed to focus on any feelings each experienced during the activity and to process these by sharing them with the group they worked with in the exercise. Having individual observers for each activity further helps with process development. Some staff groups may feel more comfortable meeting for some didactic lectures initially and then moving into experiential exercises several weeks later. If staff members can commit themselves to one to two hours per week for some group process learning, this type of model may be used. A one-day, eight-hour workshop allows for less group development, but the experience may hook students to returning or asking for more learning opportunities in group.

Videotaping as a Teaching Tool

Videotaping offers a variety of techniques to enhance process learning. The most passive form of learning with this medium is to watch a videotape of a group in action to observe specifically for process elements and then discuss these observations in a class setting. Sources of such tapes are professionally produced group sessions, such as those done by Virginia Satir (for example, "Family Therapy I: Family in Crisis," a family therapy session where the identified patient is a sixteen year-old girl). I found that focusing the students in advance by giving them a set of questions helped them to pay attention to particular process elements. Examples of appropriate questions include:

1) What interventions did the leader make to illuminate process?
2) What were elements of the "here-and-now" in the group interactions?
3) How were specific individual behaviors dealt with in the group? How did this affect the group's development?

A second level of learning by videotape involves simulations of group interactions by the students which are recorded on videotape and then viewed for analysis of group and individual process. A script with only enough information to set the scene and describe various "players" to allow for character development in the simulation prevents programming the development of the group and allows for a more natural unfolding of the group's process. A simulation activity is presented in the "Learning Activities" at the end of this section of the book. Students should probably "play" with the videotape to become desensitized to being on camera. Some warm-up experiential activities could accomplish this. Having students take turns using the camera and doing the actual taping helps sensitize them to the importance of nonverbal and how to record this on the tape. Depending on the focus of the videotaping, the instructor may act as the group leader in the scene and help facilitate the process, or students may also play this role as a way of learning to facilitate a group. The student leader does not have a script for any particular character development but is herself and uses her skill to attempt to facilitate process in the group. Students may also practice the coleadership role this way.

The most intimate learning with the videotape takes place when the students are focusing on their own subjective experiences through a series of progressively more difficult exercises on tape. Kramer (1980) developed a series of exercises designed for this purpose. An important point about video in the growth of one's own process is that the tape provides feedback to the individual who does not have the usual interactional restraints that come with attempt at face-to-face confrontation. Someone giving very honest feedback to another person frequently has difficulty with this and may not be as clear or as direct as would be the effect of a self-viewing of one's process on a videotape. Students may be asked to anticipate what they will feel on viewing themselves on tape. During and after the viewing, they may then check out their feelings. Exercises for personal awareness include pairing up and contacting or avoiding one another, playing various family member roles, and exploring one's facial expressions and the congruence or incongruence of these with one's inner feelings. The author (Kramer, 1980) suggested that such a training period could last for a year with students meeting with the same group each time. This intensive work was to prepare group therapists, particularly for those who would work with families and who needed to deal with any unfinished personal business around their own family of origin. Kramer noted that the anxiety of some students with this process led to both overt and covert resistance.

The creative possibilities for teaching group process are limited only to the instructor's imagination and understanding of his or her own process. Such teaching not only is extremely helpful to potential group leaders, but it is also very rewarding to the teacher.

REFERENCES

Caplan, G. *The Theory and Practice of Mental Health Consultation*. New York: Basic Books, Inc., Publishers, 1970.

Fife, B. "The Challenge of the Medical Setting for the Clinical Specialist in Psychiatric Nursing," *Journal of Psychosocial Nursing and Mental Health Services*, 21, no. 1 (Jan., 1983), 8–13.

Gallessich, J. *The Profession and Practice of Consultation*. San Francisco: Jossey-Bass Publishers, 1982

Hannon, J. "Group Process—Success in One Graduate Nursing Program," *Journal of Nursing Education*, 19, no. 1 (Jan., 1980), 46–52.

Kramer, J. "Using Video Playback to Train Family Therapists," *Family Process*, 19, no. 2 (Jun., 1980), 145–150.

Lambert, C. and V. Lambert. "Nursing Students and a Mental Health Consultation Program," *Journal of Psychiatric Nursing and Mental Health Services*, 19, no. 3 (Mar., 1981), 29–35.

Lammert, M. "A Group Experience to Combat Burnout and Learn Group Process Skills," *Journal of Nursing Education*, 20, no. 6 (Jun., 1981), 41–46.

Lange, F. "The Multifaceted Role of the Nurse Consultant," *Journal of Nursing Education*, 18, no. 9 (Nov., 1979), 30–34.

Langman-Dorwart, N. "A Model for Mental Health Consultation to the General Hospital," *Journal of Psychiatric Nursing and Mental Health Services*, 17, no. 3 (Mar., 1979), 29–33.

Pati, B. "Nursing Consultation: A Collaborative Process," *Journal of Nursing Administration*, 10, no. 11 (Nov., 1980), 33–37.

Polk, G. "The Socialization and Utilization of Nurse Consultants," *Journal of Psychiatric Nursing and Mental Health Services*, 18, no. 2 (Feb., 1980), 33–36.

Wilson, M. "Negotiating Group Process Experiences," *Nursing Outlook*, 28, no. 6 (Jun., 1980), 360–364.

Yalom, I. *The Theory and Practice of Group Psychotherapy*. New York: Basic Books, Inc., 1975.

TABLE 14.1
COMPARISON OF SUPERVISION AND CONSULTATION MODES

Terms

Expert— Supervisor or consultant

Recipient— Supervisee or consultee

Egalitarian/Peer—
- Expert and recipient have a well-developed knowledge base in their discipline
- Initiation of contract comes from recipient
- Either may terminate the contract between them
- Recommendations by the expert are not binding on the recipient to carry out
- Expert has no responsibility for the care the recipient is giving to clients
- Exploration of recipient's personal dynamics is not normally pursued (discussed only with recipient's permission and limited to its impact on current problems)

Administrative Authority—
- Expert has a more developed knowledge base than the recipient, who is still learning
- Contract initiated by expert and terminated with expert's approval
- Recipient obligated to follow through on expert's recommendations for clients
- Expert has accountability with agency for recipient's delivery of care to clients
- Expert routinely explores personal dynamics of recipient and its effect on client's care (part of the contract with the recipient)

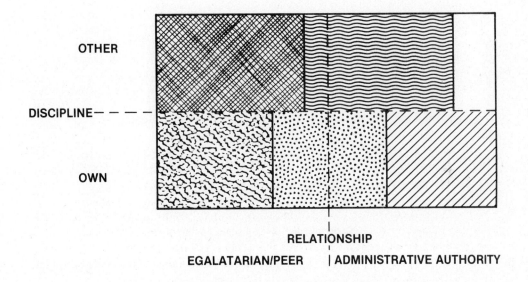

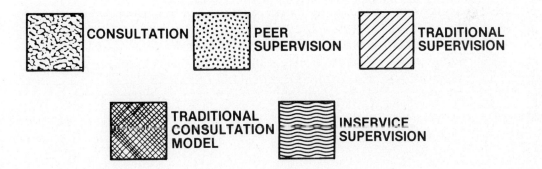

TABLE 14.2
CONTENT FOR GROUP PROCESS PAPER/ANALYSIS

I. Identifies and describes the:
   a. task role behaviors
   b. socioemotional role behaviors   performed in the group

   Indicates how these two roles were distributed among members

II. Describes behaviors characteristic of each stage of the group's movement and identifies those behaviors which were incongruent with the group's stage of development (e.g., excessive self-disclosure in the initial stage)

   Discusses process events which signified the passing from one stage to another

III. Describes the process whereby the group leader was chosen

   Discusses the style of leadership which predominated and illustrates with examples

IV. Describes any conflict between group members (distinguishes between overt and covert conflict issues and illustrates with specific process data from the group)

   Identifies specific methods used by the leader or group members to resolve conflict (overt or covert conflict) and describes the outcome

   Discusses the reason for the presence of any unresolved conflict or speculates on why all conflict issues were resolved in some way

Supplemental Learning Activities 13-14

1. *a*) Choose a peer with whom you think you could colead a group because of the "fit" the two of you might have for working together. Compare philosophies of group. Discuss any possible problems.

   b) The following is an exercise for a videotape simulation of a support group for family members/significant others of patients with terminal cancer (CA). There are two coleaders and six members. In simulating a group meeting, use the work done in "*a*" with the potential coleader to test out your relationship. The person doing the videotaping should focus on capturing the process in the group, particularly the nonverbal. Discuss the pre- and postsimulation questions.

Problem

In the pre-group interview, the members were told the following.

The group will meet for ten sessions. The purpose is to allow for sharing of feelings around their ill significant others, how the illness affects them, their understanding of what is happening, etc. Group will meet once a week on Monday evening from 7:00–8:30 P.M. Group members are expected to be on time and to notify one of the group leaders if they cannot attend. Members can expect the group leaders to respect the confidentiality of those attending the group. The group leaders have the final decision as to whether a piece of information/self-disclosure is such that the member's health would be jeopardized if the leaders did not do something with this information with regard to notifying another family member or health professional.

The group leaders want to support the members' growth and crisis-handling as much as possible. This is the group's first meeting, and only very basic procedural norms have been established (as noted above). The coleaders need to structure this first meeting in such a way that norm-setting is given major priority. They realize that the group members will be a little anxious at their first meeting.

Scene and Players

The First Group Meeting

Liz (coleader)—You are excited about the first group meeting and have shared with Jane how you hope to accomplish a lot tonight, particularly in regard to having well-defined norms made explicit before the meeting ends. You feel the group members all want to be here and will want to cooperate in getting the norms settled.

Jane (coleader)—You agree with Liz's desire to try to set very explicit norms tonight. You see the members as sincere and wanting to be in the group, but you are not sure how much you can accomplish in the first meeting. Therefore, you are cautiously optimistic and a little nervous about leading your first group.

Bob (member no. 1 whose mother has inoperable CA of the lung and is on

281

chemotherapy)—Your mother's regimen of chemotherapy has made her very physically ill. You find it difficult to visit with her because she looks like she is in so much pain. Your wife is much better at visiting and can be talkative and relaxed with your mother. You are feeling guilty and inadequate about how poorly you see yourself handling the situation and feel the need to talk about this. However, you are not sure you will feel comfortable sharing this in the first meeting.

Betty (member no. 2, Bob's wife)—You have noticed that Bob becomes very anxious when it is time to visit his mother. You are able to think about how to make her most comfortable and do so during visits. Sometimes you feel angry inside because this is not even your own mother and you have more of the burden of her illness. You love Bob's mother but resent her taking up so much energy and time in your life with Bob. You have agreed to come to this group because you see the group as a place to let off steam and really get some sympathy and understanding from others. Bob has not been able to give you much of that lately.

Barbara (member no. 3 whose son, Michael, has leukemia. It is in remission, but the extended prognosis is not good)—You have mixed feelings about attending this group even though you did express these at the time of the pregroup interview. Your husband really wants to go so you are coming primarily for his sake. Since Michael is in remission, you really cannot totally accept his disease as being terminal, and it depresses you to think of attending this group with others who have relatives with terminal CA.

Jim (member no. 4, Barbara's husband)—You really want to be here, although you sense that Barbara is coming more because of you than because she really wants to attend. You are hoping to gain a better understanding of how you can make every day that is left count in your relationship with your son. You and Michael are very close. Right now, you are not feeling depressed but hopeful about your son, regardless of how long his remission lasts.

Kathy (member no. 5 whose father is in the terminal stages of CA with a malignant neoplasm)—You have always lived at home with your dad and now must face the fact that you will eventually be alone. Your dad has always been the strong one, and you felt so comfortable in this relationship that you have never really faced making it on your own. You are scared and want the group leaders to tell you what to do.

Steve (member no. 6 whose girlfriend is in a terminal stage of leukemia)—You have known Nicole for four years and were to be married later this year. She is very weak and will probably never leave the hospital. You are particularly close because Nicole's parents were killed in an auto accident two years ago and she is an only child. Therefore, the entire burden of support lies on you. You are feeling very overwhelmed, very confused about how you can best help Nicole, and very angry at times, which serves to create some guilt feelings within you. You wonder if you are even in the right place with regard to deciding to be in the group.

Pre-Simulation Questions

- What would be an appropriate group contract for the coleaders to make with the group members?
- What are some of the problems that would arise in this first meeting: *a*) between the coleaders; *b*) among the members; *c*) between the coleaders and members?

• What are the most important norms to stress in this first meeting? In a subsequent meeting? (List important group norms and then decide which fit best with the first meeting or in a second meeting where more process is likely to occur.)

Post-Simulation Questions

• Describe the mass group process.
• What norms were established in this first group meeting? What comments by the group members led to their formation?
• Were there any anti-therapeutic group norms with which the leaders had to deal? If so, how did the coleaders deal with these?

2. Identify which process/functions each of the italicized therapist's comments serves in the group summary on page 259-260 of Chapter Thirteen.

3. Compose a written summary using the descriptive account of the group meeting in no. 2 of the "Supplemental Learning Activities" at the end of Part One (pages 151-152).

4. What would be a reason for having a consultant for your agency or the unit on which you work? What characteristics would you want in a consultant? Compose some interview questions you would ask a potential consultant.

INDEX

Couple's fair fighting techniques, 16-18
Covert rehearsal, 23
  in communications, 11
in dysfunctional communications, 13
Crisis group, 83
  compared to a social group, 84
Crossed transactions in transactional analysis, 35
Cultural artifacts in communications, 10-11
Curative factors in group experience, 208-211

-D-

Decision making, 133
Decision making *see also* group decision making
Democratic group leadership style, 95
Dependency group, 86
Desirable changes vs. life saving sanctions in
  behavior modification, 64
Directive leadership style, 95
Discount in transactional analysis, 33
Distributive group leadership style, 95
Dysfunctional communication, 12-14
  covert rehearsal in, 13
  message generation in, 13-14

-E-

Ego,
  defined, 24-25
  states in transactional analysis, 30-33
Emotional stimulation function in leadership, 103
Equifinality, 5, 6
Executive functions in leadership, 103-104
Existential influence on group behavior, 41-55
Existential theory, 42-43
Existentialist view of humans, 41

Experience,
  modes of, 9-10
    parataxic, 10
    protaxic, 9-10
    syntaxic, 10
Experiential exercises, 167-173
  sampling of, 175
Experiential learning activities,
  purposes of, 159-162
  cautions for group leaders, 162-167
  process, 157-167
  techniques, 167-173
    behavioral rehearsal-role playing, 170-172
    group member cohesion exercises, 173
    kinetic exercises, 168-169
    movement therapy, 169-170
    tension release exercise, 172
    trust and self-disclosure exercise, 172-173
    warm-up exercises, 167-168
Exploitive power of leaders, 92-93
Extinction in behavior modification, 60-61

-F-

Fair fighting techniques with couples, 16-18
Families as an interactional system, 15-16
Family crisis, behavioral assessment of, 19-21
Family therapy, goals of, 15
Feedback loop and model, 6
Fight-flight behavior role, 86-87
Figure-ground concept in Gestalt theory, 47
Free child in transactional analysis, 31-32

-G-

Gestalt,
  confluence and, 45
  contact in, 48-49

rewards and punishments in, 88-89
secondary, 1
selecting a leader in, 96
standards of action in, 87-88
task functions of, 96-97
theoretical frameworks for studying, 1-76
types of, 79-83
Growth groups, 79-81

-H-

Hooking one ego state in transactional analysis, 39-40
Hostile aggression,
defined, 16
rituals, 16
uses of, 17

-I-

Id, defined, 24
Identity for a group, 89
I'm OK–You're OK, 29
Impact agression,
defined, 16
rituals, 16, 17-18
Incomplete Gestalt, 50-52
Influence vs. control in behavior modification, 63-64
Integrative power of leaders, 93
Intellectualization, Gestalt theory and, 45-46
Interactional systems, 6
fair fighting systems, 16-18
family as, 15-16
groups as, 14
properties of, 6
Interpersonal systems, 5
Introjection, Gestalt theory and, 44

-K-

Kinesics defined, 10
Kinetic exercises, 168-169

-L-

Laissez-faire group leadership style, 95
Latent material defined, 29
Latent vs. manifest content, 29
Leadership,
defined, 92
dynamics, 92-94
experiential learning cautions, 162-167
powers of, 92-94
styles, 94-96
Leadership functions, 103-104
caring, 103
emotional stimulation, 103
executive, 103-104
meaning attribution, 104
Leadership interventions, 104-109
allowing conflict, 112-113
facilitating sharing, 105-107
initial sharing, 108
limiting self-disclosure, 108-109
maintaining a directive role, 107-108
modeling and reinforcing adaptive self disclosure, 114-115
monitoring process and content, 113-114
physical environment, 105
reinforcing acceptance of members, 107
reinforcing commonalities, 114
Learning techniques *see* Experiential learning techniques
Levels of communication, 9-12
content, 9
message unit, 11-12
metacommunication, 9

-M-

Manifest material defined, 29
Manifest vs. latent content, 29
Manipulative power of leaders, 93
Meaning attribution function in leadership, 104

Message generation in dysfunctional
communications, 13-14
Message unit in communications,
11-12
Metacommunications, 29
Models, feedback, 6
Modes of experience, 9-10
parataxis, 10
protaxic, 9-10
syntaxic, 10
Movement therapy, 169-170

-N-

Natural child in transactional
analysis, 31-32
Negative reinforces in behavior
modification, 59-60
Nonassertive behavior in behavior
modification, 66-67
Nondirective leadership style, 96
Nonverbal communications, 10-11
Nurse consultants, 269
Nursing care plan as a process, 14-15
Nurturing parent in transactional
analysis, 32
Nutrient power of leaders, 93

-O-

Open system defined, 5
Operant conditioning in behavior
modification, 58

-P-

Pairing behavioral role, 87
Paralanguage defined, 10
Parataxic distortion, 27
Parataxic mode of experience, 10
Parent in transactional analysis, 32
Peer support, value of, 215-216
Personal systems, 5
Positive reinforcers in behavior
modification, 58-59
Power defined, 92
Primary groups defined, 1

Problem framing, 134-136
Problem solving, 133
brainstorming, 141-142
creative, 138-142
steps in, 139-141
techniques for, 141-142
nominal group process, 142
steps in, 134-138
Process illumination, 241-262
Process interventions, 241-247
clues to process, 245-247
questions to illuminate process,
241-245
Projection, Gestalt theory and, 45
Property of circularity, 6, 7
Property of synergy, 6, 7
Prototaxic mode of experience, 9-10
Proxemics defined, 10
Psychic determinism, 26
Psychoanalytical theory,
anxiety and self-esteem and, 27-28
group practice and, 23-40
group psyche and, 28-29
manifest vs. latent content, 29
parataxic distortion and, 27
psychic determinism and, 26
repression and, 25-26
transactional analysis and, 29-40
transference and, 26
Psychodrama, 73, 170-171
Psychology, basic ego, 23-39
Punishers in behavior modification,
58

-R-

Racket feeling in transactional
anslysis, 35-38
Reference groups defined, 1
Reminiscing groups, 226
Repression,
acting out, 25-26
defined, 25-26
resistance and, 26
Resistance to being, Gestalt theory
and, 44-46
introjection, 44

Retroflection, Gestalt theory and, 45
Rewards and punishments in groups, 88-89
Role behavior patterns in groups, 85-87
  dependency group, 86
  fight-flight, 86-87
  pairing, 87
Role defined, 85
Roleplaying, 170-172

-S-

Scripting in transactional analysis, 38
  identification of, 39
Secondary groups defined, 1
Self awareness groups, 79-81
Self-disclosure exercises, 172-173
Self esteem and anxiety, 27-28
Self-help groups, 80
Shaping in behavior modification, 61
Social group, 83
  compared to a crisis group, 84
Social systems defined, 6
Sociodrama, 170
Spread phenomenon, 227
Staff task groups, 177-192
  communication channels, 185-187
  format, areas of practice using, 177-178
  forming of, 187-191
    definition of tasks to be performed, 187
      membership in, 187-188
      group think, 190-191
      meeting structure, 188-189
  multidisciplinary leadership in, 182-184
  multidisciplinary leadership in informal power structure, 184
  nursing staff leadership in, 180-181
  process elements, 189-191
  structure of, 178-179
    power, 179-180
  see also Task groups
Standards of action in groups, 87-88
Status in groups, ascribed and

achieved, 179
Stress,
  defined, 217
  elements of, 217
Strokes and stroking in transactional analysis, 33
Super ego defined, 25
Supervision and consultation contrasted, 265-267
Supervision and consultation modes compared, 278
Supervision process,
  coleadership and, 264-265
  individual group leader and, 265
Support group defined, 81-82
Support groups see Client support groups
Synergy, property of, 6, 7
Syntaxic mode of experience, 10
System
  closed, 5
  defined, 5
  examination of living, 6-8
  interactional, 6
  interpersonal, 5
  open, 5
  personal, 5
  social, 6
Systems,
  boundaries, of 6
  communications, 8-9
  properties of, 5-6
  interactional properties, 6
Systems theory, 5-8

-T-

Task functions of groups, 96-97
Task group, staff see Staff task groups
Task groups, 79
Tension release exercises, 172
Therapy group, 82-83
Token economy in behavior modification, 61-63
Touch in communications, 10

"Trading stamps" in transactional
analysis, 36-38
Transactional analysis (TA), 23,
29-40
complementary transactions, 33-35
crossed transactions, 35
discount in, 33
ego states and, 30-33
adaptive child, 31
adult, 32-33
adult in the child, 30-31
child, 30-32, 39
parent, 32
parent in the child, 31
free child in, 31-32
group therapy and, 38-40
hooking on ego state, 39-40
identifying script messages, 39
natural child in, 31-32
nurturing parent in, 32
psychoanalytical theory and, 29-40
racket feelings, 35-38
scripting in, 38
strokes and stroking, 33
"trading stamps" in, 36-38
transactions, 33-38

analyzing of, 39-40
ulterior, 35-38
Transference, 26
Trust exercise, 172-173

-U-

Ulterior transactions in transactional
analysis, 35-38
Unfinished business in Gestalt
therapy, 50-52

-V-

Verbal communications, 9-10
Videotaping, 260-261
as a teaching tool, 276-277
logistics of, 261
therapeutic goals and, 260-261

-W-

Warm-up exercises, 167-168
Withdrawal, Gestalt theory and,
49-50